This book is a gift from Parke-Davis.

Thank you for your generous support
of the
American Academy of Neurology
Education & Research Foundation
Geschwind Award.

BEHAVIORAL NEUROLOGY AND
THE LEGACY OF NORMAN GESCHWIND

Behavioral Neurology and The Legacy of Norman Geschwind

Editors

Steven C. Schachter, M.D.

*Director of Clinical Research
Comprehensive Epilepsy Program
Beth Israel Hospital
Assistant Professor of Neurology
Harvard Medical School
Boston, Massachusetts*

Orrin Devinsky, M.D.

*Chief of Neurology, Hospital for Joint Diseases
Director, New York University-Hospital for Joint Diseases Epilepsy Center
Professor of Neurology
New York University School of Medicine
New York, New York*

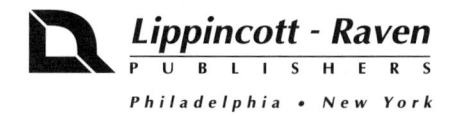

Lippincott - Raven
PUBLISHERS
Philadelphia • New York

Acquisitions Editor: Mark Placito
Developmental Editor: Mattie Bialer
Manufacturing Manager: Dennis Teston
Production Manager: Lawrence Bernstein
Production Editor: Lawrence Bernstein
Cover Designer: Brian H. Crede/bc graphics
Indexer: Susan Lohmeyer
Compositor: Lippincott-Raven Electronic Production
Printer: Maple Press

© 1997 by Lippincott-Raven Publishers. All rights reserved. This book is protected by copyright. No part of it may be reproduced, stored in a retrieval system, or transmitted, in any form or by any means—electronic, mechanical, photocopy, recording, or otherwise—without the prior written consent of the publisher, except for brief quotations embodied in critical articles and reviews. For information write **Lippincott-Raven Publishers, 227 East Washington Square, Philadelphia, PA 19106-3780.**

Materials appearing in this book prepared by individuals as part of their official duties as U.S. Government employees are not covered by the above-mentioned copyright.

Printed in the United States of America

9 8 7 6 5 4 3 2 1

Library of Congress Cataloging-in-Publication Data

Behavioral neurology and the legacy of Norman Geschwind / editors.
   Steven C. Schachter, Orrin Devinsky.
      p.   cm.
   Includes bibliographical references and index.
   ISBN 0-397-51631-2
   1. Geschwind, Norman. 2. Neuropsychiatry. 3. Clinical
neuropsychology. I. Schachter, Steven C. II. Devinsky, Orrin.
   [DNLM: 1. Geschwind, Norman. 2. Neurologic Manifestations.
3. Brain Diseases. 4. Dominance, Cerebral. 5. Behavioral Medicine.
WL 340 8419 1997]
RC344.B44   1997
616.8—DC20
DNLM/DLC
For Library of Congress   96-41088
                                                                   CIP

Care has been taken to confirm the accuracy of the information presented and to describe generally accepted practices. However, the authors, editors, and publisher are not responsible for errors or omissions or for any consequences from application of the information in this book and make no warranty, express or implied, with respect to the contents of the publication.

The authors, editors, and publisher have exerted every effort to ensure that drug selection and dosage set forth in this text are in accordance with current recommendations and practice at the time of publication. However, in view of ongoing research, changes in government regulations, and the constant flow of information relating to drug therapy and drug reactions, the reader is urged to check the package insert for each drug for any change in indications and dosage and for added warnings and precautions. This is particularly important when the recommended agent is a new or infrequently employed drug.

Some drugs and medical devices presented in this publication have Food and Drug Administration (FDA) clearance for limited use in restricted research settings. It is the responsibility of the health care provider to ascertain the FDA status of each drug or device planned for use in their clinical practice.

This book is dedicated to the memory of Norman Geschwind, M.D.

Contents

Contributors ... ix
Foreword *by Clifford B. Saper* ... xii
Preface ... xiv
Acknowledgments ... xvi

Personal Perspectives

1. A Darlin' Man ... 3
   Robert J. Joynt

2. Educator ... 5
   Kenneth M. Heilman

3. A Mensch ... 15
   Andrew Kertesz

4. Colleague ... 21
   Thomas D. Sabin

5. Advisor ... 27
   Elliott D. Ross

6. Role Model ... 31
   Stephen G. Waxman

7. Teacher ... 35
   Michael Ronthal

8. Mentor ... 39
   Bruce H. Price

9. Creative Genius ... 47
   Howard Gardner

10. International Figure ... 53
    François Boller

11. Physician ... 57
    Fritz Fairhurst

Language Disorders

12. Historical Antecedents to Geschwind ... 63
    Harry A. Whitaker

13. Norman Geschwind's Influence on the Study of Aphasia ... 71
    D. Frank Benson

14. Evolving Concepts of Anomia: Geschwind's Role 79
    Martin L. Albert and Harold Goodglass

15. Anatomy of Developmental Dyslexia: Geschwind's Last Legacy 89
    Albert M. Galaburda

16. Stuttering 101
    David B. Rosenfield

Other Disorders of Higher Cortical Function

17. The Disconnexion Syndromes 115
    Orrin Devinsky

18. Geschwind's Influence on the Study of Disorders of Attention 127
    Edward Valenstein

19. Autism and Related Disorders of Development 143
    Martha Bridge Denckla

20. Frontal Lobe Syndrome 157
    François Boller

21. Norman Geschwind and Dementing Disorders 163
    Robert C. Green

22. Apraxia 171
    Kenneth M. Heilman, Leslie J. Gonzalez Rothi, and Robert T. Watson

23. Right Hemisphere Syndromes and the Neurology of Emotion 183
    Elliot D. Ross

Epilepsy

24. Behavioral Aspects of Temporal Lobe Epilepsy 195
    Donald L. Schomer

25. Other Forms of Epilepsy 207
    Orrin Devinsky

26. Interictal Behavior in Temporal Lobe Epilepsy 213
    David M Bear

27. Neuroendocrinology of Epilepsy 223
    Andrew G. Herzog

Handedness, Cerebral Dominance, and Autoimmune Disease

28. Cerebral Asymmetries 243
    Marjorie LeMay and Steven C. Schachter

29. Handedness Measurement and Correlation with Brain Structure 257
    Steven C. Schachter

30. Left-Handed Blonds and Other Odd Correlations 271
    Stanley Coren

31. Handedness and Autoimmune Disease 287
    Peter O. Behan

Epilogue

32. Norman Geschwind (1926–1984) 295
    Albert M. Galaburda

Index 298

Contributors

Martin L. Albert, M.D., Ph.D.
Director, Aphasia Research Center
Professor of Neurology
Boston University Medical School
150 Huntington Avenue
Boston, Massachusetts 02130

David M. Bear, M.D.
Professor of Psychiatry
Department of Psychiatry
University of Massachusetts Medical Center
55 Lake Street North
Worcester, Massachusetts 01655

Peter O. Behan, M.B., Ch.B., M.D., D.Sc., F.A.C.P., F.R.C.P. (Glas) (Lond) (Ire)
Professor of Neurology
Department of Neurology
Glasgow University
Glasgow G54TF, Scotland
U.K.

D. Frank Benson, M.D.
Professor, Emeritus
Department of Neurology
UCLA School of Medicine
710 Westwood Plaza
Los Angeles, California 90024

François Boller, M.D., Ph.D.
Professor of Neurology
INSERM U324
Rue d'Alésia
Paris 75014
France

Stanley Coren, Ph.D.
Professor of Psychology
Psychology Department
University of British Columbia
2136 West Mall
Vancouver, British Columbia V6T1Z4
Canada

Martha Bridge Denckla, M.D.
Professor of Neurology, Pediatrics, and Psychiatry
Johns Hopkins University School of Medicine
Kennedy-Krieger Institute
707 North Broadway
Baltimore, Maryland 21205

Orrin Devinsky, M.D.
Professor of Neurology
Department of Neurology
New York University Hospital for Joint Diseases
301 East 17th Street
New York, New York 10003

Frits Fairhurst
56 St. Joseph Street #607
Fall River, Massachusetts 02722

Albert M. Galaburda, M.D.
Emily Fisher Landau Professor of Neurology and Neuroscience
Chief, Division of Behavioral Neurology
Department of Neurology
Beth Israel Hospital
Harvard Medical School
330 Brookline Avenue, KS-2
Boston, Massachusetts 02215

Howard Gardner, Ph.D.
Research Professor of Neurology
Department of Neurology
Boston University School of Medicine
80 East Concord Street
Boston, Massachusetts 02118

Harold Goodglass, Ph.D.
Director, Aphasia Research Center
Boston Department of Veteran Affairs Medical Center
Professor of Neurology (Neuropsychology)
Boston University School of Medicine
150 Huntington Avenue
Boston, Massachusetts 02130

CONTRIBUTORS

Robert C. Green, M.D.
Director, Emory Neurobehavioral Program
Associate Professor of Neurology
Emory University School of Medicine
Atlanta, Georgia

Kenneth M. Heilman, M.D.
Professor of Clinical Psychology
Department of Neurology
University of Florida College of Medicine
University Hospital Medical Center
Box 100236
Gainesville, Florida 32610

Andrew G. Herzog, M.D., M.Sc.
Associate Professor of Neurology
Director, Neuroendocrine Unit
Department of Neurology
Beth Israel Hospital
Harvard Medical School
330 Brookline Avenue
Boston, Massachusetts 02215

Robert J. Joynt, M.D., Ph.D.
Professor of Neurology, Neurobiology and Anatomy
Department of Neurology
University of Rochester School of Medicine
601 Elmwood Avenue
Rochester, New York 14642

Andrew Kertesz, M.D., F.R.C.P.C.
Professor of Neurology
Department of Clinical Neurological Sciences
St. Joseph's Health Centre
University of Western Ontario
268 Grosvenor Street
London, Ontario N6A4V2
Canada

Marjorie LeMay, M.D.
Associate Profesor of Radiology
Department of Radiology
Brigham and Women's Hospital and Harvard Medical School
75 Francis Street
Boston, Massachusetts 02115

Bruce H. Price, M.D.
Chief, Department of Neurology
McLean Hospital
Belmont, Massachusetts
Instructor in Neurology
Harvard Medical School
330 Brookline Avenue
Boston, Massachusetts 02215

Michael Ronthal, M.B.B.Ch., F.R.C.P.E.
Associate Professor of Neurology
Department of Neurology
Beth Israel Hospital
Harvard Medical School
330 Brookline Avenue
Boston, Massachusetts 02215

David B. Rosenfield, M.D.
Professor of Neurology
Director, Stuttering Center Speech Motor Control Laboratory
Department of Neurology
Otorhinolarlyngology and Communicative Services
Baylor College of Medicine
6501 Fannin NB302
Houston, Texas 77019

Elliott D. Ross, M.D.
Professor of Neurology
Department of Neurology
University of Oklahoma Health Science Center
920 S.L. Young Drive, 35P203
Oklahoma City, Oklahoma 73190-3048

Leslie J. Gonzalez Rothi, M.D.
Audiology and Speech Pathology Service
Veterans Affairs Medical Center
Department of Neurology
University of Florida College of Medicine
Gainesville, Florida 32610

Thomas D. Sabin, M.D.
Professor of Neurology and Psychiatry
Director, Neurological Unit
Boston Medical Center
818 Harrison Avenue
Boston, Massachusetts 02118

Clifford B. Saper, M.D., Ph.D.
James Jackson Putnam Professor of Neurology and Neuroscience
Neurologist-in-Chief
Beth Israel Hospital
Harvard Medical School
330 Brookline Avenue
Boston, Massachusetts 02215

Steven C. Schachter, M.D.
Assitant Professor of Neurology
Department of Neurology
Beth Israel Hospital
Harvard Medical School
330 Brookline Avenue
Boston, Massachusetts 02215

CONTRIBUTORS

Donald L. Schomer, M.D.
Associate Professor of Neurology
Director, Laboratory of Clinical
 Neurophysiology
Director, Comprehensive Epilepsy Program
Department of Neurology
Beth Israel Hospital
Harvard Medical School
330 Brookline Avenue
Boston, Massachusetts 02215
Professor of Neurology
University of Geneva
Geneva, Switzerland

Edward Valenstein, M.D.
Professor of Neurology and Clinical and
 Health Psychology
Department of Neurology
University of Florida
Box 100236, UFHSC
Gainesville, Florida 32610-0236

Robert T. Watson, M.D.
Neurology Service
Department of Neurology
Veterans Affairs Medical Center
University of Florida College of Medicine
Gainesville, Florida 32610-0236

Stephen G. Waxman, M.D., Ph.D.
Professor and Chairman
Department of Neurology
Yale University School of Medicine
333 Cedar Street
New Haven, Connecticut 06510

Harry A. Whitaker, Ph.D.
Department of Psychology
University of Quebec at Montreal
Montreal, Quebec
Canada

Foreword

In 1976, when I first met Norman Geschwind, it certainly never crossed my mind that one day I would have the opportunity to follow in his footsteps. I entered his office as a medical student, still fresh from my doctoral work on the connections of the hypothalamus, anxious at the thought of meeting the famous leader of behavioral neurology whose work I had pondered. I had expected to find him in a grand setting, but the room I now encountered was informal, cramped, and cluttered, and totally dominated by the warmth and energy of the man. Immediately, I was immersed in one of the most engaging, thoughtful, and enlightening (not to mention delightful) conversations of my young career. Dr. Geschwind had read my work on autonomic control by the hypothalamus and had thought about its implications for behaviors ranging from feeding to aggression. His wide-ranging conceptualizations took me to places I had scarcely before imagined.

Although I never had the privilege of training directly with Dr. Geschwind, I did manage to convince my mentor, Dr. Fred Plum, to invite Dr. Geschwind to be a Visiting Professor during the last year of my residency at Cornell. I culled through my case records for just the right patient to present to him at Grand Rounds. Finally, the appointed day arrived and I presented to him the case of a young man with complex partial seizures who worked in the hospital. He had accosted a woman in the hospital elevator and was subsequently arrested by a hospital security guard. The young man claimed that he had no memory of the event and that he had been having a seizure during the attack.

Dr. Geschwind sat down next to my patient, looked at him thoughtfully, and asked a single question: "Do you keep journals?" In the next few minutes the young man poured out his soul concerning the many volumes of elaborate diaries and journals he kept. Geschwind soon had him discussing his deep religious beliefs and strict moral code about sexual conduct. The case fit neatly into the patterns of ictal and interictal behavioral disorders that Geschwind had described in patients with temporal lobe seizures. He recommended treatment with anticonvulsants, and the young man's career was saved. To my knowledge, the patient had no further problems with sexual misconduct.

Over the succeeding years, I looked forward to seeing Norman, as by then I had come to call him, at scientific and clinical meetings. He was always ready to pique my imagination with a novel idea he had or to suggest some association between my work and some remote corner of the literature that I had never considered. I followed with anticipation the progress of his own work, which in the early 1980s was pushing into new realms, exploring the relationship between cerebral laterality and autoimmune disease and endocrine regulation.

For all of us who had anticipated many more years of this stimulation, its sudden end came as a blow. It is interesting that, at critical junctures in our lives, we retain a crystal-clear recollection of even the most trivial of surrounding events. For example, most of us (of a certain age) remember where we were and what we were doing when President Kennedy was shot. For me, hearing of Norman's death was just such a moment. I remember distinctly where I was sitting, who I was talking with, and the palpable sense of loss and frustration that the news brought. A unique and irreplaceable resource had been lost, and to this day those of us who were lucky enough to know Dr. Geschwind still miss him.

Taking up Norman's chair at Harvard and the leadership of the department that he built has had special meaning for me. It has been an opportunity to return some of the insights and opportunities that he had given to me. Behavioral neurology remains the centerpiece at our table, even though we have taken advantage of some of the advances in genetics and integrative and cognitive neuroscience to build beyond what we could have imagined at the time of Norman's death. (I have no doubt that Norman could have imagined a great deal more than we have accomplished or probably ever will be able to accomplish.)

The opportunity to follow in Geschwind's footsteps and to be ignited by the sparks of imagination that he generated was a rare and precious gift. His legacy lives in these pages, and those who read them will have the privilege of meeting and walking with, even if just for a short time, one of the intellectual giants of this century.

Clifford B. Saper, M.D., Ph.D.

Preface

When Norman Geschwind attended Harvard College and Harvard Medical School in the 1940s, there was very little academic interest in brain-behavior relationships. As a medical student, he was taught that brain disorders could result in intellectual and emotional problems but that these problems were insignificant. Much later, Dr. Geschwind suggested that more studies may have been done and papers published on brain-behavior relationships between 1870 and 1914 than between 1914 and 1970. For example, he noted that the Nobel Laureate Roger Sperry and other leading contemporary scientists had stated that almost nothing was known about the functions of the corpus callosum in the 1950s even though, by 1914, the syndromes of the corpus callosum were a standard part of teaching throughout the German-speaking neurologic world. The work on apraxia, aphasia, and alexia by Liepmann, Wernicke, and other German neurologists was also largely forgotten by English-speaking neurologists after World War I.

Therefore, to advance the state of knowledge about brain-behavior relationships, Dr. Geschwind had to rediscover our neurologic past. That he was a Jew working in the post-World War II era to recognize the contributions of German neurologists to the field of brain-behavior relationships says much about Dr. Geschwind. His Yeshiva schooling until age 12 and military service in World War II would have led him, one would think, to develop a very strong anti-German bias. But Dr. Geschwind had no interest in such bias. His efforts to understand and solve a problem had no geographic or political boundaries. With his command of eight languages, he uncovered the advances in the non-English literature for the English-speaking world and applied them to his developing view of the relationships between anatomy, neural circuitry, and behavior. As the father of behavioral neurology, he unearthed the phoenix and gave it new wings and fresh wind.

This book began in 1991, 7 years after Dr. Geschwind died, when the hospital administration decided to discard all his office charts, which contained the records of patients he had cared for at Beth Israel Hospital. One of us (SS) rescued those precious charts and spent many enjoyable hours revisiting the ideas and observations recorded in those files. A year later, during a break at an American Epilepsy Society meeting, we reminisced about Dr. Geschwind and his strong influence on each of us. We realized that his office notes and correspondence were a treasure chest that presented us with an opportunity to ask the leading figures in behavioral neurology who were his former students and associates to create a lasting tribute to Dr. Geschwind. We were overwhelmed with the enthusiastic support for this project in the behavioral neurology community.

This volume is divided into two large sections: a series of personal perspectives and four sets of chapters that are organized to reflect the different stages of Dr. Geschwind's career. The contributors include many of his colleagues, fellows, and residents from the beginning to the end of his career. They write about the impact that Dr. Geschwind had on behavioral neurology and on their own personal and professional growth and achievements.

Dr. Geschwind established an international network of colleagues to explore human behavior and set the intellectual agenda for the future by inspiring an ever-widening audience of clinicians and basic scientists to pursue new ideas and concepts. Those readers who were fortunate enough to have known him will, hopefully, smile, chuckle, nod their head, and become misty-eyed as they absorb the written memories in this book. Dr. Geschwind shone a light into the black box; those he touched in the past and those who are touched by his colleagues in the future will continue to light the way. May this book illuminate the imagination of all impressionable thinkers and honor the legacy of Norman Geschwind.

Steven C. Schachter, M.D.
Orrin Devinsky, M.D.

Acknowledgments

We would like to thank Mrs. Pat Geschwind for her generous support in exploring Dr. Geschwind's professional corespondence and previously unpublished material. We are indebted to Cecile Davis for performing the endless logistical steps in bringing this manuscript from a concept to a reality and to Cathy Somer for her careful editoral assistance. We thank Marsel Mesulam, MD, for his support and encouragement.

Jacqui Streeton, an American artist with epilepsy, drew the portrait on the front cover. Dr. Geschwind would have marvelled at her skill and valued her artistic accomplishments.

Personal Perspectives

1

A Darlin' Man

Robert J. Joynt

University of Rochester Medical Center, Department of Neurology, Rochester, New York 14642.

Norman and I had a rather improbable friendship. He was from New York City, had an Eastern European Jewish background, and was educated in the Ivy League. I am an Iowan of Irish Catholic descent and was educated at the state university. Also, Norman had about 30 or more IQ points to his advantage. We did have, however, similar views on people and institutions. The most important thing was that we did not take ourselves very seriously—I, because I was not very serious, and Norman, because he probably had a theory that you should not take yourself seriously.

NORMAN THE THEORIST

Norman had a theory about almost everything. He used to joke that his teacher, Denny-Brown, theorized about everything, but Norman did not recognize that he was the same way. When I went on rounds with him, he developed a theory, often obscure, about every patient, even those with obscure disorders that held very little interest for him. I would question Norman about some of these theories, and back would come a complicated concatenation of obscure facts that were usually convincing. However, some of his ideas were fairly simple. One time, I bemoaned the fact that I knew very little about pediatric neurology. He reached into my examining bag, pulled out the tape measure, handed it to me, and said, "There; you're a pediatric neurologist." What amazed me were the connections Norman could make between so many categories of knowledge. His mind moved nimbly around his amazing repository of information. But it was the connections, not the facts themselves, that were so astounding. He was a gatherer of facts but a master of fancy.

We first met in the early sixties when I was attending a meeting with Arthur Benton, who had already recognized Norman's innovative mode of thinking. A few years later, Norman's classic papers on the disconnection syndrome were published in *Brain*, and shortly after that, I nominated him for membership in the American Neurological Association (ANA). At that time, one had to present a thesis for membership. A senior neurologist who was a member of the membership committee telephoned me, saying, "Who is this Geschwind, and what is this disconnection syndrome he is writing about in his thesis?" I tried to explain, but he said that the membership would have to be held up until the association could get somebody to evaluate the thesis. (It must be remembered that in the sixties, behavioral neurology was considered an interesting but unnecessary part of the neurological discipline.) Norman was eventually admitted to the ANA after a year's delay. That series of papers is still among the most frequently cited in the field, and it is referred to repeatedly in this book.

I became chief editor of the *Archives of Neurology* in 1982, and I invited Norman to become one of the associate editors. His observations and reviews were superb, and his criticisms were constructive and always generous and kind. During that period, we had many lengthy phone conversations about his new project linking cerebral lateralization, learning disorders, and immunologic diseases. My first reaction was skepticism, but Norman traced the evolution of his theoretical construct, buttressed by facts and observations from a broad range of fields, including biology, physiology, endocrinology, and genetics. Responses by the reviewers to his submitted manuscript on cerebral lateralization ran the gamut from great enthusiasm to outright rejection. I used my prerogative as chief editor and accepted the article. It offered a whole new view of the role of the nervous system in controlling noncognitive function. Tragically, Norman died suddenly before his article was published.

Norman's contributions to neurology are well chronicled in this book, so I will not expand on them. His was a prodigious output spanning the field. The influence he had on his students was immense, and their influence has amplified his teachings.

NORMAN THE MAN

Norman was as generous with his time as he was with his knowledge. He would visit us in Iowa City and later in Rochester, occasionally accompanied by Pat or one of their children. Each visit was a *tour de force* in which Norman would go on rounds, speak, and consult all day long, then have a lively dinner with friends and colleagues, and, finally, come back to our house for the evening. The day was not over! Norman would settle in and touch on dozens of topics, all with great knowledge and enthusiasm. About midnight, I would bow out, but Margaret would stay on. Our children, who normally eschewed adult conversation, looked forward to Norman's visits because he included them in the discussion.

Norman always brought a present for the children. On one occasion, he arrived with a complicated game in which the plane of the playing surface could be tilted in various directions, the object being to propel a steel ball through a maze without letting it fall through a series of holes on the surface. Norman became intrigued by the challenge and would not release the game until he had mastered it. On another visit, he proudly displayed his newly acquired skill of juggling, which he had learned from reading a book on the subject. His visits also afforded the children an opportunity to speculate on what article of clothing, book, or other belonging he would forget on that occasion.

These are personal reminiscences, so they deal with only a small part of a complex man who gave so much to our field. I am certain others could write of similar experiences, for Norman was as complete a man as I have known—enthusiastic but gentle, knowledgeable but thoughtful, imaginative but pragmatic, and serious but playful.

At the time of Norman's death, I wrote:

> It is safe to say that anyone who engaged in a conversation with Norman for very long, and most conversations were long, came away with a new idea, a new view of an old idea, or a new story or joke. His remarkable enthusiasm and unvarying good humor made him an exacting researcher. His lack of guile and pretension and his generosity made him a warm friend. We are diminished both professionally and personally by his death.

The Irish have an expression for someone who is witty, captivating, whimsical, and bright: he is called a darlin' man. Norman was a darlin' man.

*Behavioral Neurology and
the Legacy of Norman Geschwind,*
edited by S. C. Schachter and O. Devinsky,
Lippincott-Raven Publishers, Philadelphia © 1997.

2
Educator

Kenneth M. Heilman

University of Florida, Department of Neurology, Gainesville, Florida 32610-0236.

Academicians have several roles. In addition to being clinicians, researchers, and administrators, they are teachers. Although Norman Geschwind's scientific contributions were extremely important in the rebirth of what he termed *behavioral neurology* (now also called neuropsychology, cognitive neuroscience, and cognitive neuropsychology), his influence as an educator is of equal significance.

In his seminal 1965 article in *Brain*, "Disconnexion Syndromes in Man and Animals," Norman Geschwind contrasted the means by which animals and human beings learn. The gift of language, including both speech and print, has provided human beings with the unique ability to share their knowledge so that each organism does not have to learn solely by personal experience. However, an educator like Norman Geschwind does more than share factual knowledge. A good educator teaches students how to observe, how to acquire knowledge, how to teach, and how to think. These are procedural skills that cannot be acquired by reading articles or texts. It takes a teacher like Norman Geschwind, one of the few people who could think aloud, to teach such skills.

The influence of an educator is difficult to assess because, unlike research findings that can be cited, that influence cannot be measured or counted. However, it increases geometrically. Not only did Norman Geschwind directly train many of today's most productive behavioral neurologists, but many of those he directly trained developed their own training programs. Therefore, he is directly or indirectly responsible for training almost every active behavioral neurologist in the United States. After he died, a memorial symposium was held for him in Boston. Bob Watson, who began his residency in Gainesville, Florida, at the same time I joined the faculty at the University of Florida, was, at the time of Norman Geschwind's death, a professor of neurology at the University of Florida. When he received the notice about the memorial symposium, he asked me if I thought it was appropriate for him to go to Boston to attend this celebration of Norman's life. I said, "Yes, by all means! He is your grandfather."

Describing the influence of an educator without sounding as if one is reading a lengthy letter of recommendation is difficult. The influence that a teacher has on individual students is a personal one. Perhaps the best means of describing that influence is to relate some anecdotes that illustrate how Norman Geschwind influenced my life. Although every student, resident, and fellow who knew him could recount different influential experiences, the basic lessons that Norman Geschwind taught were shared by all his students.

ENLIGHTENMENT

In 1967, I was a first-year resident on the Harvard Neurological Unit at Boston City Hospital. Dr. D. Denny-Brown, who had accepted me into his residency, was semiretired, but because we were residents whom he had accepted into his program, he would periodically make rounds with us and often attend our grand rounds on Saturday morning. However, in Dr. Denny-Brown's absence, Dr. Simeon Locke, a superb teacher and an astute clinician, was the acting chief of our unit.

One evening, I was called down to the emergency room at City Hospital to see a 55-year-old engineer who was brought in by his family because he was behaving strangely. Because of rheumatic heart disease, the patient had undergone a prosthetic Star Edwards valve insertion to replace a diseased valve, but the man was not taking any anticoagulants. Before calling Psychiatry, the emergency room physicians wanted to make certain nothing was wrong with his brain.

According to the history that I obtained, the patient came home around 5:30 PM and heard the telephone ring. His wife was calling to tell him that she was shopping at Filene's and would be a little late. He heard the phone ring and recognized the sound of the phone and his wife's voice. However, he could not understand what she was saying, and it sounded to him as if she were mumbling or even speaking a foreign language. He asked her several times to stop mumbling, but when she persisted, he hung up the phone. Realizing that something was amiss, she returned home. She thought he seemed fine physically, but every time she spoke to him, he claimed she was mumbling. When he started getting agitated about her mumbling, his wife phoned several of their children. They all came over to the house, and when they started talking all at once, they seemed to their father to be mumbling simultaneously. Finally he became so distraught and paranoid that they brought him to City Hospital.

When I first examined the patient, I could not get him to understand my speech. However, his hearing acuity appeared normal. He was very attentive and was trying to understand me. Out of desperation rather than reason, I wrote some messages down on a sheet of paper and showed them to him. The patient had no difficulty reading and understanding my message. The remainder of his neurological examination was entirely normal. Although I did not know what was causing this unusual problem, I decided to admit him to our neurological unit. I instructed everybody on the service to communicate with him in writing. The next day I presented him to the attending and acting chairman, Simeon Locke. After my presentation and his examination of the patient, Dr. Locke took aside the group of house officers making rounds and rebuked me. "Dr. Heilman, there is no neurological way that we can account for this man's ability to hear and understand environmental sounds but not speech. You admitted a crock." He further suggested that I call Psychiatry and get the man on the appropriate service. In my defense, I suggested to Dr. Locke that this 55-year-old man had no psychiatric history, that he had a valve that was infamous for throwing emboli to the brain, and that he was not receiving anticoagulant medication. I agreed to get a psychiatric consult, but I also asked for permission to obtain a radioisotope brain scan. Unfortunately, computer tomography was not yet available.

After grand rounds, one of the other neurology residents mentioned to me that there was someone named Norman Geschwind at the Veterans Administration Hospital in Jamaica Plains who was interested in higher cortical function. About this time I also learned that Dr. Denny-Brown would not be in town for our next Saturday grand rounds. I therefore got permission from Dr. Locke to invite Dr. Geschwind to City Hospital for our grand rounds.

Norman Geschwind had a policy of always answering and returning phone calls and letters. I had no trouble reaching him on the phone. Because he was chairman of neurology at Boston University and a world authority on higher cortical function, I was worried that he would be either condescending or arrogant. Instead, he was warm and friendly. He told me that he had trained at City Hospital and would be honored and delighted to give grand rounds.

On Saturday morning grand rounds, I presented my case to Dr. Geschwind. I was worried that I would again hear the word "crock." Instead, after Dr. Geschwind examined the patient and the patient returned to his bed, Dr. Geschwind said, "Great case—very interesting patient." He thought that this man had an embolic infarction in his left primary auditory area and that this infarction included the subcortical white matter. He went on to explain that the lesion had not only destroyed the left primary auditory area but also the white matter fibers crossing from the right temporal lobe's auditory areas to the cortex of the left temporal lobe. Although Wernicke's area, which contains the auditory images of words, was intact, it was being deprived of auditory input and therefore my patient could not comprehend speech. However, because the other perisylvian speech regions, including Wernicke's and Broca's areas, were intact, his spontaneous speech was normal. His reading was normal because he did not have to use the auditory system to gain access to the left hemisphere's language system.

Dr. Locke asked from the back how the patient could recognize the phone ringing and his wife's voice. Dr. Geschwind replied that his auditory system was not disconnected from his right hemisphere. Wernicke's area in the left hemisphere contains auditory word images. One does not need auditory word images to recognize meaningful environmental sounds or voices.

A great teacher must, above all, explain and enlighten. Since my early days in college, I had always wanted to learn how the brain works. How do we talk, read, and reason? As an undergraduate, I took psychology courses. I learned about B. F. Skinner and Freud. Whenever I asked questions about how the brain may work, I was told my questions were irrelevant and that all one needed to know was stimulus, response, and reinforcement contingencies. Similarly, when I went to medical school, I learned neuroanatomy and neurophysiology, but, again, no one explained how the brain permitted us to speak, read, and reason, and how brain diseases could influence these higher functions. When I heard Norman Geschwind explain the cerebral abnormalities that accounted for this man's disorder, I was in awe. Not only had Dr. Geschwind enlightened me, he had rekindled my curiosity. About a week after Norman Geschwind gave his grand rounds, my patient had a radioisotope brain scan that showed abnormal uptake in the superior portion of the temporal lobe approximately in the region of the left-sided primary auditory cortex, as Dr. Geschwind had predicted.

A great teacher must not only enlighten but create enthusiasm, generate interest, and produce excitement. In just one visit, Norman Geschwind had done exactly that for me. Dr. Denny-Brown's program was only a 2-year program. During the third year, one could study neuropathology or take a fellowship elsewhere. After hearing Norm Geschwind's grand rounds, I knew what I wanted to do, what I had to do. I wanted to be his fellow at the Boston Veterans Administration Hospital. However, I never got that opportunity. After Dr. Denny-Brown retired, Dr. Geschwind accepted the Putnam Professorship and became chairman of neurology on the Harvard Neurological Unit. At Boston University and subsequently at Boston City Hospital, Dr. Geschwind was able to select his residents and fellows. However, when he arrived at Boston City Hospital, he was stuck with me, and I had every intention of taking full advantage of the year and a half I was to spend with him.

FOSTERING AND PROTECTING STUDENTS

One of my first research projects was to learn the types of aphasia associated with head trauma. Together with Art Saffran and Norman Geschwind, I studied the effects of closed head trauma on language and learned that anomia was the most common deficit. The Boston Society of Neurology had a yearly meeting at which residents and fellows presented their research project findings. Norman asked me to submit the aphasia project. I had ambivalent feelings about having the project accepted for presentation. The annual society meetings were attended by giants such as Drs. Denny-Brown, Raymond Adams, and C. Miller Fisher. I was afraid that they would be severely critical of my paper.

Most of the patients I reported on at the society meeting had suffered external damage to their foreheads. In the middle of my 10-minute talk, someone in the audience raised a hand, stood up, and said, "When one gets hit in the head, there are torque forces that may occur in language areas of the left hemisphere. Based on these patients' external injuries, did you calculate the torque forces and, even if you didn't, what influence do you think torque forces had on language areas?" I had not calculated torque forces and had no idea how to do so. Nor did I have any idea how torque forces could affect our results. I did not even know what torque forces were. As I was experiencing a mild panic attack, Norm Geschwind got up and said, "Ken, that question is irrelevant to your talk. Please continue." I continued my talk, and there were no further interruptions. After my talk, some questions were raised that I could easily answer, and I received many compliments.

PERSISTENCE

Before Norman Geschwind took over as director of the unit, one of those rare vending machines that dispenses 8-ounce bottles of Coca-Cola had been installed. Because people were leaving bottles around the unit, Dr. Geschwind wanted to get rid of the machine. Ed Valenstein and I protested that several of us did not drink coffee and enjoyed our Coke. Norman then suggested the machine be replaced with one that dispenses cups of Coca-Cola, but we explained that cups of Coke were not as satisfying as bottles. In addition, we argued, cups would not solve the problem. I suspect that because Norman was a coffee drinker, he thought our argument was specious. However, being kind and interested in our welfare, he did not remove our Coke machine.

Several months after the Coca-Cola discussions, I was about to buy a soda at the Coke machine when Dr. Geschwind came into the room. We got into a conversation about an interesting patient. Some conversations with Norm Geschwind were very long, and many conversations were not really conversations. Rather, he spoke and the other person listened. If one could persist in listening, there was much to be learned. I had been up most of the previous evening and my feet were somewhat tired, so I leaned against the Coke machine while listening to Geschwind expound. The machine shifted slightly, and a partially filled bottle of Coke that had been left on top of the machine began to drip down on my neck and shoulder in the middle of Geschwind's monologue. Norman appeared to be totally oblivious of my predicament and continued talking. Every time I would start to move away from the machine, he would stop me and say, "Wait! I also wanted to mention . . . ."

I considered the possibility that the dripping bottle was some type of divine retribution. Although I initially entertained the thought that Dr. Geschwind was trying to teach me a lesson, I was later convinced otherwise. One time I had dinner at a restaurant with him and some other friends. When the waiter brought our food, we started a conversation about some aspect of neurology. After taking one or two bites of his meal, Norman started explaining something. About 30 to 40 minutes later, his entrée was bussed away, his plate hardly touched. When teaching and explaining, Dr. Geschwind became so intensely focused that food or dripping soda became irrelevant.

Some people who did not know Norman well thought he was always trying to dominate conversations or impress others. But Dr. Geschwind knew that we held him in the highest regard, and we knew that his explanations and discussions were not driven by the desire to impress or dominate but rather by a burning desire to lead, teach, and even understand. According to Ed Valenstein (also a resident whom Norman did not choose, and a Coca-Cola drinker), Geschwind's monologues, whether on rounds or informally at the Coke machine, were never dull. Whether he was talking about scientists whom he knew personally or about authors with whom he was acquainted only through their writings, his conversations reflected a very personal involvement with other scientists' intellects. Geschwind appreciated Wernicke, Liepmann, and Gowers as kindred spirits who were capable of both accurate and original clinical observations and shrewd analysis, leading to testable hypotheses. Clearly, Geschwind not only admired them but felt comfortable with them because they observed and thought as he did. He expressed reservations about scientists whose analyses were, in his view, less penetrating: he thought Hughlings Jackson and Henry Head were "overrated," and there were certain eminent contemporary neurologists whom he considered doctrinaire or wrong-headed. In every aspect of his teaching, Dr. Geschwind, by his example, engendered in his students respect and appreciation for the spirit of inquiry, the quality of observation, and the clarity of analysis that characterized both his own work and that of the people he admired, both living and dead.

Geschwind often thought aloud. Thinking aloud enabled him to sharpen his own theories and also allowed people like me to gain insight into the creative process. By thinking aloud, he got people to consider unresolved problems and develop testable hypotheses. Before attending Boys High School in New York City, Geschwind had attended the Boro Park Yeshiva in Brooklyn. Often when he thought about a neurologic problem, his reasoning maintained a Talmudic flavor: "There are two possibilities . . . ."

Several years ago, Dr. Anjan Chattergee, one of our former fellows, was interviewing an applicant to our postdoctoral fellowship program. The candidate asked Dr. Chattergee what types of skills and procedures he had learned during his fellowship. Later on, after the prospective fellow left, Dr. Chattergee told me that he had explained to the applicant that he would not learn procedures but he would learn to question, think, and postulate. After my conversation with Dr. Chattergee, I reflected on the fact that, in those long conversations, Norm Geschwind had taught me not only "what" but also "how." I think he would have been proud of our program and those of many of his former fellows and residents.

LEARNING FROM MISTAKES (IT'S OKAY TO BE WRONG)

During my internship on the medical service at Cornell, I rotated through the Cornell Medical Service at Bellevue Hospital. One month, my attending physician was the chairman of the Department of Medicine at Memorial Sloan-Kettering Institute. A patient with hemoptysis was presented to this attending physician, who had an unorthodox way of percussing the borders of the heart. Instead of putting one finger on the patient's chest and tapping it with the finger of the opposite hand, he moved across the patient's chest, tapping it with the palmar surface of his open hand. Feeling comfortable that he had outlined the borders of the heart, he did not palpate for the point of maximal impulse but after he percussed what he thought were the borders of the heart, he carefully listened to the heart on the left side of the patient's chest.

After finishing the remainder of the examination, the attending physician asked to see the patient's chest x-ray film. One of the residents put the chest x-ray on the view box so that the heart was on the right side rather than the left. The attending physician went to the view box, took down the x-ray, and flipped it over so that the heart was now on the left. The resident got up from his chair, walked over to the view box, flipped the x-ray to its original position, and said, "We believe that this man has Kartagener syndrome with bronchiectasis, sinusitis, and situs inversus with dextrocardia." The attending physician thought for a few seconds and said, "I do not recall if I mentioned that the heart sounds did sound distant to me."

One aspect of the teaching process in Boston City Hospital's Neurological Unit was the presentation of patients to the chairman by residents. After the chairman examined the patient, he made both anatomic and pathological diagnoses based on the history and examination. Of course, when the chairman made rounds, the residents would often present cases that they thought would be likely to trip up the chairman. Although it was highly unusual for Dr. Geschwind to misdiagnose a case, no physician is immune from error, and on occasion he did arrive at the wrong diagnosis. However, because he was trained by Dr. Denny-Brown, when Dr. Geschwind did misdiagnose a case, it was not because he did not do a thorough examination or because he drew the wrong conclusions based on the evidence. Rather, it was usually because a finding was misleading (a "red herring"). However, rather than give excuses or try to explain how he had been correct all along, he would usually say, "Isn't that interesting?" and then go over what had led him to the wrong conclusions and discuss how the mistake could be avoided in the future, with the hope that others would not fall into the same trap.

It is okay to be wrong, but it is important to learn from one's mistakes. Later in my internship, I rotated to the Memorial Hospital Medical Service. I again had the opportunity to watch the same internist examine a patient. He continued to percuss the chest with the open palm of one hand. Fortunately, this patient did not have Kartagener syndrome.

INFRASTRUCTURE

An academic unit needs not only teachers, students, and patients, it also needs an infrastructure, including space, salaries, laboratories, and equipment. When Norman Geschwind first came to Boston City Hospital, he brought with him several new and excellent faculty members, including the neuroanatomist Deepak Pandya. Since the time of Fleschig, it has been known that each primary sensory area projects to its modality-specific association cortex. Pandya, along with H. Kuypers, studied cortical connections in monkeys. They had demonstrated that the visual, auditory, and tactile sensory cortices converged in the region of the monkey's superior temporal sulcus and the monkey's inferior parietal lobe (Brodmann's area 7). Dr. Denny-Brown, who had been chief of the Neurological Unit before Norm Geschwind replaced him, had proposed that the human parietal lobe was important for sensory synthesis and that lesions in this region were associated with neglect, or what Denny-Brown termed *amorphosynthesis*. Because Dr. Pandya had demonstrated that the superior temporal sulcus and inferior parietal lobe region in monkeys was a multimodal convergence zone, I wanted to ablate this area in monkeys to learn if lesions in this region would be associated with neglect. I planned to train and test three or four monkeys. Pandya had learned that one of the psychologists at the VA Hospital in Jamaica Plains had several rhesus monkeys that he was not using. Pandya asked me if I would go to the Jamaica Plains VA Hospital and speak to the psychologist to seek his advice about our experimental design, to request his participation as a co-investigator, and to ask him if we could use his monkeys for our research.

I went to the psychologist's office at the VA. The psychologist asked me to sit down and explain what I wanted to do. As I started talking, he took a Boston Globe off his desk, opened the paper fully, and without folding it, started reading as I was talking. He held the paper up so I could not see his face, nor he mine. I was stunned and stopped speaking. He said, "Go ahead. Explain." I again attempted to explain the project, but he did not put the paper down. After I finished talking, he put the paper down and told me he would let Dr. Pandya know his decision. I thanked him for his time and left his office.

While I was in the psychologist's office, I wanted to pull the newspaper out of his hand, crumple it up, and tell him to go to hell. Although I did not act out (which was a change for me), I was still angry when I returned to Boston City Hospital. Dr. Pandya asked me how it went and I told him how I had been treated. I told him that I did not care what the psychologist decided and that I did not want anything to do with him or his monkeys. I said that I would rather moonlight three or four nights and buy my own monkeys. After my discussion with Dr. Pandya, I went to the Peabody Building to see some patients on the medicine service. When I returned, I learned that Dr. Geschwind had been looking for me. He told me that he was sorry about what had happened and that I could have as many monkeys as I needed for my research studies.

After such a difficult beginning I was worried that the study would not work out and shared my insecurities with him. However, Dr. Geschwind told me he thought it was a good study and that in any case it should be done. Fortunately, the study did work out. The monkeys developed neglect, and the study was subsequently published with Deepak Pandya and Norm Geschwind as coauthors.

Our Neurological Unit at City Hospital was never affluent. Dr. Geschwind's office had paint peeling off the ceiling, the same paint that had been peeling when Dr. Denny-Brown had previously occupied the office. However, Norman Geschwind made certain that his residents and fellows always had what they needed.

SETTING STANDARDS

Unlike many other chairmen of neurology, Norman Geschwind believed in teaching by invitation rather than by intimidation. He loved medicine and thought that taking care of patients was an honor, and that training and working as a resident physician should be an enjoyable rather than an adverse experience. Unfortunately, some people misunderstood his kindness as leniency.

In all the years I knew Norman Geschwind, I saw him get visibly angry only once. During my residency, the medicine service presented a patient with subacute onset of paraparesis who had been admitted the previous night. After the patient was presented, Dr. Geschwind asked the medical resident what the myelogram showed. The medical resident told Dr. Geschwind that myelography had not been done. Dr. Geschwind's face demonstrated anger, but his voice remained under control. "Why not? When a patient is paraplegic, the sun should not rise before you know the nature of the problem." The medical resident told Dr. Geschwind that he had telephoned the neurology resident on call, who told him that she would see this alcoholic in the morning when she awoke. Dr. Geschwind became furious, and now his anger leaked into his voice. He explained that there was no excuse for not providing the very best care to everybody. Although later we were all relieved to learn that the patient's paraplegia was not caused by cord compression, Dr. Geschwind remained outraged by the neurology resident's behavior. However, rather than publicly rebuke the young doctor, he chose to speak to her privately. I do not know what he told her, but I do know that he always maintained high standards of patient care. I suspect that this was one of the rare times he used a stick instead of a carrot. For the remainder of her residency at City Hospital, she was a model resident.

NO QUESTION IS STUPID

Several years after I left Boston City Hospital, Norman Geschwind and I were invited to participate in a course that was being held in California. We both had to give several lectures, and after the lectures we were scheduled to go to another location for a reception. On the way out of the lecture hall, a young woman stopped Dr. Geschwind and asked him a very naive question. I felt that if she did not know the answer, she should have looked it up before coming to the course. However, Dr. Geschwind was attentive to her question and answered it fully. She then asked another question that I thought was even worse than the first. Norman Geschwind could detect my annoyance and impatience. I motioned to him with my head that we had to go. He ignored me and gave the woman another detailed answer to her question. We then headed out of the hotel to our ride. He asked me what the rush was. I told him we were going to be late for the reception. In the car he asked me if there was anything more important than answering a student's question. I maintained that those were stupid questions. Although he admitted that some people ask questions to hear themselves talk, no sincere question is stupid. He explained that he felt it was more important for teachers to answer the naive questions of beginning students than the sophisticated questions of experienced students. Even before we got into this discussion, I knew how he felt, and although I am often impatient, I knew he was correct.

In his book *Master of the Bead Game,* Hermann Hesse notes that our educational system is inverted. We often reserve our very best, most experienced teachers for the brightest, most advanced students and put the least experienced teachers with the youngest, most naive students. Because teachers can be so influential, the most experienced ones should be assigned to beginning students and the least experienced ones to advanced students. The problem with this system, of course, is that inexperienced teachers may have nothing to offer advanced students. Fortunately, Geschwind had a lot to offer both. He enjoyed teaching both beginning and advanced students and always valued every student. That day in the car on the way to the reception, Norm Geschwind taught me that students' questions reflect their desire to learn. Their questions are not stupid, but teachers can be arrogant.

MENTORS NEVER STOP

Mentor was not only Telemachus' teacher; he was also Ulysses' advisor. Therefore, the term *mentor* means not only teacher but also counselor. After I left Boston City Hospital, Norman Geschwind never stopped being my teacher, advisor, or friend. Although he had less opportunity to instruct me directly, he was always just a phone call away. After he died, I, like many of his other residents and fellows, grieved as if I had lost a family member. Although he is physically gone, he continues to inspire me. Whenever I am writing a paper or giving a lecture, I continue to think, "What would Norman think of this?" Even when physically absent, mentors remain with their students. I miss Norm, but I am glad he is still with me.

3

A Mensch

Andrew Kertesz

Department of Clinical Neurological Sciences, St. Joseph's Health Centre, University of Western Ontario, London, Ontario N6A 4V2 Canada

As I look at the picture of a youthful Norman Geschwind in Toronto's Nathan Phillips' Square (Fig. 1) with the futuristic city hall and Henry Moore's "archer" in the background, memories of the man and the time I spent with him come alive. The time is 1969, and the occasion is the Toronto meeting of the American Neurological Association (ANA), and I am proudly showing Norman the sights. He is not an inveterate sightseer—he would rather sit in a café and talk. We drive to London, Ontario, where he gives a talk to the Department of Medicine (Neurology is only a division then). He is staying with us; his visit is "on the cheap." At dinner, he is dominating the conversation, his string of ethnic jokes unending. The others, Arthur Hudson, Charlie Drake, and Bill McInnis, don't have to make much effort. My nervousness quickly disappears as he puts everyone at ease. Occasional glances at my very proper colleagues assure me that they are enjoying his company hugely. He is hardly touching Ann's chicken paprika, he is so busy talking. His recent publication *Disconnexion Syndromes in Animals and Man* (1,2) is widely known, and he fields numerous questions about it. Norman is also sensitive to the nonprofessionals at the dinner table and we are soon back to anecdotes.

Three years before, when my family and I arrived in Boston for my fellowship with Geschwind, I called him on a Saturday to "check in" and see where I should join him on Monday. He invited us to his home that afternoon and asked if I needed a cash advance until my first paycheck. For the occasion, I had stopped at Newton Center to buy a summer suit. I need not have bothered, because everyone was casually dressed. He offered to have us stay with him until we found a house (I do not think I had told him yet that I had three preschoolers in tow). We found his generous hospitality and his unreserved kindness unaccustomed. It became obvious that he was a mensch in every respect.

Soon after I arrived and settled down to cover the ward under the direct supervision of Frank Benson, Norman arranged to have us meet with Pasko Rakic and Paul Yakovlev in the Anatomy Department at Harvard. They had described a left-to-right dominance in the medullary decussation of the pyramids in the brains of infants in their large developmental study. Their collection of anatomic specimens, from infant medullas to porpoise gyral patterns, was most impressive. Norman wanted to study the decussation of adult medullas. This was the beginning of his interest in anatomic substrates of handedness and functional asymmetry. He left the details to me. His grant covered my salary (a princely sum compared with the pittance Canadian residents received at that time), but I had to scrounge equipment from José Segarra's Neuropathology Department. In the end, we still needed more medullas, especially those of left-handers, because not many veterans who

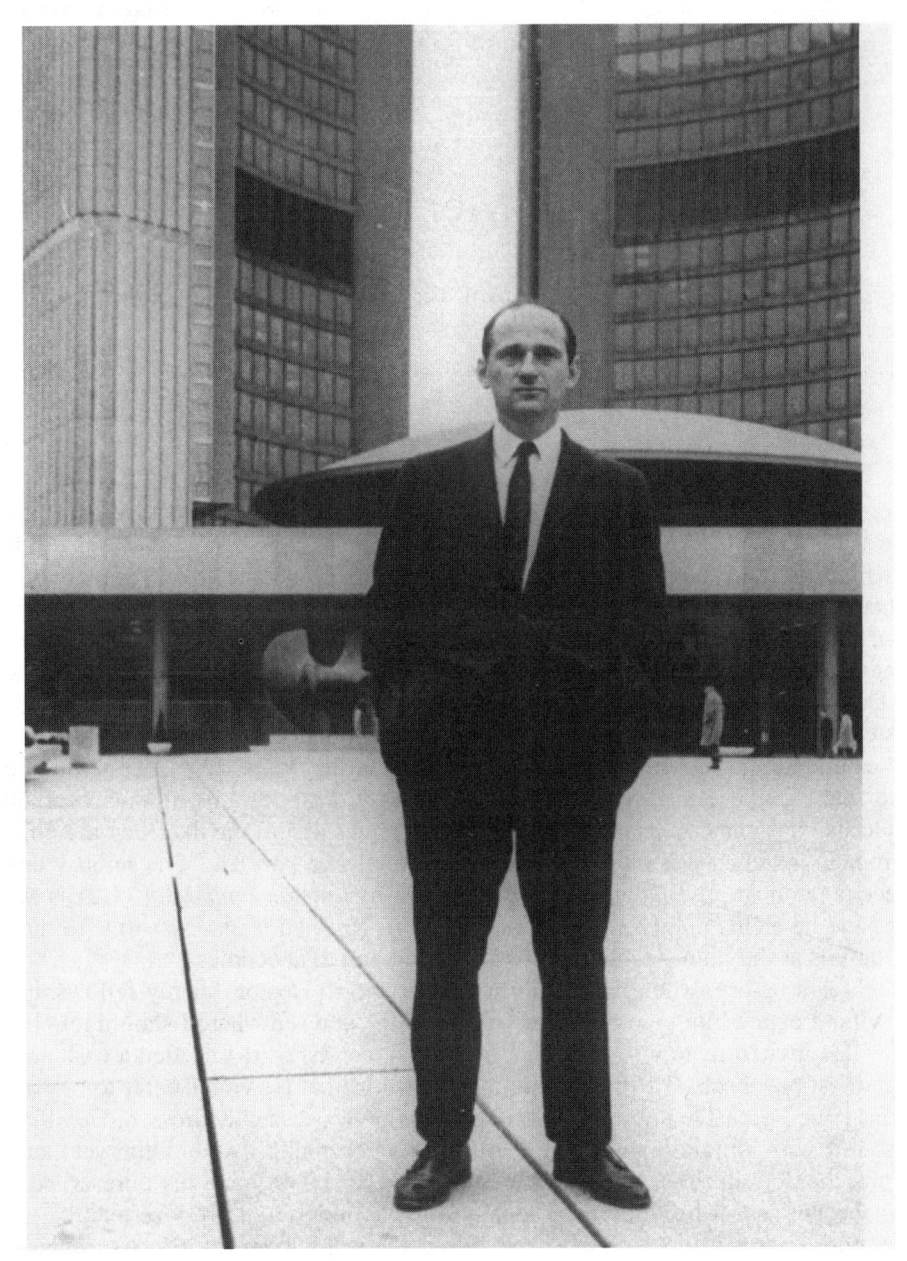

FIG. 1. Photograph of Norman Geschwind in Toronto (1969).

died around that time were left-handed. Norman encouraged me to continue in London after I accepted a staff appointment at the University of Western Ontario. He kept in touch, answered all my queries, and helped me write a paper on the relationship of medullary decussation to handedness and cerebral dominance, which was eventually published (3). Although interest in the paper was limited, Norman's paper on the asymmetry of the planum temporale, which was published in Science and described a study carried out the year before with Levitsky, became a landmark (4).

Norman's clinical approach and his familiarity with syndromes were surpassed only by the wealth of his theoretical and basic science knowledge. The well-earned reputation of the Boston Veterans Administration Hospital aphasia rounds was based partly on Norman's ability to comment on just about everything in a most erudite and stimulating fashion. This is not to diminish the contributions of others. Harold Goodglass dispensed pearls of clinical wisdom, scientific objectivity, and inescapable logic, and he launched experiments to explain clinical phenomena. Edith Kaplan could be relied upon for drama, humor, original observations, or a non sequitur, and Frank Benson held the clinical service together, being responsible for managing the patients and diagnosing their disorders, as well as for several very original research projects. The residents, fellows, psychologists, and speech therapists were all listened to carefully: everybody had an opportunity to shine. I do not remember Norman ever interrupting me, but I do recall his picking up several of my observations and dissecting them carefully, never in the form of a put-down. He may have repeated part of an examination in fascinating detail, never to point out one's omissions but always to make a clinical point. He often asked for a match to show the superiority of object use in buccofacial apraxia, and he would give a characteristic little sniff or snort of satisfaction as he explained why the patient, who previously had not even been able to imitate blowing, could now blow out the flame.

The unit was entering a dynamic phase when I was there. Both Norman Geschwind and Harold Goodglass established their own training programs. Harold was training several generations of psychologists and psycholinguists who were to become leaders in their respective fields. The fellows trained by Norman at that time included Martha Denckla (who was a very pregnant resident the year I was there), François Boller, Marty Albert, and Joe Greenberg, who were my contemporaries or preceded me by a step. Alan Rubens took over my position in 1967. Norman was appointed James Jackson Putman Professor of Neurology in 1967, taking over one of the two endowed chairs in neurology at Harvard from Denny-Brown, who retired. I was there for the time of transition. We still attended Denny-Brown's rounds on Saturday mornings and witnessed the contrast between his style and Norman's. The residents were quaking in their boots, anticipating icy scorn from the grand old man (Denny-Brown) when a mistake was made. In a way, this intimidation seemed effective in keeping the presentations concise and well prepared. However, legends abounded as to what it did to the psyche of some people. Norman transferred the professorial unit to University Hospital, Boston University, because Boston City Hospital had its problems with facilities as well as staffing.

One of the highlights of my stay in Boston was being invited by Norman to have lunch at the Harvard Club with Paul Yakovlev. On the way in, Norman stopped to chat with Leo Alexander. I shook hands and listened in awe. Paul Yakovlev was enthusiastic, entertaining, and eternally youthful. In addition to being an inexhaustible source of knowledge and information about anatomy, he was also a storehouse of anecdotes about Russian and German medicine. He was a dapper little man with a continental flourish, in contrast to Norman's casual manner, yet their scientific interest and knowledge bridged the generation gap and allowed me to witness the best tradition of clinicoanatomic analysis. The work on communicating hydrocephalus was also just published, and Norman discussed Yakovlev's ideas of stretching the leg fibers by the expanding ventricles. Another memorable event Norman took me to as a guest was the quarterly meeting of the Boston Neuroscience Association, which brought together all the greats of clinical neurology and neuroscience. The talk was the epoch-making presentation by Cotzias on the use of high-dose levodopa in Parkinson's disease. For the first time in history one could see, on film, previously immobile, wheelchair-ridden patients get up and play tennis. The jerky black-

and-white pictures were more dramatic than the smooth simulation in the movie *Awakening* that appeared decades later. Characteristically, Denny-Brown was skeptical and implied in his comments that the improvement could have been due to the concomitant physiotherapy. Norman told me on the way out of the lecture hall that this was probably one of the most important scientific achievements of the decade.

Norman was instrumental in founding the Academy of Aphasia around that time. He and Harold Goodglass joined Ron Tikofsky, Martha Taylor-Sarno, Joe Wepman, Ed Weinstein, and Hildred Schuell. I heard about the academy from Donelda McGeachy in Toronto when I was a resident there in 1964, but it was during my fellowship with Norman that I attended the first meeting of the academy in Chicago in 1966. The highlight of that meeting was Norman's talk on Wernicke. He organized the scientific program for the first meeting in Chicago, and for several subsequent ones.

Norman Geschwind's most important contribution to neurology was his revival of behavioral neurology in North America, and probably in the rest of the world as well. Although neuropsychiatry, as behavioral neurology was then known, was an important discipline at the turn of the century, growing interest in the biochemistry of muscles and nerves and the increasing importance of animal models and biochemistry in the neurologic sciences changed that. The discipline that deals with brain and behavioral relationships practically disappeared in neurology until the brilliance of Norman Geschwind revived neurologists' interest in aphasias, alexias, agnosias, and apraxias.

Norman's background was fascinating and ties in with the history of behavioral neurology. He had an undergraduate degree in psychology, and his interest at Harvard was psychiatry. But, as Norman explained, the Harvard neuroanatomy professor Marcus Singer stimulated his interest in epilepsy and aphasia, and Norman decided that a background in neurology was most appropriate for understanding these problems. When he went to England, he found that the subject of behavioral neurology was insignificant there, but after his return to the Boston VA, Fred Quadfasel, a neurologist who trained in Germany under Bonhoeffer and Goldstein (pupils of Wernicke), helped him redirect his interest to the neurologic foundations of behavior. With this background, Norman developed a training and research program with characteristic enthusiasm and spread the seeds of a discipline that has become a substantial part of neurology and continues to grow at an amazing rate. As he wrote in the introduction to his *Selected Papers on Language and the Brain* (1974), in the sixties, "the chairman of the program committee of a major neurological meeting complained there were not enough papers to fill a half-day session on behavior." Today, we have not one but two or three half days of platform papers and two or three poster sessions on behavior at the American Academy of Neurology. Furthermore, the discipline has spread to include dementia, biological psychiatry, child development, the neuropsychiatry of epilepsy, and functional imaging.

Behavioral neurology was revitalized not only by Norman's very successful training program but also by his seminal papers. He described the intellectual origins of his interest in callosal disconnections and alexia and credited Fred Quadfasel with providing him with the original reprint of Déjérine. In reviewing Déjérine's paper, he recognized the relevant recent work of Sperry to this clinical example of callosal disconnection. This led him to publish the very first modern article on human disconnection of the more anterior callosal regions. When Norman presented this case to the Boston Society of Neurology and Psychiatry in 1961, the paper created considerable interest. Norman's explanation of disconnection was met with some skepticism by Teuber, who thought that interference between the hemispheres was present as the cause of the deficit. Norman defended his position skillfully, according to the records, indicating that as long as the stimulation and response were confined to a single hemisphere, the subject performed correctly. In this paper, Geschwind and Kaplan also tried to replicate the transfer of information experiments and found that the patient could learn a maze with the left hand but not with the right, even though apraxia, agraphia, and anomia were present with left-hand performance.

The breadth of Norman's extraordinary grasp of cerebral function was displayed in his two consecutively published articles on the disconnection syndromes in animals and man (1965). There is no way to describe the content of these articles, which represent a monograph by themselves. It is surprising that, given their length, *Brain* accepted them for publication. In fact, Norman subsequently described how the editor of *Brain*, Sir Russell Brain, had expressed some misgivings about the size of the papers and some of their philosophic content but had recognized the innovative and comprehensive nature of the publications and their potential impact. These revolutionary articles have been the source of many subsequent ideas and developments in the field in the last 30 years. The two papers were probably equivalent in impact to Wernicke's 1874 article on the aphasic symptom complex. They are similar in style and expository interpretation. I still use the disconnection articles as a reference when I have a complex clinical problem or before I contemplate a study. They were certainly instrumental in my decision to spend my fellowship with Dr. Geschwind.

Norman Geschwind not only had a vast knowledge of the relevant literature in behavioral neurology but was fully conversant in psychobiology and experimental psychology. He had many friends in the neurosciences, although he was not a "neuropolitician." He was a renowned after-dinner speaker, and his outspoken, humorous delivery will be remembered by all who heard him. He was not an experimentalist: he let others do group studies. His interest in the relationship between cerebral dominance and motor learning led to extensive studies of the anatomic basis of cerebral dominance and subsequently to the discovery, with Galaburda and Kemper, of the abnormalities of brain development in dyslexia. In his later years, he explored new frontiers, in particular the relationship between left-handedness and the genetics of immunologic disease, and the association of hormonal influence and the development of cerebral asymmetries.

Dr. Geschwind's creativity was cut down at its peak by a heart attack and cardiac arrest. Although his death was a major loss to neurology and a personal loss to many of us, his work and intellect remain an extraordinary inspiration.

REFERENCES

1. Geschwind N. Disconnexion syndromes in animals and man. I. *Brain* 1965;88:237–294.
2. Geschwind N. Disconnexion syndromes in animals and man. II. *Brain* 1965;88:585–644.
3. Kertesz A, Geschwind N. Patterns of pyramidal decussation and their relationship to handedness. *Arch Neurol* 1971;24:326–332.
4. Geschwind N, Levitsky KW. Human brain: left–right asymmetries in temporal speech region. *Science* 1968;161:186–187.

4
Colleague

Thomas D. Sabin

Department of Neurology, Boston City Hospital, Boston, Massachusetts 02118.

Norman's written works remain available for all to study and enjoy, but his colleagues and students especially treasure the memories of personal contact with him. I worked for Norman during his tenure (1969–1975) as director of the Neurological Unit at Boston City Hospital and shared many cases on this busy service, usually on a daily basis. Norman enjoyed the robust clinical activity at City Hospital and often spent several hours each day discussing patients and clinical topics with his colleagues there. The nature of the service allowed Norman time to see patients, read, and reflect. Many of his important ideas took form and grew in this fertile environment.

SATURDAY CONFERENCE

The Saturday morning case discussions in the venerable Medical 9 Conference Room provided fine examples of Norman's skills as a clinician. The house staff saved their most difficult cases for these conferences. The residents invariably selected their most baffling and complicated problems, and the presentation always stopped before any laboratory data were given. Any type of neurologic case was considered fair game (although one should recall that eight of Norman Geschwind's papers were on muscle and nerve). The shrewdest residents knew that the more sophistication they demonstrated in their presentation, the more time Norman would spend in discussing the most complicated aspects of the case. An occasional presenter, fooled by Norman's gentleness, would learn that he would not tolerate sloppy presentations and fuzzy thinking. In such instances, Norman would interrupt the presenter and take great pains to persuade the person, with specific examples, that greater precision, thought, and detail might benefit the patient. His tough-minded view of history taking is reflected in the following excerpt from a note to a colleague who referred a patient to him but failed to provide promised background information: "I am forced to spend an excessive amount of time getting information at the time of the interview rather than in advance so that I cannot spend as much time directly looking for new things in the patient. Furthermore, it prevents me from being able to think about exactly what I want to look for when I see the patients who are usually, like this one, very complicated." With his powerful intellectual persuasiveness, Norman made his point effectively without ever humiliating a student, resident, or colleague.

The patient would be wheeled in at 10:00 AM, and Norman would bring out the salient findings from the examination. In spite of Norman's mild manners and scholarly appearance, even the most irascible patient, undergoing frontal lobe examination, would ultimately submit to Norman's "No ifs, ands, or buts," doing some calculations, and trying to determine whether it was the lion or the tiger that had been killed.

Norman consistently found features that had been overlooked by others, and these were not always entirely neurologic: "On the other hand, she has a strikingly short neck." He immediately pointed out, when discussing this feature of a patient, that she had said she had always been aware of how short her neck was and that people had always commented on it. Her husband had also pointed out that he had observed this feature. "She had a striking limitation of neck movement, both to the right and to the left, but no pain. . . . I must say, however, that by far the most likely diagnosis in my mind is some disorder at the foramen magnum. In support of this diagnosis are the very slow course, the strikingly short neck, the limitation of neck movement, and above all the striking reflex level with no abnormal reflexes either in the cranial musculature or at the C2, C3, or C4 level."

In another case, one of a man with probable childhood polio and recent neuropathic symptoms: "Other items of interest in his history are that the granddaughter, who is age 10, had had what appeared to be Guillain-Barré syndrome and had recovered over about a year. The patient does not think that his episode in childhood was of this nature. He has also noted that he has a diminution in his olfactory function, having lost certain odors, (e.g., that of skunk). The only other change in his health has been an allergy to clams which produces cramps and diarrhea." As the ensuing case discussion unfolded, the topics might range from the geographic distribution of left-handedness to the proper way of looking at cells in the spinal fluid. The discourse not only was wide-ranging but also was decorated with spontaneous quips, humorous insights, and detailed recollections of relevant past cases. Norman would draw an outline of the brain on the blackboard, characteristically a lateral view done in one stroke of the chalk that was in configuration halfway between a human brain and a monkey brain (Fig. 1). Gradually, he would shade in the areas of the brain involved in the case. By noon, he would interrupt his discussion, stating that he was concerned there would not be time for the second case and that it was therefore time to hear about the laboratory results in the first case. Norman consistently evoked in his listeners the excitement about neurology that originally drew us all to this specialty. Questioning and discussion would continue, the attendees meandering out of the conference room and into the corridor. Often the discussion would continue late into Saturday afternoon in the hospital parking lot.

Norman felt that it was important to teach his residents and students how to read the literature critically. In his behavioral neurology course, he assigned several papers that he viewed as seriously flawed; he wanted to make certain that his students could recognize faulty arguments, especially misleading statistical analyses. (Norman's mathematical talents were revealed in his paper on normal-pressure hydrocephalus, which appeared in the *Journal of Neurological Sciences* 1968;7(3):759–769.) Norman often stressed that statistics on the percentages of neurologic manifestations of various systemic illness such as lupus or sarcoidosis were often misleading because reports were usually prepared by internists and, therefore, the neurologic illness must have appeared as part of the systemic illness. Neurologists, he contended, should recognize nervous system manifestations when systemic signs and symptoms are absent. It was partly this view of statistics that made him a champion of individual case reports. He believed that thoroughly studying a single case was more valuable than statistically analyzing a large number of poorly studied cases, and he was fond of citing many instances in which a single case report had resulted in an incremental step forward in neurology. Some of his own case descriptions can be counted among them.

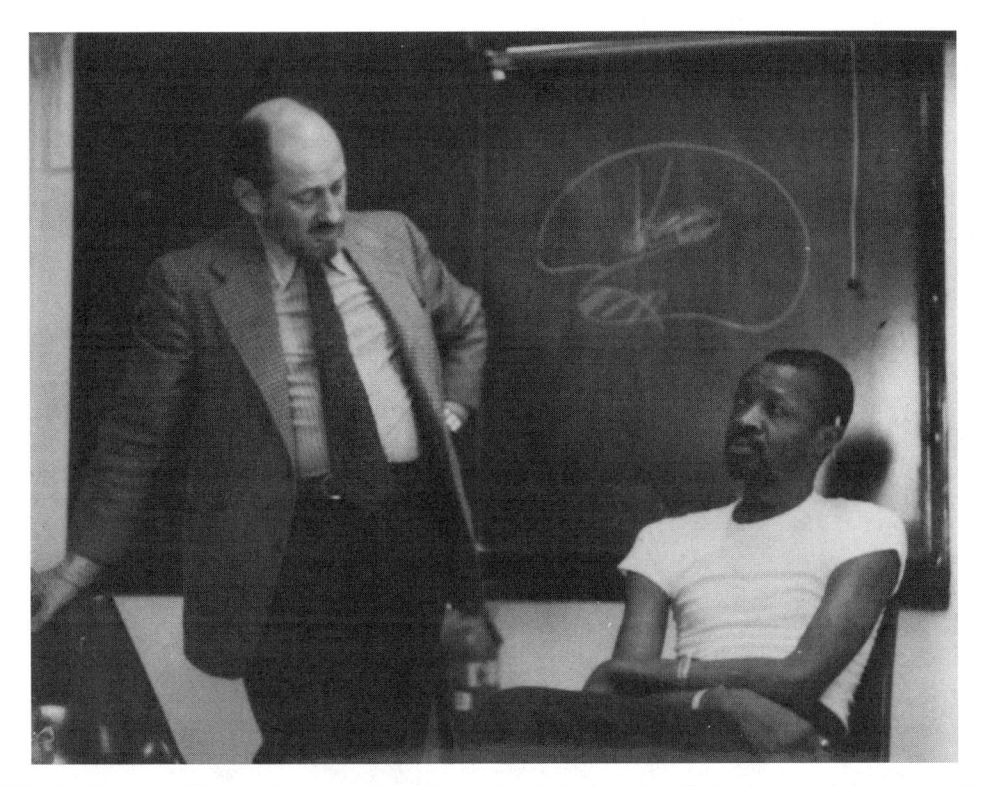

FIG. 1. Norman Geschwind examining a patient during the Saturday conference on the Boston City Hospital Neurological Unit (1979).

Norman felt strongly that neurologists should learn about rare diseases because, otherwise, "Who could possibly diagnose them? Should we call in a nurse practitioner specializing in rare diseases?" He pointed out that rare diseases were often treatable and that their recognition would, at the very least, prevent inappropriate, costly, or dangerous treatments or tests from being done. He also argued that the understanding of the natural history of such diseases would very likely promote insights into more common ailments.

Norman's bedside evaluations were always meticulous and complete; although long, they were never boring to watch because of his masterful use of his observations in sculpturing subsequent parts of the assessment. The discussion wove together all these observations into a diagnostic formulation that might include the significance of the patient's multiple religious conversions or the possible influences of the patient's intrauterine environment. Norman's clinical approach reflected a mode of thought that underpinned his contributions to neurology. His works did not reflect a single flash of insight but an accumulation of knowledge in astounding detail, in which Norman saw elaborate and profound interrelationships. He was known for his lengthy discourses and typically spent more than 2 hours discussing a single case. These sessions not only served patient care and teaching but also were an integral part of his creative process. Those who viewed Norman's lectures as iterative missed the new thread in the conceptual tapestry that appeared in each discussion of a topic. Details—and he had a prodigious memory for them—were as vital to him (a naturalist of nervous system disease) as the small differences in the Galapagos flora and fauna were to Darwin. Each patient was important to him because he believed that clinical problems were one of the most important ways of determining how the human nervous system worked: "The interictal behavioral features in temporal lobe epilepsy provide a unique window into the human limbic system." Those who did not have the opportunity to hear his full elucidation of the topic might be mystified by a part of the story given in isolation, but those who had the opportunity to hear the 3-hour version could not help being persuaded by the marvelous interlocking of so many observations. Anything short of a full hearing was unfair to Norman's contributions.

NORMAN'S "JUNIOR COLLEAGUES"

Norman took a great personal interest in his residents and followed their careers, particularly their scholarly publications, with the most intense interest. During the period at City Hospital he pointed with pride at the high percentage of his residents who went into academic neurology. The list of neurologic residents on the unit during those years includes:

David Bear	Michael Biber	Remi Bouchard
Louis Caplan	Thierry Deonna	Stephen Depperman
Joseph Donnelly	Howard Fields	Albert Galaburda
Patrick Griffin	Andrew Herzog	John Hooge
Angkana Indarakoses	Glen Jamison	Eduardo Karol
Kyung Sae	Kim Frank Ludwig	Robert Marin
Jaime Mejlszenkier	Marsel Mesulam	James Nealis
Edgar Oppenheimer	Nicholas Panagiotis	Eberto Pineiro
Mark Platt	Frisso Potts	Michael Remler
Elliott Ross	Edward Schima	Brooke Seckel
Benjamin Seltzer	William Sheremata	Taranath Shetty
Everard Siller	Denis Simard	Thomas Stanley
Lawrence Tomasi	Edward Valenstein	Jesus Velez-Borras
Stephen Waxman		

Norman was also exceedingly interested in the education of medical students, whom he treated as junior colleagues. He was concerned about the fact that medical students learned almost all their clinical skills from persons who were only a year ahead of them in their training. He thought that students should spend more time with senior faculty. To this end, he took time from his hectic schedule, often early on Saturday mornings, to have weekly sessions with the medical students. Phone calls from students had, next to those from his patients, the highest priority for returning. He made an extra effort always to be available for appointments with students in his office.

Despite Norman's traditional, methodical approach to physical findings and differential diagnoses, he was ever alert for new relationships. In his last years, he became fascinated with the frequency with which developmental anomalies in the nervous system were reflected in the skin and its appendages. I showed him a woman with late-life chorea, which could have been a possible recurrence of childhood Sydenham's chorea. He analyzed the movement disorder but was also struck by the patient's head of black hair with two white streaks arising from her hairline, much like the bride of Frankenstein. After leaving her, he smiled and produced a characteristic gesture, placing his hand at his forehead; then suddenly he extended his arm in mock epiphany and said, "Premature graying right over her caudates."

Norman was never at a loss in a teaching situation. In his early years at Boston City Hospital, he was called upon by Paul Rosman to make a monthly visit to the Child Neurology Service. I once had to locate him during one of these rounds, and I found him in the nursery, begowned and surrounded by pediatricians. He was standing beside an incubator with a newborn in it, holding the pediatrics staff spellbound by a discussion of aphasia.

He was most canny in using keen insights into the nuances of everyday behavior to make indelible impressions on his students. On one occasion, he tried to explain that the syndrome of denial and lack of concern over the existence of a left hemiplegia was a relative phenomenon. He went on to note that if he asked an older person how he or she was feeling, the person might say, "Well, thank you," in spite of myopia, dental cavities, hemorrhoids, graying hair, and extensive hair loss. People tend to ignore these maladies, he pointed out, because they are relatively unimportant. So it was with a patient under discussion who, although he did not deny his hemiplegia, was inappropriately unconcerned about it.

WEDNESDAY "BRAIN-CUTTING"

"Brain-cutting" sessions on Wednesday afternoons were another weekly high point for Norman's staff. Here, with Flaviu Romanul, Don Price, Larry Embree, and Tom Kemper serving successively as neuropathologists on the unit, Norman found another medium for his clinical acumen. He viewed these sessions as a major opportunity for feedback on his residents' progress in the mastery of neurology. His own discussion of the case began with a detailed reply, rebuttal, or amplification of the comments previously made by the junior discussants. He also allowed the students to discuss these cases, and the senior secretary, Portia Tholl, gave the selected student discussant a copy of the protocol, with strict instructions that it not be shared with anybody else. The student also received a handout that was written by Norman on how to discuss a clinicopathologic conference (CPC).

This document begins: "The natural tendency of students to carry out a sequential line-by-line analysis should be avoided since a major characteristic of the well-trained clinician is the ability to place differing weights on certain pieces of information and often to deliberately disregard certain of the data."

Brain cuttings are inevitably a time when one occasionally must accept one's errors. Norman always did this with humility and grace, using the opportunity to point out the line of argument that might have led to the correct diagnosis. He once wrote in a consult: "At the time I saw him, I had to admit that I had no idea what his diagnosis was. At any rate, the postmortem showed a remarkable set of findings." Indeed, he seemed always eager to hear criticisms of his ideas as long as they were offered sincerely. He once related to me that when the wife of a colleague talked about her husband, she attributed almost God-like qualities to him. He said he felt sorry for this colleague, because "he was losing one of the great benefits of marriage." He explained that Pat, his wife, had just told him, when he was describing a forthcoming lecture, "Oh, Norman you aren't going to talk about that old stuff again," and this spurred him on to develop some important new ideas for the forthcoming lecture.

Norman seemed to be a person devoid of malice. The worst thing I ever heard him say about anyone was that he was a person of "modest intellect." Norman tried to avoid some committees and administrative problems, but he always accepted tasks related to teaching, and thus he came to be on the house officers' committee at Boston City Hospital and on the curriculum committee at Harvard. He was interested not only in the specifics of day-to-day teaching but the general approach to teaching medicine at all levels. Some of his ideas on what a medical education should include were posthumously published in an article entitled, "Even Homer Sometimes Nods—On Cerebral Technological Obsolescence," which appeared in the Harvard Medical Alumni Bulletin for the spring of 1985.

•2•

THE ROLE OF THE SPECIALIST

Norman was adamant about the fact that clinicians would increasingly need specialized knowledge to assimilate effectively the fruits of basic science into medical practice. He also believed that care by highly skilled specialists should be cost effective. He thought that a single, lengthy, "more expensive" visit with a good neurologist could take care of most headache problems, contrasting this with multiple, brief, "less costly" visits to nonneurologists, producing a barrage of tests and long-term polypharmacy. He thought that the difference in outcome from practice of neurology at the very highest level as compared to practice at the journeymen level was very small—five or six cases per year. This estimate of the "cost of excellence" was a warning to us of the ascendancy of today's pressure to use a strategy of combining both nonspecialists and no testing. When a resident's only defense for ordering a test was that an academic service needs to find out everything, Norman was quick to point out that in an academic setting, the priority is teaching physicians how to take care of patients properly and that doing unnecessary or risky testing was contrary to this highest academic priority. In a consult, Norman wrote about a multiple sclerosis patient with absent reflexes in the lower extremities: "Obviously, this issue might be settled by actually measuring nerve conduction velocities. On the other hand, when one considers the unpleasantness of the procedure and the lack of implications for therapy, I am not sure I would want to proceed with any further studies, at least at this time."

I cherish the time I spent with Norman on the Boston City Hospital Neurological Unit. He was one of those rare persons who have a lifelong impact on their colleagues.

5
Advisor

Elliott D. Ross

Department of Neuroscience, University of North Dakota School of Medicine, Fargo, North Dakota 58102.

When I entered medical school at Boston University in 1964, my goal was to be a surgeon. However, after two surgical rotations, I was more interested in my patients' medical problems than their surgical treatment. In my fourth year, I was introduced to the fascinating behaviors exhibited by psychiatric patients and considered a career in psychiatry, but I rapidly became disillusioned because the attending physicians were analytically oriented and never once discussed their patients' behaviors in terms of the brain. Instead, they talked about schizophrenic mothering, toilet training, and other issues that seemed irrelevant to me. Toward the end of the rotation, after I had stopped going to formal teaching rounds, one of my fellow students urged me to attend a special teaching session: a patient was being presented with severe depression and temporal lobe epilepsy and "some neurologist named Geschwind" was the discussant. Begrudgingly, I went to the rounds, and Dr. Geschwind expounded eloquently for over 2 hours on temporal lobe epilepsy, interictal personality disorders, depression, and schizophreniform psychosis (1–3). It was a spellbinding experience that sealed my fate—I would become a behavioral neurologist and train under Dr. Geschwind. From then on, I attended Dr. Geschwind's ward rounds and formal lectures whenever possible and read and reread many times his extraordinary disconnexion papers (4).

I finally began my neurology training at Boston City Hospital in 1973. Not only was the program blessed by having Dr. Geschwind as chairman, but the quality of residents he recruited was outstanding: Brooke Seckel, who ultimately became an academic plastic surgeon, and Ben Seltzer were a year ahead of me; Steve Waxman (currently chairman of Neurology at Yale), Andy Herzog, and Jesus Velez-Borras (currently chairman of Neurology at the University of Puerto Rico) were fellow residents; and Marsel Mesulam and Al Galaburda were a year behind. Even the residents who went into private practice, such as Ed Schima and John Hooge, were incredible sources of knowledge. In addition, Tom Sabin, Ira Sherwin, Tom Kemper, Dee Pandya, Simeon Locke, and Simmons Lessell provided further academic sustenance, and we were exposed periodically to special guest lecturers, such as Derek Denny-Brown, Jerry Lettvin, Hans Kuypers, Paul Yakovlev, Mort Mishkin, and Carelton Gadjusek. It was an incredible academic and clinical milieu for residency training.

ALWAYS RESPECT YOUR PATIENTS

As head of the Neurological Unit, Dr. Geschwind set the standards of operation, mostly by example. He always emphasized that, regardless of the situation (including scholastic pursuits), one's clinical responsibilities always came first, and all patients were to be treated with respect. This precept often tested our mettle because our patient population consisted mainly of indigent, down-and-out alcoholics. Often, these patients were so ill that taking a history was not possible. (For example, the most common presentation for brain tumor was coma.)

My most instructive patient in regard to respect was "Ralph." He had been banished by his wife to the basement of their house because of bizarre behaviors with which we rapidly became acquainted after his admission to our ward. Although Ralph could walk unassisted, he would just stare unresponsively at whomever attempted to engage him in conversation. He would periodically retire to the utility room and sit on the sink counter drinking the contents of urine specimens while toasting anyone who walked by. Once in a while, he would completely undress, casually amble down the hall, look intensely with a wild and bug-eyed demeanor at some object or person, and then immediately follow this behavior with projectile vomiting. On the day we presented his case, I, as senior ward resident, accompanied Dr. Geschwind to Ralph's bedside, followed by the other residents and medical students. As we turned the corner, there was Ralph standing naked in the middle of the corridor with his wild, bug-eyed facial expression. Before I could produce a word of warning, Ralph's projectile vomitus struck Dr. Geschwind in the chest. The rest of us plastered ourselves against the wall as Ralph blithely walked pass and continued to vomit. We finally captured him and placed him in bed. Meanwhile Dr. Geschwind was carefully washing off his tie and shirt at the sink. After he had finished and replaced his white coat, Dr. Geschwind approached Ralph in a most respectful manner, formally introduced himself, and extended his hand. Amazingly, Ralph shook Dr. Geschwind's hand and rounds resumed. After interviewing and examining the patient, Dr. Geschwind discussed the case (out of Ralph's earshot) in terms of the Klüver-Bucy syndrome, and he casually remarked that Ralph was without a doubt the most demented patient he had ever seen who could still walk.

Dr. Geschwind always reinforced the idea that each patient was unique, and that all patients, from those with higher cortical deficits to those with simple compression neuropathies in the foot, offered us an opportunity to discover something about the nervous system. Every aspect of neurology was important. In all my years as a neurologist, I have never seen anyone perform a more detailed muscle and nerve examination than Dr. Geschwind. He also insisted that we read the literature relevant to our patients and that we not accept his or any other attending's interpretation of a case without first checking the literature. His reason for this admonishment was that he himself could be wrong, and if he was wrong, it was our responsibility to let him know so that he could learn from his mistakes. Needless to say, in the 3 years I spent with Dr. Geschwind poring over the literature, I never discovered errors in his scholarship.

PURSUE YOUR QUESTIONS

The most telling aspect of Dr. Geschwind's mentorship was the large percentage of residents he trained who pursued academic careers. After I became director of Resident Training in Neurology at the University of Texas Southwestern Medical Center at Dallas, Norman and I had a discussion about the general quality of residents and their lack of interest in academic pursuits. He commented that at a recent American Neurological Association meeting, he had had a similar conversation with Drs. Robert Fishman, Stan Appel, and, I believe, Bud Roland. Only 20% of their residents went on to academic careers, despite spending time in the laboratory. They were astounded to learn that almost two thirds of Norman's residents continued in academia. Although his program lacked a major basic research program, Norman explained that he endeavored to make clinical neurology so fascinating that his residents, upon completing their training, had no choice but to embark on an academic career if they wished to pursue their many unanswered questions about the nervous system.

In addition to making clinical neurology fascinating for students and residents, Dr. Geschwind was always available to answer questions, see difficult patients, and engage in sophisticated and detailed discussions about neurologic issues that went beyond the scope of formal rounds. Although he was a Putnam Professor, he never let ceremony or rank interfere with his commitment to teaching. Everyone felt important and welcomed when entering his office. When I was struggling to write my first paper (5), he took each draft and corrected not only the thematic flow of ideas but also errors in spelling, syntax, and paragraph construction. The drafts were full of penciled comments, corrections, and suggestions. After six edits, the paper was finally ready for submission. When I thanked him for his help and commented that I was embarrassed that he had spent so much time on the paper, much like an English teacher, he responded that he considered this to be an important obligation. He assured me that writing papers would become easier over time, especially if I had something worthwhile to publish. He then admitted that he also found writing difficult and that six or seven drafts were usual for him.

CONCLUSION

In looking back over my academic career, what is most striking is the pervasive influence Norman had, first as a mentor and finally as a friend and colleague. But even more important is that Norman engendered such good will in persons of diverse scientific disciplines that at almost every critical juncture in my research career, someone with connections to him helped provide me the correct direction. Although Norman passed away more than 10 years ago, when I reflect on scientific and ethical issues or administrative and teaching obligations, I always consider, even if only briefly, what advice Norman would have offered if he were still alive.

REFERENCES

1. Slater E, Beard AW. The schizophrenia-like psychoses of epilepsy (in 5 parts). *Br J Psychiatry* 1963;109:95–150.
2. Bear DM, Fedio P. Quantitative analysis of interictal behavior in temporal lobe epilepsy. *Arch Neurol* 1977;34:454–467.
3. Waxman SG, Geschwind N. The interictal behavioral syndrome of temporal lobe epilepsy. *Arch Neurol* 1975;32:1580–1586.
4. Geschwind N. Disconnexion syndromes in animals and man (2 parts). *Brain* 1965;88:237–294, 585–644.
5. Ross ED, Jossman PG, Bell B, Sabin T, Geschwind N. Musical hallucinations in deafness. *JAMA* 1975;231:620–622.

*Behavioral Neurology and
the Legacy of Norman Geschwind,*
edited by S. C. Schachter and O. Devinsky,
Lippincott-Raven Publishers, Philadelphia © 1997.

6
Role Model

Stephen G. Waxman

*Department of Neurology, Yale Medical School,
New Haven, Connecticut 06520-8018.*

One of the most wonderful things about academic medicine is the tradition of mentorship: both the experience of having a mentor and the opportunity to be a mentor to others. I learned this explicitly from my wife, Merle Waxman (1), but I learned it implicitly from one of my more pivotal teachers and role models, Norman Geschwind. Norman Geschwind became my mentor in July of 1972, when I returned to Boston from the Albert Einstein College of Medicine in New York, where I had chosen to study in the combined M.D.–Ph.D. program. I had picked Norman Geschwind's residency (indeed, I viewed it not as the Boston City Hospital Neurology Residency but as Norman Geschwind's program) because of its emphasis on clinical neurology and behavioral neuroscience. The choice had been made especially easy by Norman. Although it was only toward the end of my clinical rotations in medical school that I decided to do my residency in neurology rather than psychiatry, Norman welcomed me enthusiastically to the world of neurology and, in fact, rapidly emerged as a major figure in my intellectual growth.

It is hard to forget Professor's Rounds with Geschwind—they were uplifting, provocative, and challenging experiences. During my time at Boston City Hospital (1972–1975), these rounds were held every Tuesday morning in the neurology library on Med-9 (the ninth floor of the Medical Building) at Boston City Hospital. The room itself had an informal and somewhat shabby, yet clearly imposing, ethos to it: it had been the training ground for many neurological luminaries. Photographs of these giants surrounded us in the neurology library, peering down through small eyes as if to ask, "Will you ever walk in our footsteps?" Not an easy act to follow.

Despite his small size, Geschwind dominated rounds, shifting his eyes, along with the dialogue, from medical student to house officer to student again, at each juncture injecting his own provocative and incisive comments. In his rounds, he found even the most mundane patient interesting, and every medical student, every clerk, every house officer felt as if his or her opinions were important. Rounds often continued on the neurology ward. Geschwind was, of course, a master at the bedside and managed to find (or create) something interesting and instructive in every patient. Geschwind's belief that it was crucial for house officers to commit themselves and, having done so, to defend their views, irrespective of how unconventional or provocative they might be, produced a scintillating atmosphere. Ideas reverberated throughout the ward at incredible speed.

THE INTERICTAL SYNDROME

One of these ideas, which first came to my attention in 1972, concerned the behavioral changes that occur in patients with limbic epilepsy [at that time, Geschwind referred to the seizure disorder as temporal lobe epilepsy (TLE)]. When I first heard his description of the voluminous, pathologically detailed writings by patients with TLE, I did not believe him. My entreaty to him for a reference that I could read about the subject was met with a puff on his pipe and a shrug of his shoulders: "It's not in the literature, Steve, but these patients are a dime a dozen." It was this simple discussion that led me to take a careful interictal behavioral history from my patients. The results, which provided clear documentation that patients with limbic epilepsy had an unusual, pathological tendency to produce voluminous writings, were written up and published in two papers (2,3) that are still widely quoted and are more fully discussed in Chapter 26. This syndrome, to my mind, is reproducible, interesting, and important. It met with mixed reviews, some rave ("Geschwind . . . and Waxman galvanized the neurological world") (4) and some highly critical. Our joint papers continue to be cited as much as some of my more recent, avant-garde molecular studies. Attribution for the initial observation continues to be confused, as references to the Waxman-Geschwind syndrome, the Geschwind-Waxman syndrome, and the Geschwind syndrome reflect. My role was to listen, to read, to coin the term *hypergraphia,* and to collect and describe the patients that appeared in these papers—the idea was Norman's. Thus, over a decade ago, I pointed out that the term *Geschwind-Waxman syndrome* is more apt than the converse (5).

I worked with Norman for three years after finishing my residency, first as assistant professor, then as associate professor. Then, in 1978, I moved to Stanford. It was there, nearly a decade after we published the first descriptions of the interictal syndrome, that one of my residents, Harmeet Sachdev, confronted me and asked whether the interictal syndrome of TLE was a common one. By now, I knew how to answer, and although I had no pipe to puff on, I replied, "They're a dime a dozen." The next day, Sachdev was back in my office, sufficiently provoked to ask how we could prove it. We put together a small study in which he sent a stamped return envelope, together with a request to write "as much as you wish, in any form, on any kind of paper," to all patients who had been discharged over a six-year period with the diagnosis of epilepsy or seizure disorder. I predicted that we would be able to pick out the patients with TLE by weighing the responses. The results of this study were published in 1981 (6), and indeed, they showed a very strong tendency for patients with TLE to reply more frequently and with more extensive writing. The responses from patients with TLE (mean: 1,301 words) were more than ten times as long as those of patients with other forms of epilepsy (mean: 106 words). Two patients returned responses that were longer than 4,000 words, and both of these patients had bitemporal EEG foci.

DISTAL SENSORY LOSS

Norman Geschwind was a truly eclectic man. Who would have expected this master of behavioral neurology to teach me about peripheral nerve disease? It was Geschwind who first pointed out to me (although the idea may have been Tom Sabin's) that distal sensory loss (i.e., stocking–glove sensory loss) in peripheral neuropathies does not necessarily imply distal pathology. He suggested that the stocking–glove pattern of deficit might be explained by random scattering of multifocal, microscopic lesions along the entire trajectory of the axons within a nerve. If lesions were placed randomly, a longer fiber would be more likely to have a lesion somewhere along its length.

Because at that time I had just begun to become interested in demyelination, this hypothesis was exciting to me. Working nights and evenings in the laboratory of Jerry Lettvin at the Massachusetts Institute of Technology together with Michael Brill, a graduate student, I did a number of computer simulations to test this hypothesis. At that time, all that was available to us was a PDP LINC-8 computer, which we used for free after 10:00 PM. Largely as a result of slow peripherals, the computations took much longer than they would now (Mike, who smoked at the time, was able to take more than a few puffs while we waited for the results). Our results showed that a random scattering of abnormalities (e.g., sites of conduction block) provided a condition that could cause distal sensory deficit, with the longest fibers being involved at the earliest stages (7).

We also examined the possibility that weak interactions between nerve fibers could produce a situation in which small increments or decrements in membrane potential could bring a given fiber closer to, or farther from, threshold. We predicted that this situation might produce axon–axon interactions similar to the weak coupling between nonlinear oscillators that had been a familiar problem in engineering since the time of Huyghens, who observed the entrainment of the pendulums on the wall of a watchmaker's shop. Our simulations did not provide unequivocal evidence, but they were consistent with the idea that axon–axon interactions might play a role in the generation of paresthesia in peripheral nerve disease. Jerry Lettvin, in the final manuscript, added a graphic description of the proposed physiologic events:

> One imagines that an impulse, coming to a partial block, either halts there or is aided in passage by an impulse in a neighboring fiber. If it is so aided, the two fibers carry impulses in phase and will be even more effective with respect to a block in some third fiber a little farther up the path. In this way, a coherent front forms, subverting the information available from the fibers separately into the meaningless chant of a group in lockstep . . . similar to the "pins and needles" of paresthesia.

GESCHWIND AS ROLE MODEL

It is hard to describe Norman Geschwind without at least briefly acknowledging the associations he helped me to forge, the introductions that he made for me. Tom Sabin, Jerry Lettvin, Ian McDonald, Ian Simpson, Paul Yakovlev, and Derek Denny-Brown, among others, were all introduced to me by Norman Geschwind. Elliott Ross, Marcel Mesulam, Al Galaburda, and I shared the conference table in the library that was a focal point of Geschwind's program, and we became lifelong associates as well as friends.

I felt close to Norman throughout our years together. But it wasn't until years later that I understood what had transpired between us. Recognition came in a conversation with Merle. "Role modeling," she said, "that's one of the things Norman provided for you. It's one of the reasons that you are the person that you are."

Perhaps the most important gift that Norman gave me was a glimpse of his life: physician, scholar, father, and husband. Even in his most private moments, Norman Geschwind, by his very presence, signaled that these various beings could coexist, cooperatively and pleasantly, in a single person. Norman Geschwind taught me much about being a neurologist and a neuroscientist but even more about being a whole person.

REFERENCES

1. Waxman M. Mentoring, role modeling, and the career development of junior faculty. *J Coll Sci Teaching* 1992;22:124–127.
2. Waxman SG, Geschwind N. Hypergraphia in temporal lobe epilepsy. *Neurology* 1974;14:629–637.
3. Waxman SG, Geschwind N. The interictal behavior syndrome of temporal lobe epilepsy. *Arch Gen Psychiatry* 1975;32:1580–1586.
4. Sacks O. *An anthropologist on Mars*. New York: Alfred Knopf, 1995.
5. Waxman SG. Norman Geschwind. *J Neurol Sci* 1985;69:113–115.
6. Sachdev HS, Waxman SG. Frequency of hypergraphia in temporal lobe epilepsy: an index of interictal behavior syndrome. *J Neurol Neurosurg Psychiatry* 1981;44:358–360.
7. Waxman SG, Brill MH, Geschwind N, Sabin TD, Lettvin JY. Probability of conduction deficit as related to fiber length in random-distribution models of peripheral neuropathies. *J Neurol Sci* 1976;29:39–53.

7
Teacher

Michael Ronthal

Department of Neurology, Beth Israel Hospital, Boston, Massachusetts 02215.

Norman Geschwind spent the last 9 years of his life at Beth Israel Hospital in Boston. During these productive years, he established the Division of Behavioral Neurology, with Marcel Mesulam at its head, and the Epilepsy Unit with Donald Schomer as the electrophysiologist and Howard Blume as the neurosurgeon specializing in temporal lobectomy. Albert Galaburda pursued research in brain asymmetries and the cytoarchitectonics of the human cortex, and Andrew Herzog studied the endocrinopathies of patients with temporal lobe seizures. The clinical service was organized initially by Simeon Locke, and I succeeded him.

Norman presided over a weekly departmental clinical meeting, conducted a weekly Professor's Round, and was always present at the weekly radiology round. Every Saturday morning, he would make "walk rounds" with the residents.

PROFESSOR'S ROUND

The highlight of the week was always Professor's Round. Norman sat at the head of a rather long table in the conference room. Chairs were at a premium, so many of us stood, sometimes for as long as 2 hours, just to be there. Although he was not a religious man and believed only in science, it is possibly because of his Talmudic forebears that there was an almost Yeshiva-like atmosphere. The bare bones of the session would be a case presentation, preferably by the medical student; a short trip to the bedside, where the patient would be examined by Norman; and then a discussion of the findings and a final diagnosis, with recommendations for further management. The "flesh" on those bare bones was succulent indeed.

Geschwind insisted on meticulous history taking and on the use of words with specific meanings, to avoid ambiguity. He "banned" certain words—*expressive aphasia* particularly provoked him. His reason was that it was imprecise and had become a wastebasket for all sorts of language disturbances. Far better to be specific and call the aphasia syndrome Broca's or Wernicke's aphasia.

Norman was fascinated by clinical associations and familial disease. Two extremely rare or superficially unrelated events in the history would set him off. For every patient, he wanted to know the family history, not just of neurological disease but of all illnesses. The coincidence of left-handedness, early gray hair, and autoimmune diseases was his favorite example. We presented a 38-year-old man who had epididymitis with fever and a week later had his first temporal lobe seizure, which was caused by a glioma—which to Norman was not a coincidence at all! His audience would be treated to a discussion of the many similarities found in the function of testicle and brain.

Norman's clinical examinations of patients were superb. Rarely was a patient presented to him in whom he did not elicit some subtle sign that had been missed by all previous examiners. He was at his best, however, when examining patients with aphasia. What had previously seemed somewhat obscure he made simple and straightforward—and his audience went away with the feeling that at last they, too, had mastered the subject and were fledgling aphasiologists.

Another favorite topic of Norman's in the field of behavioral neurology was the confusional state. One of his points was that in this state, previously dour patients became unconscious humorists. He told an anecdote about such a man, a trustee of the hospital, who had become ill and was in a confusional state. When Norman asked the man where he was, the trustee replied, "I'm in the Temple." Norman then asked the patient what he meant, and the man explained that the Temple was a place of greater hope than Beth Israel Hospital!

Norman was a humble man. He freely admitted that he might be wrong. Each patient, either his own or those of other neurologists, was reevaluated on the premise that all previous diagnoses might be incorrect. He allowed discussion from all quarters ("It's funny you should ask that!"), he would take up all sorts of questions posed, and then, after seeming to ramble for a while, he always returned to the original problem. It was the "rambling" that distinguished him: he was able to discuss almost any subject—medical, ethical, or unrelated to the practice of medicine—in depth and, above all, wisely.

His favorite educational tool was the anecdote, and he perfected the art of using it to illustrate a point. Many and varied were his stories. Even for those who had been around for years, the retelling of the tales held a strange fascination.

One of Norman's teaching points was that migraine is a familial disorder and that the march or progression of somatic symptoms is a rather slow affair. All his students will remember Norman's story about a patient who became slowly paralyzed on the beach and subsequently recalled that his brother had experienced exactly the same phenomenon. There was also the story of the man with hyperhidrosis who rusted his rifle!

Temporal lobe epilepsy, Geschwind believed, was one of the keys to answering the question, How does the brain work? He was convinced that, quite often, the interictal behavior disorder found in patients with temporal lobe epilepsy was missed simply because the right questions were not asked. As an example, he would quote the patient who, when asked whether or not he was religious, replied simply, "No." When pressed further, it turned out that the patient had "tried them all" and had fallen out with his rabbi, who was "theologically unsound." There was the story of the baseball coach who sustained a head injury, after which posttraumatic temporal lobe seizures developed. When the patient was asked if he wrote, again the answer was no. It turned out, however, that the man, who was almost illiterate before the accident, was now obsessed with the idea that he, indeed, *had* to write—although he had never really had the wherewithal to do so, and he ruminated on this theme all day.

When Norman was a resident at Boston City Hospital, he diagnosed a patient's posterior fossa tumor and tonsillar herniation entirely on the basis of her headache and head tilt. The patient, who was too busy to see a physician during the week, had visited many of the emergency rooms of Boston hospitals on Saturdays or Sundays. She had been repeatedly turned away and told to come back on a weekday. Then one Sunday she was fortunate to appear at Boston City Hospital when Norman was on call.

He never forgot a patient. From time to time, to make a point, he would resurrect patients he had known long before, recalling even their names and origins.

Another of Norman's favorite subjects was the management of cerebrovascular disease. He was never convinced that any form of prophylaxis, other than control of hypertension or anticoagulation if a cardiac embolus was diagnosed, was of any value whatsoever. He delighted in reviewing the statistics on carotid endarterectomy and would establish over and over that there was no proof at that time that the operation helped. In fact, he would point out, it often did the opposite, and he practiced what he preached.

Occasionally, Norman was stumped. When that happened, or if he was unable to answer some question on the spur of the moment, the questioner could expect an answer, perhaps by mail, sometimes weeks later, when the problem had been forgotten by everyone—everyone, that is, except Norman. On one occasion, he was asked to see a patient with an obscure endocrinopathy. For a couple of weeks, he seemed to vanish, and then, on one of those memorable Professor's Rounds, he gave an exposition of neuroendocrinology and general endocrinology that was astonishing—he appeared to have mastered the whole field! It was perhaps as a follow-on to that period that he wove his hypothesis about testosterone and the brain.

Although it was in the field of behavioral neurology that his expertise was considered to be undisputed, Geschwind was completely at home in most subspecialties. Normal-pressure hydrocephalus was but one of these. He pointed out that the first case of this syndrome was in fact described in a patient with a third ventricular colloid cyst. Further, a radionucleotide cisternogram was abnormal if, in the presence of large ventricles, the isotope did not, at the very least, get into the ventricles. This fact would spur yet another anecdote—the story of the physicist who kept increasing the sensitivity of his detector to demonstrate that the radioactivity had lingered in the ventricular system, when, by conventional means, the isotope had already been cleared. This led to a false diagnosis—a "grave error."

Norman had special ways of handling special problems. Perhaps the most valuable of these, and one that he repeatedly demonstrated to be a winning strategy, was his management of patients with "functional" disease. The medical student assigned to such a patient would be told to spend an afternoon just "talking" with the patient. No specific probing or searching questions were allowed. Invariably, on the following day, the student would recount the trigger for the patient's psychopathology.

On the subject of intracranial bleeding, Norman would ask the question, Why don't we guaiac the cerebrospinal fluid? The point was that continuous bleeding or oozing was extremely unusual in the central nervous system. Intracranial bleeding was a sudden, self-contained episode, perhaps followed by recurrent episodes of the same rather than a continuous leak. Norman had in fact described a patient with hemosiderosis of the brain and postulated a slow ooze from a choroid plexus tumor, the only source of oozing.

Norman found gross hysteria "always fascinating." His teaching point about hysteria was that it is a syndrome of the socially unsophisticated, often of uneducated migrants to the big city. It was possible to review the various migrant and ethnic groups, who over the years had successively moved to Boston, and demonstrate a high incidence of hysteria in those groups, just as Charcot had done in Paris.

WEEKLY ROUNDS

The weekly departmental clinical meetings were always well attended, both by the staff and by other interested physicians, often nonneurologists. At these meetings Norman was "on show." He would examine the patient, and then a discussion would follow. If uninterrupted, he was quite capable of talking for hours, and always to an enthralled audience.

He would demonstrate his mastery of the history of neurology and encyclopedic knowledge of the literature. He could quote obscure papers dealing with experimental neurophysiology as well as the classics of clinical neurology. His off-the-cuff dissertations, which were liberally spiced with humor and anecdote, were marvelously alive.

During neuroradiology rounds, Geschwind was at his sparkling best. He was a master raconteur, and friendly banter was the order of the day. The neuroradiologists averred that the rounds with Norman were the best in the city. With it all, he drove home the teaching points so that they would never be forgotten: calcification in a tumor made metastatic disease very unlikely, lumbar disk disease could cause pain even without root irritation, the best way to visualize subtle disease on the computed axial tomography scan was to "squint" and so blur out the artifact.

Norman's formal presentations at grand rounds were gems. He utilized all the strategies of an accomplished public speaker, entertained while he taught, and made difficult concepts easy to understand. When he himself was not the main speaker, he would lead the discussion and was always capable of presenting an entirely novel way of supporting or refuting any particular argument. In later years, his subjects included brain asymmetries, and the coincidence of left-handedness, early gray hair, scoliosis, and autoimmune diseases; but every now and then, he would be asked to talk on an old behavioral favorite and his audience might be treated to a review of, say, apraxia.

Every Saturday morning Geschwind would meet with the Beth Israel residents for rounds. The audience for these rounds, however, soon swelled to include virtually all the residents in the program as well as students and staff. The format was supposed to be a leisurely walk from bed to bed. Every patient Norman saw held special interest for him, and often the round would come to a halt with the very first patient while Geschwind pointed out subtle signs and clinical associations. He believed that patients, in general, enjoyed being used as teaching subjects in this way, and he would relate the story of the patient who asked why *his* bed had been passed by so quickly. Norman respected the wishes of any patient who specifically asked not to be a teaching subject; however, he believed that it was, in the long run, better to be a patient in a teaching hospital than in a nonteaching institution—often the medical student attached to the patient would come up with a suggestion or diagnosis that had quite escaped the student's instructors.

On the other hand, it was the belief of the students and staff that the greatest advantage for these patients was to be in the hands of Norman Geschwind.

Behavioral Neurology and the Legacy of Norman Geschwind,
edited by S. C. Schachter and O. Devinsky,
Lippincott-Raven Publishers, Philadelphia © 1997.

8
Mentor

Bruce H. Price

Department of Neurology, McLean Hospital, Belmont, Massachusetts 02178.

My first encounter with Norman Geschwind ended in a men's room. It was 1980, and we were in Keystone, Colorado. Dr. Geschwind had just delivered a controversial talk on interictal personality changes in temporal lobe epilepsy. Some listeners were quietly persuaded, but others were furious with him, citing his lack of statistical data, overreliance on anecdotes, and tendency towards verbosity. I listened to him for 30 minutes while he held court. The group surrounding him gradually dwindled, and I timidly introduced myself, asked a question, and never got another word in edgewise. He started walking while he was talking, so I took my cue and followed him. It was apparent that he was oblivious to his surroundings. Mesmerized by his thoughts, I suddenly found myself standing next to him in a men's room, where he was using the urinal while continuing his discourse. Amy Vanderbilt never prepared me for this situation! Modestly, I took two steps away from him. Unaware of any anatomic correlation with brilliance, I focused my eyes straight ahead instead of downward. He finished his task, zipped up his pants, and continued talking without interruption. I then realized that this was no ordinary person. My life had changed. My intellectual imprinting had begun.

My final encounter with Norman Geschwind occurred 4 years later near the Kirstein Building elevator at Beth Israel Hospital in Boston. This time, I asked Dr. Geschwind a question about schizophrenia. Ten minutes into his monologue, he recalled a rather obscure article from Japan that suggested that male schizophrenics had smaller and more asymmetric testicles than nonschizophrenic men. I remember thinking, "Who but Norman Geschwind would have found that article, marked its significance, and recalled it years later?" I asked him how he had developed this encyclopedic talent. He shrugged his hands and shoulders, saying, "Maybe I'm crazy, maybe I was born different. I don't think I'm that much smarter than other people. It's just that my memory is a little better."

Only at Dr. Geschwind's memorial service did I hear of a possible explanation. Growing up poor in Brooklyn, Norman and his brother would make daily trips to the general store, where one brother quickly read the newspaper while the other diverted the storekeeper with conversation. The two brothers would then return home and report the news to their family, sparing them the expense of buying the paper. On the next trip to the general store, the boys would switch roles. Memory is still incompletely understood. Why does it vary among people? Is there an anatomic basis? Can environmental events in childhood have a lasting impact? Can we develop its acuity over time? Upon Norman Geschwind's death, his family, I'm sure in deference to his ever-inquisitive nature and insatiable thirst for knowledge, donated his brain for future study. Perhaps one day, Norman, we'll understand.

REVELATIONS

To explain the development of Norman Geschwind's philosophical outlook and method, passed on to his students by example, it is best to excerpt his own words (1):

> Like most neurologists of my generation, I had been trained to an overwhelming skepticism toward the view that there were highly characteristic aphasic syndromes associated with different lesions of the brain. Even more forcefully, I had accepted the view that any attempt at "explaining" the syndromes on the basis of anatomy was a futile endeavor. Although Sir Charles Symonds had, during my years at Queen's Square, stood almost alone against this view, I had been so caught up in the standard approach that I disregarded his perceptive teachings.
>
> By 1961, I found myself perplexed by the general rejection of anatomical approaches in contemporary writing, contrasted with their support by so many of the great classical neurologists. I therefore decided to study the ideas of the classical "localizationist" school by reading their own writings rather than by reading the interpretations of later hostile authors. It was my intention to decide for myself whether the repudiation of the classical views was indeed justified.
>
> The very first paper that I read turned out to have a major impact on my thinking. It was Déjérine's paper describing "the first post-mortem on a case of pure alexia without agraphia. . . ." The impact of the paper was multiple. In the first place, the description was so lucid that it was immediately clear that this "pure" syndrome must exist, despite the insistence by some modern writers that these selective syndromes "could no longer be seen" (a statement implying that the earlier description had been grossly in error). Indeed, it was most obvious that Déjérine's standard of examination was superior to that of most modern students of aphasia. Furthermore it was a shock, but a salutary one, to discover that even so masterful a paper had been neglected by later writers, or grossly misquoted. . . . I also realized that the standard accounts of localization had considered the doctrine of centers, but had generally totally neglected the classical stress on connections between cortical regions.
>
> Within a few weeks of reading this paper I saw my first case of alexia without agraphia, and only a few weeks after that the callosal case later published by Edith Kaplan and myself. . . . I was again made aware not merely of how inadequate most of the histories of the higher functions were, but also that important confirmed scientific observations could almost be expunged from the knowledge of contemporary scientists. My presumption is that this must occur in other fields as well. The reasons for this phenomenon were fairly standard: neglect of work written in a foreign language, neglect of work done by someone in a different field, excessive reliance on the authority of certain towering individual figures.

From these revelations, Norman Geschwind's first seminal work emerged in 1965, *Disconnexion Syndromes in Animals and Man* (2). Before this, the primary emphasis in the study of human behavior was on psychology, not neurobiology. This monograph restored anatomy to neurology, underscored the importance of connectional anatomy, integrated experimental animal work with human case reports, and generated testable hypotheses. Geschwind boldly concluded that every behavior had an anatomy. The discipline of behavioral neurology, firmly rooted in neurologic tradition, was catapulted forward.

HISTORY, SCIENCE, PROGRESS

To understand Norman Geschwind, one must also understand his interpretation of world history, its impact on science, and the need for scientific revolutionaries. Addressing the paradox between Germany's political upheaval in the 19th century and its upsurge in scholarship, he wrote, "Periods of confusion are sometimes more conducive to that passion and freedom which is so essential to great scholarship than are periods of undisturbed tranquility. The professor who lives under the threats of major disturbances consequent on political upheaval may well feel it worth his while to be daring in the precious periods available to him for research and may not see the use of those cautious attempts to climb the academic ladder that are more likely to take precedence in periods of relative quiet. The many German scholars who made their positions even more untenable by their participation in forbidden political activities must also frequently have paid little attention to the long-range effects of their scholarly works on their formal academic careers" (3).

"Few scientists create revolutions, and the revolution in aphasia occurred in the 1860s with Broca and in the 1870s with Wernicke. Most people who advanced their field must disagree with their predecessors to some extent and in some measure destroy the past; they must also disagree with their contemporaries and so increase chaos. Usually a field is least usefully active when it is apparently least chaotic" (4). Norman Geschwind, always provocative, never afraid of taking risks, practiced what he wrote.

THE INSPIRATION OF CARL WERNICKE

A person's choice of heroes often reveals his or her own convictions. Carl Wernicke was a particularly admirable figure to Norman Geschwind. In fact, they shared similar traits, triumphs, and tribulations. Geschwind regularly alluded to Wernicke's life. "In 1874 . . . he published his epoch-making work on aphasia, *Der aphasische Symptomencomplex*, subtitled *Eine psychologische Studie auf anatomischer Basis.* This 72-page monograph was to set the tone for research in aphasia over the next forty years. . . ." (3). Why was Wernicke's work so important? "Not only did he provide new evidence for the localization of aphasia but also set forth a theory which tied these phenomena to existing neurological knowledge. He thus made possible the development of a scientific approach to aphasia. On the basis of this theory, it was possible to predict the existence of syndromes not previously seen and to devise experimental means of testing hypotheses. No one had previously supplied this. Little wonder that the appearance of this paper by an unknown 26-year-old physician, with less than 4 years of clinical experience and only 6 months' study of anatomy under Meynert in Vienna, was considered so astonishing" (3). "He was . . . without previous publications, unknown, without academic rank, of an undistinguished family, in a provincial university, without the support of major well known figures" (5).

Geschwind cited another reason why Wernicke's importance extended beyond his work on aphasia. "He had the ability, not common to all distinguished figures, of developing great students" (3). Lichtheim, Déjérine, Karl Bonhoeffer, Otfrid Foerster, Lissauer, and Liepmann were all pupils of Wernicke. Again, Geschwind practiced what he wrote.

Norman Geschwind was also acutely aware of the political intrigues within academia. "Following the publication of Wernicke's early master-work in 1874, he left Breslau to work in Berlin at the Charite Hospital under Westphal. But within 2 years he was dismissed because, as Liepmann put it, 'he came into conflict with the direction of the Charite in a nonscientific and nonofficial situation, which was intensified by Wernicke's obstinacy. . . .'" (6). "Wernicke went into private practice with no academic connection. A possible appointment in Heidelberg was lost when he fell ill for 6 months. He applied for an appointment at Dalldorf, the Berlin Municipal Mental Hospital, but was turned down. . . . Finally, in 1885, an appointment at Breslau was realized. . . . The years at Breslau were to have a bitter end, however. Wernicke had used the Municipal Psychiatric Hospital as a source of most of his clinical material. He had tried fruitlessly for some years to have a university clinic built but had repeatedly been refused on economic grounds. Liepmann records his repeated complaint, only too familiar to those in academic life, that '12 million (marks) are granted without any further question for a warship, but the paltry million for a clinic is not to be had. . . .' [6]. The clinic's connection to the hospital was severed; Wernicke was permitted to use patients for demonstrations in clinical lectures to students, but even this privilege was later withdrawn" (3). As summarized by Geschwind, "At least the marked decline in the workload of the department had the advantage of giving him considerably more free time to finish his *Foundations of Psychiatry* [7]. It seems clear, however, that he lacked the ability to convince himself of the benefits of adversity" (3).

Even such antagonists as Kurt Goldstein, a former pupil of Wernicke's, were influenced by him. Over 50 years later, Goldstein wrote the following words about his early experience with Wernicke: "His way of examining patients and his demonstrations were so elucidating and stimulating that we who had the good fortune to attend his clinics were deeply influenced in our further consideration of neurological and psychiatric problems. We could never forget him. His influence can be seen in the work of each of his many pupils, not a small number of whom became men of stature in their own right in the profession. . . ." (8). No truer words could be used to describe Norman Geschwind's teaching skills. He, too, inspired many men and women of subsequent stature.

THE VALUE OF CASE REPORTS

Norman Geschwind passionately believed in the power of anecdotes and case reports. In response to the frequent criticism that clinical observation is anecdotal and unreliable at best, he responded in the following manner:

> Many of the neurologic journals made it clear that three types of papers will be refused: "obscene articles, plagiarized articles, and single-case reports. . . ." The argument that [clinical observation] is inadequate or anecdotal is curious. Why was Darwin so successful in its use? Why did Broca and Wernicke and Liepmann and Gowers and Charcot and Déjérine use it so well and make such important contributions? Has it suddenly lost all validity? The fact is that science is a field of discovery, a fact not understood by the granting agencies who award grants only to those who will predict what they will find. There is no way to predict the unexpected. Chance favors the prepared mind, but one must spin that little wheel. One must go out into the clinic to see the chance experiments of nature. Nature continues to carry out experiments which none of us would think of or could do. We are obliged to read these. Furthermore we are lucky because this field is still adventurous. If the sea is not fully charted, all the more exciting the discoveries. Furthermore, the issue goes deeper. We have a moral obligation. The mechanisms of disease are too important not to be learned, since any such case may give clues as to treatment. . . . Even when we have no understanding of them, it is vital that they be recorded so that future investigators can study them.
>
> The single case will increasingly become our fate. If you own a unique computer, you surely do not want a repairman who has a circuit diagram of some standard model. Every human is surely different from another, each is a special model and many will be very different from the average. Without single-case analysis we will never understand many patients. It is furthermore becoming clear that the individual history of development of each person *in utero* and in early life will change the pattern of the brain. We have to learn more and more about these things to understand each case." (9)

I think Dr. Geschwind would uphold these statements today. It remains true that one or two extremely well-described and well-studied cases can be more illuminating than a series of patients buried in statistical analysis, without individual variations taken into account. Case reports have yielded major insights into amnesia, aphasia, hemineglect, constructional difficulties, hemispheric asymmetries, prosodic disorders, dissociation and temporal lobe epilepsy, and left-sided neurologic signs in depression. Geschwind understood that the voyage of discovery often begins with case reports. This insight explains his fascination with each patient he examined, his ability to turn a seemingly mundane case into a fascinating one.

COGNITION AS A MULTIDISCIPLINARY ENDEAVOR

To understand complex human behaviors, Geschwind preached and practiced a multidisciplinary approach. "The realization that the conceptual nature [of cognitive science] cuts across so many areas should perhaps make us all realize that inspiration may come from areas that appear at first glance to be totally remote. This new society is concerned with psychology, mathematics, computer science, linguistics, philosophy, the social sciences, and of course, the neurologic sciences" (10). He strongly argued for cross-fertilization between neurology and other related fields. "Suppose one looks at those fields in which psychology and linguistics have made their most brilliant contributions—aphasia, memory, inattentional syndromes, alexia, constructional disorders, temporal lobe epilepsy. But what about those fields in which our psychological or linguistic knowledge is most inadequate—schizophrenia, childhood autism, many other childhood disorders? The message is clearer than you may be aware. Linguistics and psychology have been most effective in those areas in which we have the most detailed neurologic knowledge, and least effective on the average in those where neurologic knowledge is lacking. Neurolinguistics has only flourished since aphasia again became anatomical. It is not that neurology is more important than linguistics or psychology, but without it the linguist or the psychologist never knows the real borders of the problems" (9).

It is no surprise that the introduction to his *Selected Papers on Language and the Brain* included the following foreword: "His research . . . presents a fascinating and provocative examination of fundamental questions which will concern not neurologists alone, but also psychologists, physicians, linguists, speech pathologists, educators, anthropologists, historians of medicine, and philosophers among others, namely all those interested in the characteristic modes of human activity, in speech, in perception, and in the learning process generally" (1). A tribute to his far-ranging approach, he spawned countless investigators across many disciplines, from speech therapy and brain rehabilitation, neuropsychology, and neuroanatomy, to immunology and neuroendocrinology.

THE VALUE OF CONTROVERSY

Although Norman Geschwind would often argue his viewpoints tenaciously, he understood and welcomed controversy. Prefacing his article "The Development of the Brain and the Evolution of Language" (11), he wrote, "This paper remains one of my favorites, although the speculations in it may well be wrong, since it is perhaps the only theory in existence which tries to relate the mechanisms of some, although not all, aspects of language specifically to the structure of the brain. As I have said, the theory may be wrong, and it has been criticized quite harshly. I would welcome some really cogent criticisms, since these might well serve either to refine the theory or to be replaced by a more sophisticated neurological picture" (1).

Geschwind understood that controversy was the fuel that drove science forward. Describing the scientific dispute during the late nineteenth and early 20th centuries between the holists, mosaicists, and localizationists, he wrote: "If the holists were excessively outspoken, they were certainly not unimportant and they left their permanent seal on our thinking about aphasia; they studied new areas, fostered therapy, and forced refinement of clinical observation and anatomy. They had a profound effect on the course of the stream but did not establish a new channel. The mosaicists were also useful. If their anatomy had no link to psychology, their researches could be used by others who were more oriented in that direction. They made fundamental advances in our knowledge of the gross and fine anatomy of the cortex. . . . It is perhaps comforting to consider that the activities of highly skilled and intelligent men are rarely totally wasted, even when wrong" (3).

NEUROLOGY AND PSYCHIATRY

Norman Geschwind's exhortations influenced my recent career decision. "The largest group of neurological patients have behavioral problems. Those who believe that this is rare do a disservice. But if even an ordinary neurology service has these problems, how much more in mental hospitals!? We must move that way. We have a service to provide. No one else can. We see many cases who would otherwise be neglected" (9).

His teachings have served me well in my worlds of behavioral neurology and neuropsychiatry at McLean and Massachusetts General hospitals. I attempt to pass them on to those students, residents, and fellows I now train. As part of their orientation, I recommend a chapter Norman Geschwind wrote in 1975 entitled, "The Borderland of Neurology and Psychiatry: Some Common Misconceptions" (12).

> While it has become fashionable to acknowledge the existence of an area of overlap between neurology and psychiatry, this common ground unfortunately bears more resemblance to a no-man's-land than to an open border. While neurologists tend to mutter darkly about the failure of psychiatrists to be aware of the brain as the organ of the mind, psychiatrists, perhaps somewhat defensively, have stressed their awareness of the whole man, biologic as well as psychologic. Unfortunately, few members of either group have in fact really interested themselves in the borderland area, and too frequently interactions between them are educationally disappointing, whether at the level of mutual consultation or in the interchange of residents for training. It is hoped that this situation will be corrected in the next few years, but until then both psychiatrists and neurologists will often have to acquire the necessary knowledge themselves. [Geschwind firmly believed that this cross-disciplinary study of mental life could thrive like any other domain of rational investigation.]
>
> Another common failure in taking histories or examining patients, even when done by a physician, is the tendency by some to make dynamic interpretations of the patient's behavior right from the initial contact. The possibility of organic diagnosis is almost excluded when the patient is approached in so closed-minded a fashion. It should furthermore be kept in mind that the mere fact that a patient's behavior is concordant with his personality dynamics does not mean that the disorder is psychogenic.
>
> Neglect of the fact that every behavior has an anatomy may lead in some cases to incorrect psychodynamic explanations of changes in behavior that are not dependent on past experience. One should not, however, make the equally serious error of concluding that, since all behavior takes place in the brain, all disorders of behavior must be organic, a view sometimes expressed in the vivid, but, in my opinion, erroneous aphorism that "behind the crooked thought lies the crooked molecule." No one can deny that learning is one of the major functions of the brain, and it is reasonable to assume that normal learning processes can lead to difficulties in adjustment.
>
> I have tried to discourage the notion that simple rules of thumb enable one to separate the organic from the functional. I have also attempted to show that not only is the organic disease erroneously diagnosed as functional, but it is also common to misdiagnose treatable functional disorders as irreversible organic disease. Above all, I have tried to convince the reader that in order to be an effective diagnostician, one must learn the natural course and clinical pictures of the different syndromes, just as one would have to do in any branch of medicine.

Geschwind reinforced the message that there are no simple methods to exclude neurological causation in disordered behavior. A normal magnetic resonance imaging or computed tomography scan, electroencephalogram, or cerebrospinal fluid (CSF) examination does not exclude neurologic possibilities. He thought CSF analysis was vastly underutilized. He preached that detailed history, clinical judgment, and knowledge of brain–behavior relationships were the keys to further diagnosis and understanding. He impressed upon me the value of detailed postmortem examinations and their discussion in a clinicopathologic format.

Geschwind forcefully taught how attentional matrix was the foundation of the mental state examination. He relished examining patients in acute confusional states, demonstrating the remarkable array of secondary memory, language, and constructional disorders. He was wary of using a single measure of intelligence, and he taught the significance of asymmetry, anomalies, and dissociations as well as subtle findings in the elementary neurologic examination. When examining dyslexic patients, he was quick also to elicit many of their superior compensating talents. He demonstrated how the mental status examination, when used well, could be sharply illuminating. If the examination was not administered or interpreted well, he would often smile as the examiner induced a confusional state in himself or herself more often than in the patient.

THE INSPIRATION OF NORMAN GESCHWIND

I never found Dr. Geschwind truly satisfied with his own explanations. He believed in reinventing and expanding himself as necessity dictated. Hence, he learned five foreign languages so that he could read various articles in their original languages, not their translations. In the last decade of his life, he studied endocrinology, immunology, and genetics to further understand brain development. To him, the journey was of utmost importance. He taught that a topic should take one where it needs to. He opposed traditional thinking and insular approaches. He demonstrated an intellectual ability to change and adapt as needed.

Geschwind cautioned against preconceived notions. "One must cultivate naïveté and remember that there are no coincidences. One must abandon common sense, unusual explanations are better. Don't believe review articles. Don't measure too quickly, measure everything. The pressure to standardize exams and nomenclature avoids thoughts and new observations" (9).

It was his sweeping and optimistic view of the human race, his belief in science as a liberating tool, his insatiable curiosity, and his far-reaching speculations that filled amphitheaters wherever he lectured. He allowed one to laugh while learning. He convinced his pupils that they too were part of the historic struggle for biologic truths. His greatness as a teacher was not as a conveyor of facts but as an exemplar of the joy of scholarship. His door and mind were always open, he was full of good cheer, and he had few of the pretensions so often seen in someone of his stature. In my opinion, these attributes best explain the compelling effect he had on those he touched.

I was the last behavioral neurology fellow fully trained under Norman Geschwind's tutelage. I fervently wish this were not true. Strangely enough, though, I no longer grieve for those he left behind. Instead, I grieve for those who never knew him, for those who have no idea what they missed, for those who would have been so inspired by his presence. Perhaps this book will convey the spirit of this remarkable mentor.

REFERENCES

1. Geschwind N. Selected papers on language and the brain. In: Cohen RS, Wardofsky MW, eds. *Boston studies in the philosophy of science,* vol 16. Boston: D Reidel, 1974;1,2,19.

2. Geschwind N. Disconnexion syndromes in animals and man (2 parts). *Brain* 1965;88:237–294, 585–644.
3. Geschwind N. Carl Wernicke, the Breslau school and the history of aphasia. In: Carterette EC, ed. *Speech, language, and communication,* vol 3: *Brain function.* Berkeley, CA: University of California Press, 1963;1–16.
4. Geschwind N. The paradoxical position of Kurt Goldstein in the history of aphasia. *Cortex* 1964;1:214–224.
5. Geschwind N. Wernicke's contribution to the study of aphasia. *Cortex* 1967;3:449–463.
6. Liepmann H, Wernicke C. In: Kirchoff T, ed. *Deutsche Irrenarzte,* vol 2. Berlin, Germany: Springer, 1922; 238–250.
7. Wernicke C. *Grundriss der Psychiatrie in Klinischen Vorlesungen,* 2nd ed. Leipzig, Germany: Thieme, 1906.
8. Goldstein K, Carl Wernicke. In: Haymaker W, ed. *Founders of neurology.* Springfield, IL: Charles C Thomas, 1953.
9. Geschwind N. *What is behavioral neurology?* Presented to the Behavioral Neurology Society at the 35th Annual American Academy of Neurology meeting, San Diego, CA, April, 1983.
10. Geschwind N. Neurological knowledge and complex behaviors. *Cognit Sci* 1980;4:185–193.
11. Geschwind N. The development of the brain and the evolution of language. In: Stuart CIJM, ed. *Monograph series on languages and linguistics,* vol 17. Washington, DC: Georgetown University Press, 1964:155–169.
12. Geschwind N. The borderland of neurology and psychiatry: some common misconceptions. In: Benson DF, Blumer D, eds. *Psychiatric aspects of neurologic disease.* New York: Grune and Stratton Fine, 1975;1–8.

9

Creative Genius

Howard Gardner

Harvard Project Zero, Harvard Graduate School of Education, Cambridge, Massachusetts 02138.

Many people today have become quite interested in the phenomenon of creativity—the creativity of scientists, artists, financial experts, advertising copywriters, and even politicians. As one who monitors the area of creativity, I note as well the accumulation of books, articles, television programs, workshops, and other symptoms of growing interest in the topic. Yet, despite this almost prurient curiosity about the topic, most of us have not had the opportunity to observe a highly creative person firsthand. We read about Freud or Einstein, we watch films of Woody Allen or Martha Graham, and we listen assiduously to interviews with Francis Crick or Barbara McClintock. From these scattered hints, we try to understand the intriguing phenomenon of a single person who changes the way in which others think about or experience the world.

I was fortunate to have been a colleague and friend of Norman Geschwind, one of the indisputably creative scientists of our era. I learned much about creativity from observing him; and some of what I have learned has been useful to me as I have thought more broadly about the dimensions of creativity (1). In this chapter, I attempt to capture the interplay in my own thinking about Norman Geschwind as a creative scientist and the more general phenomenon of creativity.

DIMENSIONS OF CREATIVITY

Three general points serve to introduce this discussion. First of all, there are many different kinds of creativity, ranging from the creativity involved in leading a political revolution, à la Mao or Lenin, to the creativity entailed in producing a work in a genre, the way that Keats and Rembrandt repeatedly did. Even within the sciences, there are numerous forms of creativity. Darwin and Piaget were masterful observers who were able to draw powerful generalizations from their initial observations. Einstein could conceive of thought experiments and then design crucial empirical and theoretical tests of what he had envisioned. Albert Michelson and Roger Sperry were brilliant experimentalists. Even when one thinks about Nobel laureates in the area of brain and behavior, it is clear that Roger Sperry, Konrad Lorenz, Herbert Simon, and David Hubel are distinctly different from one another. Norman Geschwind's own creative genius spanned observation and theorizing; he was not primarily an experimentalist. As Antonio Damasio once pointed out, Norman Geschwind's laboratory was inside his head.

A second point recognizes that many different factors contribute to individual and group creativity. In addition to possible genetic predispositions, one must take into account developmental, family, school, cultural, social class, and motivational factors, among others. For this reason, creativity can never be understood simply from the point of view of a single discipline, be it neurology, genetics, or sociology. Clearly, Norman Geschwind's accomplishments reflect this range of factors; and it is perhaps appropriate that he himself was superlatively gifted in the way that he could range across disciplines and families of disciplines.

A third point is that creativity should not be confused with other virtues. A person can be highly intelligent without being creative, highly successful without being creative, and creative without being "right" in the long run. It is heuristic to think of creativity as the capacity to come up with ideas, problems, solutions, and the like that are initially novel but that are ultimately acceptable in at least one domain or discipline or culture. Creative ideas or products change domains; that is the acid test. One can immediately see that persons with superbly high IQs may have neither the inclination nor the capacity to change domains; that persons who are widely acclaimed may exert no appreciable effect on domains; and that persons may affect domains in the short term but in ways that are ultimately seen as wrongheaded or unproductive.

Because Norman Geschwind's ideas have already affected several domains, we know that he was creative, rather than "merely" successful or "merely" intelligent; only time will tell whether he discovered basic truths, in the manner of a genius.

VARIABLES IN SCIENTIFIC CREATIVITY

In light of these preliminary considerations, I have isolated four variables that figure importantly in the area of scientific creativity. Perhaps no one of them is critical in itself, but the combination of them surely signals that the person is "at promise" for leading a creative life. Norman Geschwind illustrates these factors well, in consort as well as in isolation.

To begin with, Norman Geschwind was a man of great raw intellectual power. No matter how one defines intelligence (or intelligences), it is clear that Norman stood out in terms of the power and penetration of his logical/mathematical ability. His verbal skills were legendary—speaking, writing, readily mastering languages, reading at a prodigious rate, exhibiting impressive sensitivity to how language works and how it breaks down. Norman had equally powerful gifts in the area of logical/mathematical thinking; he began as a mathematics major in college and never lost the habit of thinking about issues in a logical, rational, and often mathematical way.

Norman was less outstanding in the realms of spatial thinking and in the use of his hands—in this way, he did not resemble many bench-top scientists. But his *interests* swept across all domains. For example, although he confessed to very little competence in music, he encouraged people like me to study music, he collaborated with Tedd Judd and me in the study of a composer who had become verbally alexic (2), and he frequently attended concerts (including one just hours before his untimely death). Clearly, Norman wanted to keep learning about everything until the very end of his life.

In addition to his polymathic intellect, Norman also had a kaleidoscopic capacity to draw on his knowledge. Virtually everything that he knew—and he knew more than just about anyone else I have ever met—was available at his cerebral fingertips. Any new observation or fact could kindle a startling chain of associations, a new pattern, as that kaleidoscope went famously to work and to play. I suspect that if one had been able to perform a positron emission tomography scan on Geschwind's brain in operation, one would have beheld a uniquely beautiful series of pictures.

Working hand-in-glove with intellect are the personality structures of the individual. Norman Geschwind displayed in abundance all the personality traits that are concomitants of great creativity—a driving personality, a high degree of energy, clearly focused attention, perseverance, a willingness to take risks, and a reassuring amount of self-confidence. Those in search of creative role models had no better option than to spend time in the presence of Norman Geschwind. Moreover, like the creative people described by Howard Gruber (3), Norman had an expansive network of enterprise—a large number of persons and projects that he helped to sustain and that in turn kept him fully occupied.

But although Norman resembled the textbook case of the creative personality, he also gave us a whole ensemble of bonuses. He was wonderfully funny; he was a pleasure, a treat, a perpetual feast to be around. He was without a trace of vanity or self-importance. One could never tell a person's status simply by observing his or her encounters with Norman from afar; Norman would spend hours with a naive undergraduate even as he would put a pretentious senior scientist in his place. He set an enviable standard for collegiality, responding to letters and phone calls promptly, almost always answering requests favorably, putting himself out for others in ways that were not necessary and that should have filled more of us—the unbridled requesters—with embarrassment. Perhaps it is best to say that Norman made us feel that he was one of us although, deep down, we knew that he was one of the immortals.

Contrary to what the language hints at, people are not intelligent or creative in general—they exhibit these virtues in specific domains or disciplines. Norman Geschwind was a true scholar and could probably have made contributions in an ensemble of domains, ranging from mathematics to history to linguistics. But his chosen domain was behavioral neurology, and it was there—and in neighboring disciplines—that he was to make his enduring contributions.

Norman's relation to the domain of behavioral neurology was peculiar. He did not invent the field, and he did not for the most part pull it in wholly original directions. Rather, he rediscovered a tradition that had existed a century earlier but had mistakenly been allowed to become dormant. To revivify the wrongly discredited works of persons like Wernicke, Lichtheim, Liepmann, and the "diagram makers" was an act of courage in the days when doctrines of holism and equipotentiality reigned supreme.

Of course, Norman Geschwind did not just direct his undereducated contemporaries to consult the dusty journals on the shelves of the medical libraries. He described new cases that either confirmed the traditional descriptions or that modified them in fresh and illuminating ways. His work on the disconnection syndromes had become classic within a decade of its original publication. His papers on the aphasias, the apraxias, the alexias, temporal lobe epilepsy, and many other neuropsychological syndromes and conditions brought classic typologies in touch with newly observed phenomena and contemporary modes of analysis. He himself was in contact with the outstanding scientists in Russia, Europe, the Orient, and the Americas; and he brought the rest of the community of brain and behavior in touch with these same authorities. Under his founding leadership, the Aphasia Research Center at Boston University and the Boston Veterans Administration Medical Center and then the neurology units at Boston City and Beth Israel hospitals became international centers. For years, there were but a few behavioral neurologists and neuropsychologists who had not been trained by Norman Geschwind; and even those who had not been trained at his scintillating rounds flocked to his lectures and combed the new journals for his writings—and, eventually, for the writings of his students.

Toward the end of his life, Norman Geschwind embarked on what may well have been his most important work—a pioneering effort, undertaken in conjunction with Peter

Behan and Albert Galaburda, to tie together information on genetics, laterality, fetal development, sex differences, hormonal systems, immune disorders, and an array of cognitive skills and disabilities. Even to list these domains is to be daunted; and only someone of Geschwind's intellectual courage and kaleidoscopic thinking could have undertaken this effort, let alone brought it to an amazing degree of readiness in a tragically short period of time (4). In all probability, the details of this ambitious synthesis will need to be revised; but, as is so often the case in science, the set of issues raised by Geschwind and his colleagues will endure.

Indeed, few efforts of the past decade have sustained more discussion and empirical work than the investigation of what is often termed the Geschwind hypothesis. I regard this synoptic work as perhaps the first full-blooded instance of what has since come to be called cognitive neuroscience.

A final dimension of the phenomenon of creativity is often overlooked—the dimension called the *field* (1,5). Whatever the talent of the person and the state of readiness of the domain, a creative effort cannot come to be seen as such without the collaboration of those persons, institutions, award panels, and the like that render judgments of quality.

The field recognized Norman Geschwind's talent at an early age. He was appreciated as a student at Harvard College and the Harvard Medical School; he won more than his share of fellowships, residencies, grants, and prizes; he was appointed the James Jackson Putnam Professor of Neurology at the Harvard Medical School in his early forties; and he was widely appreciated across the globe at the time of his death. Part of this success has to do with Norman's choice of fields: he was wise enough to be born in New York City when it was a unique cauldron of creative vigor, and to be at Harvard, at Queen's Square, Moscow, and on the European continent at times when intellectual breakthroughs were happening. Of course, the field was also fortunate that Norman Geschwind presented himself for its consideration.

But I want to stress another aspect of the field. Even as Norman helped to reorient the domain of behavioral neurology and its neighbors, he was crucially important in helping to shape its concomitant fields. Norman's judgments about work, his taste with respect to issues worthy of study, and his ability to shape discussions and standards were remarkable and, to my way of thinking, remarkably beneficent. Norman Geschwind exerted this effect by his writings, his choice and development of students, his engagement at scientific meetings, and, perhaps especially, by his lectures. Nearly everyone who heard Norman Geschwind concurred that he was one of the great scientific lecturers of the age. He could discuss complex issues in a straightforward way, bring new excitement to a discussion, and respond to even the most vexing questions with insight, appropriateness, and timely wit. By his effect on others, directly and indirectly, he almost single-handedly and single-mindedly redirected the standards of what lines of work were important and how such issues could be addressed in an intellectually rigorous way. Indeed, as happens in such cases, Norman exerted a powerful influence even on those who staunchly disagreed with his claims.

Norman Geschwind stood at the center of what Margaret Mead once called a cultural cluster—"whose defining characteristic is at least one irreplaceable individual, someone with such special gifts of imagination and thought that without him the cluster would assume an entirely different character—a genius who makes a contribution to evolution not by biological propagation but by the special turn that he is able to give to the course of cultural evolution."

NORMAN GESCHWIND: EXCEPTIONAL SCIENTIST AND HUMAN BEING

I trust that, in terms of the criteria that I have defined, Norman Geschwind emerges as an exceptional person, one who embodied creativity of a very high order. His combination of probing intellect, driving yet generous personality, substantive reorientation of behavioral neurology, and shaping of the field of judges places him centrally in that privileged group of scientists who have made a difference in our time.

For those who knew him, Norman exceeded these criteria, for he is irreplaceable in two respects: as a scientist with whom one craves further interaction on a myriad of rich issues, and as a marvelously warm, empathic, and humane human being—the kind of person who is rare in any domain and virtually without peer in the hard-driving and often cutthroat domain of scientific research.

We have but one consolation. Great minds endure not through their genes but through their ideas and their personal examples. Norman Geschwind's ideas fueled a generation of talented researchers in several disciplines spanning the brain and behavior, and his personal example has sustained, and will continue to sustain, all those who were privileged to know him directly, and perhaps even some who knew him only through his reputation. As one who has since studied many creative people drawn from a galaxy of domains, I have encountered no one who so well combined intellectual brilliance and personal decency.

REFERENCES

1. Gardner H. *Creating minds: an anatomy of creativity seen through the lives of Freud, Einstein, Picasso, Stravinsky, Eliot, Graham, and Gandhi.* New York: Basic Books, 1993.
2. Judd T, Gardner H, Geschwind N. Alexia without agraphia in a composer. *Brain* 1983;106:435–457.
3. Gruber H. *Darwin on man.* Chicago: University of Chicago Press, 1981.
4. Geschwind N, Galaburda A. *Cerebral lateralization.* Cambridge, MA: Harvard University Press, 1987.
5. Csikszentmihalyi M. Society, culture, and person: a systems view of creativity. In: Sternberg R, ed. *The nature of creativity.* New York: Cambridge University Press, 1988;325–339.

10
International Figure

François Boller

INSERM U324, Centre Paul Broca, 75014, Paris, France.

The purpose of this chapter is to evoke an important aspect of Norman Geschwind's legacy by showing the influence he had on behavioral neurology and neuropsychology* in countries outside North America, particularly Italy and France. This will be exemplified through his participation in the International Neuropsychological Symposium.

The International Neuropsychological Symposium is a yearly meeting at which a relatively small number of neurologists, psychiatrists, neuropsychologists, and persons in related fields discuss various topics relevant to neuropsychology. So far, all 40 symposia have been held in Western Europe or adjacent countries (e.g., Israel, Tunisia, and in 1995, the Czech Republic). The first meeting, convened by Henry Hecaen (Paris), Hans Hoff (Vienna), and Oliver Zangwill (Cambridge, England) was held in Austria in 1951. At each symposium, several topics (usually three) selected in advance are discussed by a small number of presenters who have been invited to speak by the topic organizer. Approximately half of the time is devoted to an exchange of views among all participants. It appears that the frontal lobe was one of the topics in 1972 and in 1981; both topics were organized by Brenda Milner. We have no evidence that Norman Geschwind participated in either of these two meetings. The symposium is worth mentioning, however, because it illustrates another important aspect of Norman Geschwind's life and legacy.

The symposium was at first very "Eurocentric," but it has become much less so over time. Its current chairperson is Michael Goldberg from Bethesda, Maryland, and over one third of its current members are from North America. Among the first symposium attendees from the United States were three persons who, in different ways, have shaped the fields of behavioral neurology and neuropsychology in the United States. They were Hans-Lucas Teuber (head of the Department of Psychology at the Massachusetts Institute of Technology from 1960 to 1977; he, like Norman Geschwind, died prematurely), who first attended in 1958; Arthur Benton (who is still active in the field of neuropsychology in Iowa City, Iowa), who attended in 1962; and Norman Geschwind. We have records of Norman Geschwind's participation in the 1964 sym-

---

*There is no question that Norman Geschwind (and most U.S. neurologists after him) did not like the term *neuropsychology* to be applied to their field. Even though I understand some of their reasons, I will freely use the word in this chapter, following the definition provided by Henry Hecaen, the man who gave its modern meaning to the term: "La neuropsychologie est la discipline qui traite des fonctions mentales superieures dans leurs rapports avec les structures cerebrales" (1,6–8). In most countries outside the United States, *neuropsychology* is the preferred label for the discipline of those who study brain and behavior relationships.

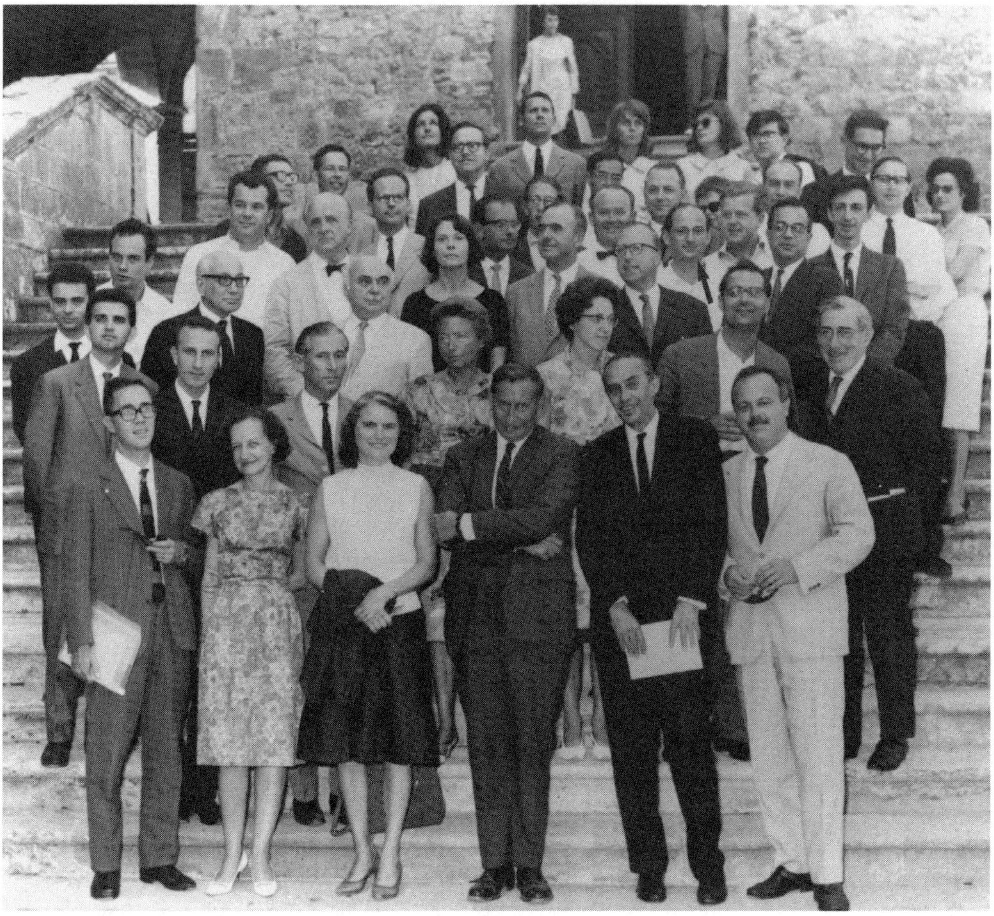

FIG. 1. Group picture taken during the 1964 meeting of the International Neuropsychological Symposium (San Gimignano, Italy). At least 9 of the 45 attendees were from North America. From left to right: 1. Ennio DeRenzi; 2. Brenda Milner; 3. Martha Wilson; 4. Hans-Lucas Teuber; 5. Henry Hecaen; 6. Carlo Gentili; 7. unidentified Italian neuropsychologist (Loperfido?); 8. Edoardo Bisiach; 9. Clemens Faust; 10. Ilse Gloning; 11. Elizabeth Warrington; 12. Marcel Kinsbourne; 13. F. Grewel; 14. Pietro Faglioni; 15. Hans Hoff; 16. Franz Gunther von Stockert (father of Theodore); 17. Josephine Semmes; 18. Anton Leichner; 19. unidentified Dutch neuropsychologist (B.G. Deelman?); 20. Norman Geschwind; 21. Klaus Poeck; 22. William Wilson; 23. Colwin Trevarthen; 24. unknown; 25. unknown; 26. Hans Spinnler; 27. Rudolph Quatember; 28. Heinrich Scheller; 29. Luigi A. Vignolo; 30. Karl Gloning; 31. Eric Lenneberg; 32. Davis Howes; 33. unknown; 34. unknown; 35. Malcolm Piercy; 36. François Boller; 37. George Ettlinger; 38. Ron Myers; 39. unknown; 40. travel agent; 41. unknown; 42 unknown; 43. Sue Oxbury; 44. John Oxbury; 45. unknown.

posium (Fig. 1), at which he spoke on the disconnection syndromes, one year before his seminal *Brain* articles.

During the 1964 symposium, Dr. Geschwind met Ennio DeRenzi, Luigi Vignolo, and other members of the "Milan group." This meeting marked the beginning of his strong influence on the development of Italian neuropsychology (1). He was one of the first members of the editorial board of *Cortex,* the journal founded by Ennio DeRenzi in 1964.

Many Italian researchers trained and performed research in the services Geschwind directed (DeRenzi, Vignolo, Savoiardo, Denes, Cappa, and Boller, to mention only a few). In 1966, Norman Geschwind remarked, upon the arrival of a plane from Milan carrying Vignolo, Savoiardo, and Boller, all headed to the neurology service he then directed at the Boston Veterans Administration Hospital, "Here comes il Draino del Braino Italiano." The brain drain may not have been permanent, but the witty remark is worth its weight in pasta.

Norman Geschwind's participation in the symposium also exemplifies his very strong ties with two of its original founders. The first was Oliver Zangwill [without whose urging, the disconnection paper "would never have been written" (2)]. The second was Henry Hecaen, who became a frequent visitor to Geschwind's service, as were Athanase Tsavaras, Michel Poncet, François Michel, and many others. Later, Martin Albert and I participated actively in the INSERM Unit founded by Hecaen in rue d'Alesia (now Centre Paul Broca), which represents a development of these ties. Further ties with the French school are demonstrated by his personal rapport with François Lhermitte, François Chedru, and later, Jean-Louis Signoret.

Norman Geschwind's legacy is felt in many other countries, of course. Several students and fellows (John Meadows and David Neary come to mind, but there were many others) came from the United Kingdom, which had seen the beginning of his scientific career (3). Klaus Poeck, who can be said to have been the founder of modern neuropsychology and neurolinguistics in Germany, was a frequent visitor to Norman Geschwind's service. They may sometimes have disagreed (4), but they certainly respected each other. Theodore von Stockert was also a fellow there.

Current neuropsychology research in the Netherlands is certainly influenced by the relation between Geschwind and the Boston group and Robert Haaxma, now in Groningen, the Netherlands. Similarly, the strong ties with Antonio Damasio during his formative years have influenced, at least indirectly, Portuguese neuropsychology. Geschwind's influence extends to Switzerland through Ted Landis, to Canada through Andrew Kertesz, to Australia through Bruce Tomlinson, and to Japan through Atsushi Yamadori.

Geschwind's influence over research carried out in other countries was facilitated by his extraordinary gift for foreign languages. He spoke perfect French, and his ability to read German as used by 19th century neurologists allowed him to go back to the original literature, a very significant factor in his intellectual development (5). In addition, he enjoyed speaking and reading Italian. He amazed many Italian neurologists when, in 1966, he gave a course at the University of Milan in nearly perfect Italian and announced that he would take questions put to him in Italian without need for a translator but would then reply in French. He could go even further: having been asked to give a course in Brazil, he took a short "immersion course" and delivered his lectures in fluent Portuguese. I do not know whether his courses at Amman University in the early 1980s were delivered in Arabic.

Norman Geschwind participated as a member and, several times, as a topic organizer in many meetings of the International Neuropsychological Symposium between 1964 and 1984. The last picture in my possession (Fig. 2) goes back to the meeting held in Calcatoggio, Corsica, in 1980, 16 years after the San Gimignano meeting. As Figure 2 shows, several of the same persons attended both the 1964 and the 1980 meetings. A number of them (and countless others not shown in this picture) owe much of their intellectual development to Norman Geschwind.

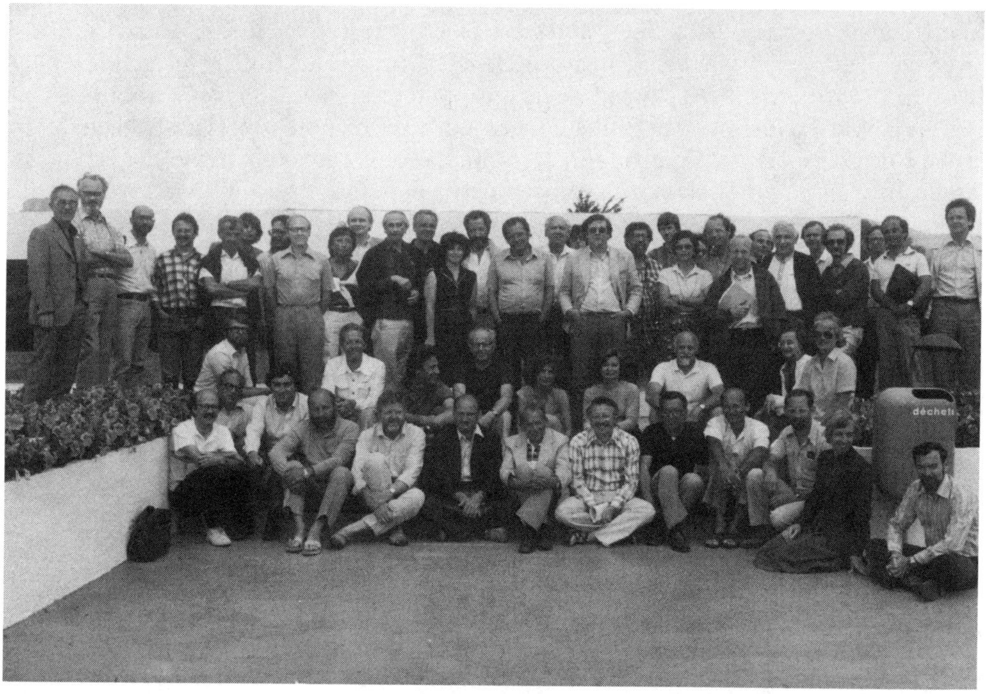

FIG. 2. Group picture taken during the 1980 meeting of the International Neuropsychological Symposium (Calcatoggio, Corsica). At least 15 of the 52 attendees were active in North America at the time. From left to right: Sitting: 1. Gus Buchtal; 2. William Wilson; 3. Bruno Preilowski; 4. Carlo Marzi; 5. Carlo Umilta; 6. Jacques Paillard; 7. Klaus Poeck; 8. François Boller; 9. Norman Geschwind; 10. Luigi A. Vignolo; 11. Harold Goodglass; 12. Marie-Claire Goldblum; 13. Morris Moscovitch; 14. Sue Oxbury; 15. Gianfranco Denes; 16. Robert Haaxma; 17. Brenda Milner; 18. unknown; 19. Martha Wilson; 20. Sue Corkin; 21. Patrick Rabbitt. Standing: 22. Ennio DeRenzi; 23. Steve Russel; 24. Klaus Heeschen; 25. Walter Huber; 26. Etienne Perret; 27. Edgar Zurif; 28. Athanase Tsavarras; 29. L. Taylor; 30. Michele Brouchon; 31. unknown; 32. Henry Hecaen; 33. Giovanni Berlucchi; 34. Felicia Huppert; 35. Rudolph Cohen; 36. Gil Assal; 37. Oliver Zangwill; 38. Dorothea Weniger; 39. John Oxbury; 40. Charles Gross; 41. Wolfgang Hartje; 42. Maria Wyke; 43. Marie Louise Kane; 44. Marcel Kinsbourne; 45. Nelson Butters; 46. Michel Poncet; 47. Jean-Louis Signoret; 48. Daniel Beaubaton; 49. Walter Sturm; 50. unknown; 51. Giorgio Innocenti; 52. Paolo Nichelli.

REFERENCES

1. Grossi D, Boller F. Sviluppo della Neuropsicologia Italiana moderna. In: Denes G, Pizzamiglio L, eds. *Manuale Italiano di Neuropsicologia.* Milan, Italy: Zanichelli. 1996;16–34.
2. Geschwind N. Preface to the reprint of *Disconnexion syndromes in animals and man.* In: Cohen R, Wartofsky M, eds. *N. Geschwind's selected papers on language and the brain.* Dordrecht, the Netherlands: D Reidel, 1974;105 (*Boston Studies in the Philosophy of Science*, vol. 16).
3. Geschwind N, Simpson J. Procaine amide in the treatment of myotonia. *Brain* 1955;78:81–91.
4. Strub R, Geschwind N. *Gerstmann syndrome without aphasia. Cortex* 1974;10:378–387.
5. Geschwind N. The paradoxical position of Kurt Goldstein in the history of aphasia. *Cortex* 1964;1:214–224.
6. Hecaen H. *Introduction à la neuropsychologie.* Paris, France: Larousse, 1972;327.
7. Bruce D. On the origin of the term "neuropsychology." *Neuropsychologia* 1985;23:813–814.
8. Benton A. Neuropsychology: past, present and future. In: Boller F, Grafman J, eds. *Handbook of neuropsychology,* vol 1. Amsterdam, the Netherlands: Elsevier, 1988;3–27.

11
Physician

Frits Fairhurst

56 St. Joseph Street, #607, Fall River, Massachusetts 02722.

During my days at Beth Israel Hospital, it still had that locker-room decor: linoleum floors, institutionalized colors on the walls, stainless steel elevators that seemed larger than life, and ever-flickering, buzzing fluorescent lights. Many people remember Seven North Neurology, but few talk about the unit candidly (at least, patients don't hear about its history). They *do* sometimes make comments about how crazy or serious the happenings were up on Seven North. In many ways it was a fertile place for change—a change that was led by Dr. Norman Geschwind, one that would protect the rights of patients with temporal lobe epilepsy (TLE) and frontal lobe epilepsy. His emphasis on support networks replaced the neglect, the harsh treatment, and the blame mentality that had so often characterized the care of persons with epilepsy in "the old days." He also supported the nurses who were fighting for more authority in the care of their patients by trying to institute primary care nursing. Often, they became deeply and emotionally involved in their patients' care. Frequently I could hear nurses arguing with doctors until they finally got their way; I believe their courage to do this came from Dr. Geschwind's influence.

I was admitted to Seven North in 1981. I had severe seizures that were considered by some to be purely an emotional disorder. I was next to a woman who had a shunt in her head and a brain tumor. As I drifted in and out of seizures, I could feel her presence. She could still hear me. I thought I heard her speak to me once, comforting me. One day, she motioned to her family. Her gesture made all the difference in the world to them before she died; perhaps it indicated that she was, on some level, aware, and that she understood and appreciated them.

I had another friend on the unit who was blind, diabetic, and epileptic. Relationships between patients with epilepsy always seemed to have a certain warmth and innocence about them. After all, we were often blamed for things that went wrong—we were the "possessed" and unmanageable. Yes, a remarkable innocence would come to me, perhaps caused by my own vulnerability, but I do not recall ever being harmed by these friendships.

We patients were never treated as freaks by Dr. Geschwind. We were all important individuals in his sight. It could only have been through his consent that my illustrations and drawings were allowed to be hung around me. His attitude toward us set a precedent for others to follow on the Neurological Unit; it had to do with valuing scientific study for its potential to enhance life, not merely to analyze it.

A man whose low profile to patients made him seem shy, Norman Geschwind, M.D., came into my life as he did to those of many others, bringing to bear his critical eye, his keen insight into acute and chronic states, and a superb mental acuity. His diagnosis of my case came soon. I was still in limbo, in and out of extended dream states that I know

now were psychic lands of unreality. Outside the door to my room, I could hear the murmuring of the medical team (that all-invasive and intrusive collection of professional bodies learning through experience). Norman, as I would like to call him at this moment, came close to the bedside and took my hand, not in a clinical manner, but in a communicative one. His presence on that day, the simple fact of his "being there," gave me hope. Nobody else had been able to give me hope before in quite the same way. His astonishing gnome-like features immediately reminded me of *The Hobbit* by Tolkien. Usually I would overreact to any change in the environment, but Dr. Geschwind's calm, discerning manner made me feel protected. He stared into my eyes for what seemed like minutes and then said something positive to me about my creativity before he departed. Then I heard his voice outside the door, and he said clearly, "This man has TLE . . . with . . . ." As he moved down the corridor, the rest of Dr. Geschwind's statement faded out until he raised his voice to give one loud order: "Only one person at a time should enter his room!" From his voice, I discovered that a powerful concern for my well-being now existed that never had before.

Platoons of medical students, residents, and attending physicians were led through the Neurological Unit by their mentor, Dr. Geschwind, who exposed them to patients whose lives were very different from their own and whose disorders he knew could only be treated by an approach that integrated neurosurgery, neurology, and behavioral neurology. As he walked down the hallway, he could barely be seen, surrounded as he was by medical students. Often, they would leap to absolute conclusions as they argued modalities of treatment for epilepsy. Dr. Geschwind was a taskmaster and always set the students straight about their misconceptions. He had a knack for inspiring others with his insightful observations, and all these inspired physicians became familiar faces to the patients. These doctors and many others would learn from his contributions and continue his work, progressively and proactively pursuing, in their medical studies and writings, the complex interactions of brain, body, mind, and consciousness. Dr. Geschwind's research left open many questions in areas of medicine, ranging from endocrinology to neuropsychology, questions to which answers are essential for the optimal management of epilepsy.

It was under Dr. Norman Geschwind's leadership that Dr. David Bear began to advocate for the rights of people with epilepsy. I don't know if Dr. Geschwind knew it, but the members of the TLE support group took hits from other hospital "professionals" outside the unit. But those potshots were worth it if they meant standing up to the challenges faced by TLE patients on both fronts, the internal and the external. For example, after having a seizure in the waiting room for psychology outpatients, I was prohibited from sitting in the waiting room with the other patients and made to stand out in the corridor (how reminiscent that was of my grammar school years, when, because of a flushed face, I was placed in an oversized straight-backed chair with my feet dangling in the corridor). Medical professionals forget that they are like everyone else, and when doctors refuse to accept how much the condition of their patients changes them, they create an undue degree of internal stress. We patients all hoped that the growing body of information about seizure disorders would ultimately be applied to the promotion of happier and healthier lives for persons with epilepsy in our society. Dr. Geschwind did not want people to suffer.

In a word, Dr. Geschwind was prescient. He left his legacy for all those future medical scientists who would be curious and gifted enough to meet the challenge. Many of his students are now talented epilepsy researchers. When Dr. Geschwind died, I was taken aback. Now I visit his gracious image, in the form of a black-and-white photograph, located at Beth Israel Hospital in the breezeway between the main entrance and the Rabb Building. There is a little shrine there to honor his memory.

Those times were bleak for many of us with epilepsy; however, we knew by his words and actions that Dr. Geschwind offered real hope for change. Before his inspiring leadership fostered a transformation in their thinking, medical professionals had an archaic, hands-off approach to the investigation and treatment of seizure disorders. Dr. Geschwind's teaching, research, and writing, along with the work of his students and staff, began to undermine this prevailing "textbook" view of epilepsy.

Now a patient of Dr. Geschwind's students, I have been managing to live with my epilepsy for a good decade. Seizures still intervene, but as a writer, I draw solace from my belief that Dr. Norman Geschwind embraced the epileptic artist as the most enigmatic and most complex epileptic persona. I don't know if all persons with epilepsy are aware of the substantial inroads he made toward securing our safety and rights.

As we head toward the turn of the century, a warning must be issued. The search for better medicines, more thorough management, and improved diagnostic techniques must not be hindered, especially in the treatment of epilepsy. I worry that epilepsy patients, who have been helped so much by Dr. Geschwind, shall once again be buried in the recesses of society's consciousness by changes in health care reimbursement. Doctors and nurses must be alerted to the multidisciplinary care that persons with epilepsy require, and not revert to the so-called tried and true (but neglectful) clinical methods of the past. Dr. Norman Geschwind emphasized the importance of a humane approach to all persons with epilepsy, regardless of their symptoms.

Language Disorders

12

Historical Antecedents to Geschwind

Harry A. Whitaker

Laboratory of Cognitive Neuroscience, Department of Psychology, University of Québec at Montréal, Montréal, Québec, Canada H3C 3P8.

USING HISTORICAL STUDIES

Norman Geschwind's work in the 1960s (1,2) was influential in kindling an interest among neurologists and psychologists in the historical contributions of late 19th and early 20th century neuroscientists, notably those of Wernicke, Liepmann, Goldstein, and Déjérine, whose models of brain function had, over the intervening half-century, slipped from their former prominence. One of the tangible, albeit indirect, consequences of Geschwind's interest in history was the establishment of the history section of the American Academy of Neurology. The founding of the International Society for the History of Neuroscience in 1995 is evidence that the interest continues and is growing. Geschwind's use of history was quite straightforward: the connectionist model of brain function that he had come to believe in had clear origins in the work of those earlier scientists. It was good scholarship to recognize that indebtedness, and it was interesting and entertaining, all of which we should consider a first "use" of history: finding the roots of scientific concepts and uncovering the background of contemporary ideas.

Concomitant with searching out roots is the more difficult task of placing historical contributions in their proper context, to understand what might have been dictated by necessity, what might have been a limiting factor because of the then-dominant scientific paradigms, where there were true breaks with tradition and where not, what knowledge was built up incrementally through one or more trends, and what accidents of popularity, influence, social pressure, and the like might have led to one event rather than another. Consider, for example, why Broca focused on disorders of speech production *(langage articulé)*. At least part of the reason is that before the 1860s, one did not talk about the "comprehension" of language. Language was *constructed* as speech output and the rest, what would have or could have been discussed under the notion of comprehension, fell under the notion of mind, which at the time was in the province of philosophy, religion, and nascent psychiatry (the alienists). Since the 1820s, the medical as well as the phrenologic journals had been filled with case reports of expressive language impairments arising from stroke and trauma, with and without autopsy evidence of the involvement or lack of involvement of the frontal lobes (3). The works of Bouillaud, Lallemand, Broussais, Dax, and Lordat are more familiar; however there were dozens of obscure medical practitioners publishing these reports; Alexander Hood was one such lesser-known researcher (4), about whom more will be said later. Beginning at least as early as 1866 with the publication by Theodor Meynert of a case report of receptive aphasia with jargon (5), followed by the dissertation of Arnoldus van Rhijn on aphasia in 1868 in which the notion of "disconnection" was introduced (6), in turn followed by the publication of Bastian's symmetrical model of language input and output in 1869 and Schmidt's case of receptive aphasia in 1871, the stage was set for the reconstruction of language by the neuroscience community to include comprehension, seen in the work of Hughlings Jackson and Wernicke starting in 1874. Two exemplary models of historical analysis of the trends in the neurosciences as well as insightful expositions of the varying milieu are to be found in the work of Harrington (7) and Clarke and Jacyna (8). A third, monumental contribution to this subject is Finger's recent text (9), a compendium of the origins of neuroscience from the earliest written records—nearly a third of the chapters bear directly on neurolinguistic issues.

PITFALLS IN HISTORICAL RESEARCH

Establishing priority is both interesting and challenging. It is intellectually entertaining to learn that Roberts Bartholow, in 1874, was the first person to electrically stimulate the human brain with an electrode inserted directly into the cortex, regardless of what one may think about the ethics of this experiment, for which Bartholow was publicly berated in a British medical journal (10). When the electrode was pushed deeper into the cerebrum, possibly into the basal ganglia, or the thalamus, but most certainly subcortically, the subject of this experiment cried out; otherwise, Bartholow did not elicit speech, nor did he test to see if electrical stimulation could interrupt speech. On the other hand, establishing priority is typically a very tricky enterprise. Consider the following, quoted from David Caplan (11, p. 46): "The 1861 paper by Broca is the first truly scientific paper on language–brain relationships." Caplan supports that conclusion (here, as elsewhere, Caplan successfully integrates historical with contemporary research) with three claims: that Broca presented a detailed case history with "excellent gross anatomical findings at autopsy," that Broca had the insight that the gross brain convolutions are constant anatomic features that may be related to particular psychologic functions, and that Broca's primary conclusion that expressive speech depends on a small part of the inferior frontal gyrus is a good first approximation that we generally accept today. Clearly, priority in this example is a matter of scholarly judgment. What, then, can one make of the fact that Alexander Hood, in 1824, did a better job of analyzing expressive language functions and correlating them to frontal lobe anatomy? Hood postulated a lexical–phonologic level, a phonologic–articulatory level, and a motoric level for expressive speech, based upon the speech and language impairments that he observed in stroke patients. The oddity is that he used the phrenologic model of Gall and Spurzheim (4,12,13). What, then, can one make of the fact that excellent clinicopathologic studies of aphasic cases may be found in the 17th century autopsy studies of Wepfer (14), studies that are so good that one may verify the left hemisphere localization of language from them, or of the fact that Lallemand and Bouillaud, in 1824 and 1825, published dozens of autopsy reports on patients with aphasia? What, then, can one make of the fact that the classic neuroanatomists of the late 19th and early 20th centuries virtually abandoned the possibility of systematically describing gyral geography because of its evident individual variability, a variability that currently plagues positron emission tomography (PET) researchers, who need to co-register sites of PET activation with magnetic resonance images in order to compare results across subjects? And finally, what can one make of the fact that the autopsy of Broca's patient in 1861 actually demonstrated a very large left hemisphere lesion encompassing frontal, parietal, and temporal cortex? Broca "inferred" that the third inferior frontal part of this large lesion was the one responsible for the patient's aphemia by estimating the degree of necrosis and trying to back-correlate that with the patient's medical history.

What is important to appreciate here is that it is not a question of disputing the facts but a question of how one chooses to interpret the historical record. The view I prefer is that (a) Broca inherited a tradition of clinicopathologic correlation that already presupposed that different brain regions had different functions, (b) Broca was theoretically constrained by a construct of language that placed psychologic pre-eminence on speech production, (c) Broca was immediately challenged and certainly intrigued by the debates (involving many famous members of the French scientific community, such as Gratiolet, Bouillaud, Auburtin, and Flourens) concerning the role of the frontal lobe in speech and therefore was predisposed to see the age of that lesion and, most important of all, (d) Broca had the position, power, and prestige to take advantage of a serendipitous clinical observation.

WHAT NOT TO DO

Although some historical "facts" are subject to interpretation, as we have seen, some are just plain right or wrong, and it behooves us to get them right. It is quite another matter, however, to commit the unpardonable historical sin of *presentism*. Consider the following quotation from John Morton (15, p. 40): "We have a number of lessons to learn from history. If we are lucky we can avoid making the same mistakes as thinkers in the past." The *mistake* made by the "diagram-makers," according to Morton, was to confuse the goal of representing the elements of language processing in the brain with the goal of determining the localization in the brain of these elements. Needless to say, Morton assures us that "the same mistake will not be made again. . . ." (15, p. 61), leaving this reader with the clear impression that his logogen model has at last revealed the truth about language *(veritatem patefacere*—Cicero). There is a fine line between science and religion, and Morton's rhetorical style makes it hard to tell if the line has been crossed. That is of less concern at present, however, than the notion of an historical "mistake." Following the scientific paradigm of the day is simply not a mistake; to evaluate an earlier paradigm using the principles of one's own paradigm is *presentism*—judging the past by today's standard. Most historians regard presentism as an unproductive and misleading approach to the study of the past.

On the other hand, scientists do make mistakes, past and present company included, and some of the historical errors in brain–language relationships are quite interesting. Consider Franz Joseph Gall's localization of language functions *(sprachsinn und wortsinn)* in the anterior inferior frontal lobe. The craniologic method, after Gall, of relating skull protuberances (the "bumps") to hypertrophy of the underlying brain regions, in turn due to above-normal development of the faculties that are expressed by those same regions, is an unexceptional scientific method. We may find it humorous, but it is a clear and falsifiable hypothesis. And in fact, one could argue that Flourens' experiments that demonstrated that animals in whose cerebellums he had created lesions still exhibited copulatory behavior, which thus provided evidence against Gall's localization of the reproductive faculty in the cerebellum, were one of the principal reasons why many scientists rejected craniology and later phrenology. Gall refused to accept Flourens' evidence—the scientific community, particularly Bouillaud, accepted it. So far, this is all legitimate scientific debate. On the other hand, Gall's argument that a well-developed language faculty would cause a protuberance of the inferior anterior frontal lobe, which in turn would make the eye sockets shallow—thus, persons with superior verbal skills were said to have "cow's eyes"—was not successfully challenged by the scientific community, even though in fact it should be regarded as a mistake, an error in reasoning using the craniologic method. It was well known at the time that the backs of the eye sockets do not abut the frontal lobe—a great deal of sinus cavity lies between the two. It is quite impossible that a frontal brain bump could impinge upon the eye sockets. Curiously, from the standpoint of good science, Bouillaud not only accepted *this* localization but championed it unceasingly right up to 1861, when Broca's publication seemed to vindicate Gall's model. Evidently, it was the accumulating evidence that frontal lesions typically led to speech disturbances, documented by Lallemand, Bouillaud, and others from the 1820s on, that kept the phrenologic language model alive until the great paradigm shift of the 1870s.

Another error, not fully appreciated until recently, was committed by Lichtheim, one of the diagram-makers discussed in Morton's chapter. Laubstein (16) has elegantly shown that this "paradigmatic diagram-maker" produced a neurolinguistic model that is ambiguous with respect to some predictions of language disorders, that fails to predict some language disorders that had already been described, that is internally inconsistent and, finally, that cannot be falsified, all in terms of the 19th century paradigm within which Lichtheim operated. This is the kind of analysis of the diagram-makers' diagrams that goes to the heart of the basic model-making assumption of that period and of our own: the correlation between aphasic language data and the components of the processing model of language used to account for such data. There is nothing to be gained in pointing out how our forebears differed from us; there is much to be learned from analyzing how they developed and tested hypotheses.

PSYCHOLOGIC VERSUS NEUROLOGIC MODELING

Having argued that what Morton says is the diagram-makers' "mistake" should not be considered a mistake, I will next examine the actual claim that Morton makes: Did the diagram-makers confuse the psychologic (processing elements) with the neurologic (localization of elements) goals of their neurolinguistic enterprise, as Morton asserts? Baginsky (1871), the first diagram-maker discussed by Morton, believed he was basing his model on the "physiology of speech formation"; he did not stipulate specific anatomic sites for each of his language "centers," maintaining that "we do not yet have a precise conceptualization" of this relationship (17). Kussmaul, the sixth diagram-maker discussed by Morton, claimed that his colleagues, particularly Wernicke, were mistaken in trying to localize the various speech centers to specific regions of the brain. Kussmaul was "acutely aware of the limitations of the localizationist approach to linguistic processes" (17, p. 509); "...extraordinarily removed from strictly anatomical and physiological considerations, Kussmaul the physician achieves an understanding of the psychology of language in terms of the concepts which constitute the core of present day models, eg, the distinction between various levels of representation . . . their respective autonomy yet interconnection, and the notion of linguistic processes" (17, p. 497). The same may be said of Elder (18) and Grasset (19), both mentioned by Morton, as well as of Bastian (20), who, though not discussed by Morton, was one of the best known of the British diagram-makers of the period. As Paul Eling (20) remarked: "In general, characterizing the work of these classical aphasiologists with a few short statements and adjectives does not do justice to the careful analytic description and argumentation of these scientists."

In fairness, it ought to be noted that Morton's questionable analysis of the model-theoretic assumptions of Baginsky, Kussmaul, Elder, and Grasset may not be entirely his fault; he relied on Moutier's 1908 dissertation as his secondary source material. Moutier was the student of Pierre Marie, notorious for his antipathy toward anyone who fractionated language into its component elements and thus anyone who believed that there were several different types of aphasia, obviously the main tenet of the diagram-makers. Ironically, and history sometimes has a penchant for the ironic, it was Pierre Marie who proposed that the insula (island of Reil) was a functional component of expressive language (Marie's quadrilateral). George Ojemann and I (24), about two decades ago, finally established empirically that the insula can be language cortex (electrical stimulation of the insula elicited naming errors), and recent work by Nina Dronkers (25), using the lesion-overlap technique, suggests that insular lesions lead to apraxia of speech, a view quite consistent with Marie's view, as Dronkers has noted. To return to the question of psychologic versus neurologic modeling, Marie's fundamental objection to the localizationists/diagram-makers was a psychologic one (viz, the dictum *l'aphasie est une*). In Marie's view, the reconstruction of language in the 1870s to include comprehension now became reconstructed again such that comprehension (including understanding and the lexicon) now *was* language, and speech production was relegated to the status of motoric output.

To this day, neurolinguistics has wrestled with the motor component of the expressive aphasias. In the 1960s and 1970s, this was one of the major theoretical disputes between the Mayo school (Darley, Aronson, Brown, et al.) and the Boston school (Geschwind, Goodglass, Benson, et al.), a dispute which, with the benefit of two decades of hindsight, squarely addressed and never resolved the different demands of a psychologic versus a neurologic model of language.

GAPS IN THE STORY (1600–1900)

As entertaining as it may be to learn that pharaonic medicine circa 3000 B.C. recognized temporal lobe injuries as leading to aphasia (8), this knowledge was not passed on to later cultures. Comments in the Hippocratic texts—which do have historical continuity with the present through the reintroduction of Greek texts via Arabic texts in the early Renaissance—refer to what we would likely label dysarthria or aphasia, and additionally to right-sided paralyses sometimes associated with speech disorders; it is debatable whether these neurolinguistic observations were systematically understood (21), although several recent historians have argued that the epilepsy commentaries indicate that the Hippocratic physicians did understand the connection between unilateral brain lesions and symptoms lateralized to the contralateral side of the body. From the period of Plato and Aristotle through the time of Galen and up to the Renaissance, many observations on the loss of speech and language associated with either intrinsic brain disease or traumatic injury were written. However, based as they were, for the most part, on theories of meningeal or ventricular function, these accounts differ substantially from our concepts of brain function, as is very well documented in O'Neill's scholarly text (21). Benton and Joynt (22) pointed out that most of the "classic" aphasias had been described (*observed* would be more apt terminology) by 1800. O'Neill demonstrated that, at least through the Renaissance (at the beginning of the 17th century), these observations were hardly part and parcel of any general, coherent theoretical model of brain–language relationships (21).

The dominant brain function model before the Renaissance was "ventricular theory," derived from Galen and elegantly modified by Descartes, among others; basically, this model was based on fluids and fluid flow, for the obvious reason that thoughtful early scientists realized that something in the brain must move in order for it to be responsible for functions—something passes from sense organs to effectors, and the animal spirits were as good a candidate as any available. One marvels at medieval and early Renaissance discussions of memory disorders after damage to the fourth ventricle, which are models of clinicopathologic correlation despite the casual disregard of the actual neuroanatomy. However, by the end of the Renaissance, ventricular theory had been disproven by, for example, the cases reported by Johannes Schenck (1530–1598) in 1584, cases concerning patients with fourth ventricle damage in whom memory was spared, and patients with damage to the cortical substance in whom the fourth ventricle was intact but memory was impaired (14). O'Neill's summary of early neurolinguistics ends at the 17th century, leaving us with a number of gaps in the story from the Renaissance to the 20th century, gaps that are only partly filled in by current research on persons who have actually made substantial contributions to the development of neuropsychology and neurolinguistics.

Little has been written (14) about the 17th century brain scientist Johannes Jakob Wepfer (1620–1695); for our interests here, his posthumously published book, *Medical-Practical Observations of Affections Inside and Outside the Head* (1727), is most relevant. In it, Wepfer discussed 13 well-described cases of aphasia, often noting *paralisys in dextri lateris, cum loquelae impedimentum* and yet never drawing the self-evident conclusion that left-hemisphere lesions and right-sided paralysis were associated. Perhaps the fever from which he died overtook him before he completed his work; perhaps the reason for his silence on the matter of laterality was that his contemporaries, particularly those in the church, might have viewed such localization as too materialistic. Galileo was "processed" less than 30 years before, and the squares of Europe still smelled of the stakes of the Inquisition (14).

Although David Hartley (1705–1757), an early 18th century village doctor practicing without the benefit of a medical degree, neither wrote on language nor studied patients with brain damage, he was one of the first to explicitly propose a brain-based model of psychologic functions (23). (Thomas Willis, a contemporary of Johannes Wepfer, had proposed the rudiments of such a model in the 17th century.) Hartley's psychologic theory was taken from the associationism of Locke and it later became the dominant neuropsychologic model of the 19th century. His physiologic theory was based on elements in gentle vibration he called *vibratiuncles* [analogous to Willis' corpuscles; both were directly borrowed from Isaac Newton (8,23)], which allowed him to account for the transmission of sensory images into the brain, the control of motor operations by the brain, and attentional and memory mechanisms in the brain. Presaging the thinking of neuroscientists of the 19th century, Hartley's vibration theory led him to a concept of domain-specific localization of function.

Much has been written about Franz Joseph Gall's (1758–1828) contribution to neuroscience (3,4,7–9,12,13,20), but not much is known about the roots of his ideas. Christine Grou, in her unpublished doctoral dissertation, demonstrated a close parallel between the faculty psychology of Thomas Reid (1710–1796) and the faculties of Gall and Spurzheim and also a commonality between the (hundreds of) physiognomic characteristics proposed by Johann Kaspar Lavater (1741–1801) and the phrenologic faculties. Gall's idea that growth patterns of the cortex, hypertrophy or atrophy, would impress themselves on the inner table of the skull and thus be "readable" as bumps on the outside of the skull was directly borrowed from Lavater. The great 18th century naturalist Charles Bonnet (1720–1792) proposed a vibration-based theory of memory reminiscent of Hartley; Bonnet also proposed a doctrine of localization of function in the brain that clearly influenced

Gall (the latter cites the former in several of his books). Nonetheless, the details of Gall's indebtedness to those 18th century scientists remain to be elucidated. On the other end, we have worked out a few of the connections between craniology/phrenology and the development of neuropsychology in the period from 1820 to 1860 (3,12), and we have also begun an analysis of how the early phrenologists helped to found the doctrine of clinicopathologic correlation of language impairments (4); little is known about phrenology's contribution to other aspects of neuropsychology and psychiatry. Craniology/phrenology was quite clearly an early personality theory (compare its roots in physiognomy); whether and in what respects it may have influenced the development of personality theory in modern psychology as well as psychiatry are not well worked out.

CONCLUSION

The historical analyses discussed in this chapter can help us realize that the neurolinguistic models proposed by Geschwind and his followers, as reflected in later chapters in this book (a) have precursors, (b) are contextually influenced by the scientific milieu, and (c) are relative to the assumptions and constraints of the paradigms we happen to currently accept. And they can amuse.

REFERENCES

1. Geschwind N. Carl Wernicke, the Breslau school and the history of aphasia. In: Carterette EC, ed. *Speech, language, and communication,* vol 3: *Brain function.* Berkeley, CA: University of California Press, 1963;1–16.
2. Geschwind N. Disconnexion syndromes in animals and man. (2 parts.) *Brain* 1965;88:237–294, 585–644.
3. Whitaker HA, Grou C. From craniology to neurology in 19th century France: how the localization of language became the test case. *Psychol Can* 1993;34(2a):435.
4. Whitaker HA, Grou C. Spurzheim's legacy: the case of Adam M'Conochie (1824). *Neurology* 1991;41:239.
5. Whitaker HA, Etlinger SC. Theodore Meynert's contribution to classical 19th century aphasia studies. *Brain Lang* 1993;45(4):560–571.
6. Eling P. *Arnoldus van Rhijn on aphasia: a forgotten thesis.* Paper presented to the International Society for the History of the Neurosciences meeting, Buffalo, NY, May, 1966.
7. Harrington A. *Medicine, mind and the double brain.* Princeton, NJ: Princeton University Press, 1987.
8. Clarke E, Jacyna LS. *Nineteenth-century origins of neuroscientific concepts.* Berkeley, CA: University of California Press, 1987.
9. Finger S. *Origins of neuroscience.* New York: Oxford University Press, 1994.
10. Whitaker HA, Ojemann GA. The early history of electrical stimulation of the human brain: from Bartholow (1874) to Penfield (1928). *(In preparation.)*
11. Caplan D. *Neurolinguistics and linguistic aphasiology.* Cambridge, England: Cambridge University Press, 1987.
12. Grou C, Whitaker HA. Le cerveau: petite histoire de la localisation des fonctions. *Interface* 1992;13(5):14–21.
13. Zola-Morgan S. Localization of brain function: the legacy of Franz Joseph Gall (1758–1828). *Ann Rev Neurosci* 1995;18:359–383.
14. Luzzatti C, Whitaker HA. Johannes Schenck and Johannes Jakob Wepfer: clinical and anatomical observations in the prehistory of aphasia and cognitive disorders. *J Neurolinguistics* 1996 *(in press).*
15. Morton J. Brain-based and non-brain-based models of language. In: Caplan D, Lecours AR, Smith A, eds. *Biological perspectives on language.* Cambridge, MA: MIT Press, 1984;40–64.
16. Laubstein AS. Inconsistency and ambiguity in Lichtheim's model. *Brain Lang* 1993;45(4):588–603.
17. Jarema G. In sensu non in situ: the prodromic cognitivism of Kussmaul. *Brain Lang* 1993;45(4):495–510.
18. Whitaker HA. William Elder (1864–1931): diagram maker and experimentalist. In: Hyman L, Li C, eds. *Language, speech and mind.* London, England: Routledge, 1988;163–174.
19. Dos Santos G, Nespoulous J-L, Whitaker HA. Grasset's polygon. *(In preparation.)*
20. Eling P, ed. *Reader in the history of aphasia.* Amsterdam, the Netherlands: John Benjamins, 1994.
21. O'Neill Y. *Speech and speech disorders in Western thought before 1600.* Westport, CN: Greenwood Press, 1980.
22. Benton AL, Joynt R. Early descriptions of aphasia. *Arch Neurol* 1960;3:205–221.
23. Aubert D, Whitaker HA. David Hartley's model of vibratiuncles seen as a contribution to the localization theory of brain function. *History Philos Psychol Bull* 1996;8(1).
24. Ojemann GA, Whitaker HA. Language localization and variability. *Brain Lang* 1978;6:239–260.
25. Dronkers N. Presentations at meetings of the Academy of Aphasia, 1992 and 1993.

13

Norman Geschwind's Influence on the Study of Aphasia

D. Frank Benson

UCLA School of Medicine, 710 Westwood Plaza, Los Angeles, California 90024.

To say that Norman Geschwind exerted a major influence on the development of aphasia in the 20th century is merely to state the obvious. The century is nearing completion, and even superficial reflection clearly demonstrates that his works have effected major changes in the study and understanding of acquired language impairment. His accomplishments are significant. Geschwind stands with (or against) Marie as the most influential figure of this century in the field of aphasia.

CHIEF CONTRIBUTION TO THE FIELD

Geschwind's contributions to the study of aphasia were produced over a relatively short period. In the foreword to his collected writings on language (1), he commented that his major papers in the field had been published in just over 11 years, a fairly accurate dating of his attention to acquired language impairment. Although he had become immersed in the field for several years before publication of the first paper in this collection (2), his major interests had changed well before the last of the papers in the collection was finally published (3). Geschwind maintained an interest in language disorders and wrote a number of influential review papers in the years that followed, but it was during a single decade, approximately 1960 to 1970, that he focused his attention on the problems of language.

Geschwind's crowning achievement was to return the brain to an important place in the investigation of language functions. His vigorous insistence that the investigator of aphasia should correlate the disordered language parameters with the findings of the standard neurological exam, with related behavioral abnormalities, with data from neuropathological case studies, and with the relevant neuroanatomy of the cerebral hemispheres reversed the holistic approach to the study of aphasia that had prevailed for most of the century.

To gauge the importance of Geschwind's influence, one must appreciate the state of aphasia investigation in the preceding half-century, particularly the decades immediately following World War II. Starting with Broca and the European aphasiologists who followed, a strong inclination to correlate individual behavior patterns with specific localization of lesions within the cerebral cortex had developed. This activity coincided with, and was actually one of the most exciting aspects of, the neuropathological explanation of disease processes that flowered in Germany and was strong in France, the United Kingdom, and the United States in the last half of the 19th century. Based primarily on individual case studies of aphasic symptomatology, many of the suggested correlations were excessively precise but nonreplicable. All involved correlation of language abnormality with location of lesion in the hemispheric cortex; subcortical disorders had not yet been recognized as a source of neurological symptomatology. A mosaic pattern of postulated hemispheric centers evolved. Although many valuable observations were recorded and a basic classification of acquired language impairment was formulated, the claims of precise centers for specific language functions were excessive and, in many instances, untrue.

A strong reaction to this mosaic approach to the explanation of language function arose, particularly after the challenge raised by Pierre Marie early in the 20th century. Through the efforts of a number of influential clinical investigators, such as Jackson, Goldstein, and Head, a less fragmented, central language function was postulated. Aphasia was considered to be the result of damage to the language system, modified by additional impairments of neighboring functions (e.g., motor, visual, auditory, or somesthetic abilities). The variations so obvious in aphasia symptomatology were thought to represent the influence of these neighboring complications; the aphasia itself indicated a disturbance of the language function. Although this holistic view may be adequate for many types of investigation—for example, psychologic and linguistic—and even for aphasia rehabilitation as it existed at the time, it is severely limited by the absence of correlation with brain functions. In this approach, the brain is truly a black box.

When Norman Geschwind first studied aphasia, the holistic approach prevailed; within just a few years, his publications altered the prevalent view of aphasia. It is fully accurate to state that the major influence Geschwind exerted on the study of aphasia was to initiate the change from holistic to brain-oriented language investigations. The brain was again recognized as an important factor in aphasia.

Controversy continues concerning these approaches; both are useful, and both warrant serious consideration. For many psychologists, linguists, and speech pathologists, the holistic approach is fully adequate. For neuroscientists, the importance of the brain to human language is obvious. By stressing the importance of various portions of the brain to language, Geschwind introduced aphasia and related language dysfunctions to the newly burgeoning field of neuroscience. The return of the brain to a position of significance in the study of language ranks as Geschwind's major contribution to the field.

PRIMARY INTELLECTUAL STRENGTHS

To accomplish his contributions to the study of aphasia, Norman Geschwind drew on a number of intellectual strengths. The first was his competence in the clinical evaluation of aphasic patients. Under the guidance of experienced colleagues such as Fred Quadfasel, Davis Howes, and Harold Goodglass, Geschwind developed a method to evaluate language function and, more pertinent, language dysfunction at the bedside. He combined carefully thought out language testing with an equally careful neurological evaluation. To these he added the demonstration of a number of related neurobehavioral findings, stressing such problems as ideomotor apraxia, the Gerstmann syndrome, and color-naming disturbance. The anatomic correlates of the neurological examination, plus those of the related behavioral problems, represented valuable adjuncts to the primary language evaluation for purposes of localizing the site of disease with a given type of language disability.

A second significant strength was a distinctly superior grasp of neuroanatomy. He not only used the basic neurologist's knowledge of neuroanatomy but maintained an active interest in anatomic research and carefully studied the areas of structural damage in the relatively few individual patients with language disorders whom he was able to follow to postmortem study. By combining his neuroanatomic knowledge with data from his clinical observations of these patients, he was able to uncover definitive neuropathological correlations for several varieties of language disturbance, a powerful tool.

In addition to these basic clinical skills, Geschwind had an extensive knowledge of the original aphasia literature. Almost all reports that described the early approaches to aphasia were written in German and French; their translation demanded a considerable scholarly effort. In translating the older German literature, Geschwind received considerable assistance from Dr. Fred Quadfasel, who had been trained in Germany. Geschwind ranked, without question, as one of the most knowledgeable persons in the United States or Europe on the writings of the 19th century aphasiologists. Although many of the 19th century writings were excessively localizationist, the case reports often provided good neuropathological correlations and became useful building blocks for a 20th century theory of the neuroscience of language.

Finally, the most important of Geschwind's intellectual strengths was his basic intelligence. He had a superb memory coupled with an exceptional ability to correlate diverse material, allowing him to ferret out, amalgamate, and emphasize important features. With the comprehensive knowledge of language function, clinical neurology, and neuroanatomy that he was gaining, Geschwind rapidly became a powerful creative force in language investigation. Within just a few years of developing an interest in the field, his brain-based approach influenced all studies of language, and it remains strong to this day.

SPECIFIC CONTRIBUTIONS TO THE STUDY OF APHASIA

Although Geschwind's major contribution was to return correlation of focal brain dysfunction with specific language dysfunctions, he strongly championed certain disorders that, by themselves, came to represent important contributions to the study of aphasia. In truth, most of these disorders were not discovered by Geschwind; they had been observed and described in the past. Most had not, however, been presented with sufficient strength to be broadly accepted and were lost or ignored in mid-20th-century descriptions of language disorders.

One of Geschwind's most important yet almost universally overlooked contributions was his reintroduction of repetition of spoken language in aphasia testing. Repetition testing, which has become a standard procedure, was, a mere three decades ago, virtually unknown in the English-speaking world in formal language evaluation. Repetition had been recognized as a significant language parameter by the early European aphasiologists, but their knowledge had never been adequately translated into English. Even in the European countries where repetition was originally accepted, the procedure had fallen into disuse and was reintroduced through Geschwind's influence. In the 1950s, repetition was used only to monitor articulation, not as a probe of a significant language function. Geschwind insisted that repetition in language testing was important and demonstrated that several types of aphasia, recognized and described by the 19th century aphasiologists, could not be uncovered without including competency in repetition among the language parameters tested.

The most immediate and obvious use of repetition as an assessment tool is to demonstrate the existence of conduction aphasia, a disorder considered by most mid-20th-century aphasiologists to be nonexistent, a product of the excessive localization practices of the 19th century. Conduction aphasia, as originally described in the 19th century and rediscovered by Geschwind, features a notable impairment of the ability to repeat despite otherwise relatively intact language. It is now universally recognized that conduction aphasia represents a distinct clinical entity with distinct neuroanatomic implications; unless repetition is compared with other language functions, conduction aphasia cannot be demonstrated. Geschwind not only reintroduced a key language test but championed the existence of a distinct type of aphasia.

Conversely, the presence of significant aphasic disturbance but preservation of the ability to repeat spoken language also represents a major type of language disorder that was well recognized by the late 19th century. Although this problem had been outlined and studied by the early European aphasiologists, it was totally lost in the holistic approach. Geschwind provided a powerful demonstration of these disorders (called transcortical aphasias) with several reports in which he described a carefully studied case of isolation of the speech area (mixed transcortical aphasia). The patient described in these reports was totally aphasic (nonfluent, anomic, alexic, agraphic, and without any verbal comprehension) except for a relatively intact ability to repeat spoken language. The anatomic basis for this dramatic phenomenon represents a cornerstone of the neural basis of the transcortical aphasias. The rediscovery and acceptance of these unusual aphasias was directly related to the emphasis given to repetition testing by Norman Geschwind.

Another major reintroduction to the language literature by Geschwind concerned alexia, acquired impairment of the ability to comprehend written or printed language. Two types of alexia—alexia with agraphia and alexia without agraphia—had been demonstrated in the 1890s by Déjérine and accepted by a number of his contemporaries. The distinctive features of the two alexias were almost entirely buried by the holistic view in the early 20th century. By reviewing Déjérine's original paper on alexia without agraphia (2), combining the information it contained with a case that he had evaluated personally (4), and noting the site of neuropathology common to both (5), Geschwind reintroduced the premise that two dramatically different types of alexia with discretely different loci of structural neuropathology can be distinguished. His interest in this subject led him to prepare a chapter on alexia for *Handbook of Neurology* (6), a chapter that became a prime reference source for most research on acquired reading disturbances. Almost all current studies of alexia derive from Geschwind's reestablishment of a neuroanatomic correlation for acquired reading impairment.

Geschwind's most important contribution to the study of language is his disconnection theory (7). Although this theory has many aspects, some of which apply to other aspects of behavior, the importance of this work to the study of language abnormality cannot be overemphasized. Nineteenth century theories of acquired language disturbance stressed cortical involvement, depicting a mosaic of cortical areas associated with specific language functions. There was almost no acknowledgment that the various neocortical "centers" were connected. In reintroducing brain functions to the study of aphasia, Geschwind greatly enhanced the validity of neuropathologicoclinical correlations by noting that the cortical areas were connected by both long and short subcortical pathways, and by demonstrating that damage to these pathways could produce language disturbance. The idea was not new, but it had not been emphasized previously. Geschwind's disconnection theory greatly strengthened the neurological approach to language function and was almost immediately accepted. It is now obvious that a number of language dysfunctions are based on disconnection, not on focal cortical damage. For instance, both conduction aphasia and alexia without agraphia are disturbances of connecting pathways, not specific cortical areas, and the understanding of apraxia was greatly aided by Geschwind's restatement of the importance of cerebral pathways to these functions. The split-brain literature of the 1960s demonstrates the importance of the corpus callosal connections for behavior; recognition and acceptance of this work was dependent, to a considerable extent, on the disconnection theory formally proposed in 1965. All aspects of brain/behavior correlation have been greatly enhanced by the increased power provided by the disconnection theory.

Finally, Geschwind provided an additional impetus for language investigation by introducing a system for classifying the various types of aphasias based on anatomic/behavioral correlations. This classification is, of course, neither solid nor absolute; no absolute nosologic system can exist in medicine. The classification, which was developed at the Boston Veterans Administration Hospital under his guidance (8), has provided a strong structure for aphasia research and remains an important aspect of ongoing language research.

INFLUENCE ON COLLEAGUES

The importance of Geschwind's work on language study was rapidly recognized, and a number of neurologists gathered to work with him. This group, together with psychologists and language therapists working together at the Boston Veterans Administration Aphasia Research Center, ultimately became known as the Boston school. Although never formally organized, the Boston group had and continues to have a strong influence on the study of aphasia; the approach they advocate stemmed from Geschwind and continues to be influenced by his teaching. Geschwind's work on localizing, classifying, and describing types of aphasia attracted a number of disciples, many of whom have continued his research and have added to the world's knowledge of aphasia. Included in the group that have worked in this field are Benson, Kertesz, Rubens, Heilman, Damasio, Alexander, Naeser, and many more.

Geschwind also had a considerable influence on the origination and course of the branch of psychology now called neuropsychology; that discipline has grown remarkably in the past two decades. Without actively practicing psychology, Geschwind influenced, by his comprehensive knowledge of brain-related activities, a number of key persons who defined and developed the field. Among those who worked with and were directly influenced by Geschwind were Goodglass, Kaplan, Butters, Cermak, Weintraub, Spiers, Gardner, and Benton. In fact, almost all practicing neuropsychologists have been affected by his contributions.

Another relatively new field—psycholinguistics—and the directions taken by many investigators in that field reflect Geschwind's influence. A number of acknowledged leaders in psycholinguistics have worked with the Boston group, including Albert, Goodglass, Hecaen, Zurif, and Blumstein.

Aphasia therapy was not one of Geschwind's major interests, but he gave his full support to the aphasia rehabilitation program at the Boston Veterans Administration Aphasia Research Center. The program prospered. Many of Geschwind's brain/behavior correlations were noted and utilized in the development of language therapy techniques in the program. Such persons as Sparks and Helm-Estabrook were strongly influenced by Geschwind, and many other language therapists acknowledge his contributions to the field.

Finally, Norman Geschwind had considerable influence on European investigators of language function. He traveled to Europe frequently and, even more often, was host to innumerable scientists from a broad variety of nations. Norman developed strong friendships and professional relationships with DeRenzi, Vignolo, Hecaen, Poeck, Behan, Simpson, and Yamadori, among others. Many of these investigators spent at least some time working with Geschwind, and all spent many hours discussing approaches to language function with him. His impact on the field was truly international.

CONTRIBUTIONS TO NEUROLOGICAL SCIENCE AND NEUROBEHAVIOR

Language was not accepted as a significant aspect of the newly developing neurological sciences until Geschwind's influence became felt. The development of a body of knowledge that demonstrated neuroanatomic/behavioral correlations allowed a neuroscientific approach to the function of language and thence to many other cognitive functions. Geschwind introduced neuroscience to studies of human higher brain functions and vice versa.

Through numerous lectures and overview articles he wrote for widely read journals, Norman presented his ideas on brain/language correlations. Even after his own interest in language research had waned, Geschwind wielded considerable influence on language investigation through his clinical and scientific discussions. In addition, he continued to produce excellent overview articles on language function. They appeared in such widely distributed periodicals as *Science* (9), *The New England Journal of Medicine* (10), and *Scientific American* (11). He also contributed important overview chapters to such major textbooks as *Clinical Neurology,* volume 1 (Baker and Baker, editors) (8), *Handbook of Neurology* (6), and *Textbook of Medicine* (Beeson and McDermott, editors) (12). These writings became standards in the field. All neurologists and neuropsychologists, plus a vast number of specialists in related clinical and academic pursuits, have been exposed to and influenced by Geschwind's writings. And a large number, quite possibly a quorum of specialists in the field, have heard Norman's inspiring discourses on language and related disorders.

Geschwind was also instrumental in having language dysfunction and related problems accepted as significant topics for discussion at a number of national and international meetings. Most particularly, and almost single-handedly, he developed the behavioral neurology section of the American Academy of Neurology (AAN). Starting from almost nothing, he built both the platform and the course presentations of neurobehavioral topics, including language, at the annual meeting. When he first took over the behavioral neurology section of the AAN meeting, it consisted of only 2 hours each year, usually the final 2 hours on Saturday morning, and was attended by only a handful of the dedicated. The previous director of the behavioral neurology section complained that there was no interest in the topic and that no one submitted papers on behavior. That section has undergone explosive growth; multiple half-day sections are devoted to neurobehavior and additional sections are devoted to related neurobehavioral problems including dementia. An even larger number of posters are presented on these topics. A healthy number of special courses on topics related to neurobehavior are included at each meeting and are, in general, well attended. Similar neurobehavioral topics are now included in other national and international neurological meetings. The behavioral aspects of neurology have become a fully accepted and truly exciting aspect of neurology. The present high degree of interest in brain/behavior as a neurological and neuroscientific topic can be traced largely to the influence of Geschwind.

SUMMARY

Norman Geschwind produced 60 items (scientific papers, chapters, reviews, and one volume of his collected writings) that dealt with language. Seminal contributions from this extensive bibliography have been cited in the text, but the reader is encouraged to look further. Geschwind was an accomplished writer as well as an inspiring teacher.

In my opinion, Norman Geschwind ranks as the single most influential figure of the 20th century on the study of aphasia. Even those persons who promote very different approaches to the field acknowledge his tremendous influence. His introductions and reintroductions to the field now have a permanent place in the study of the brain's participation in language function. The fact that all of his significant works on aphasia were published within a relatively short period of time is a testament to his genius. Norman Geschwind went on to have a considerable impact on several other aspects of the study of the brain and behavior, but during the short span that he devoted to the subject of acquired language dysfunction, he produced ideas that will stand forever.

REFERENCES

1. Geschwind N. *Selected papers on language and the brain.* Boston: D Reidel, 1974.
2. Geschwind N. The anatomy of acquired disorders of reading. In: Money J, ed. *Reading disability.* Baltimore: Johns Hopkins University Press, 1962;115–129.
3. Geschwind N. El lenguaje escrito y sus desordenes. In: Caceres A, ed. *Lenguaje y audicion.* Lima, Peru: Editoral Juridica, 1973;49–56.
4. Geschwind N. Alexia and color-naming disturbance. In: Ettlinger G, ed. *Ciba Foundation symposium on the functions of the corpus callosum.* London: J & A Churchill, 1965;95–100.
5. Geschwind N, Fusillo M. Color-naming defects in association with alexia. *Arch Neurol* 1966;15:137–146.
6. Benson DF, Geschwind N. The alexias. In: Vinken PJ, Bruyn GW, eds. *Handbook of neurology,* vol 4. Amsterdam, the Netherlands: North-Holland, 1969;112–140.
7. Geschwind N. Disconnexion syndromes in animals and man. (2 parts.) *Brain* 1965;88:237–294, 585–644.
8. Benson DF, Geschwind N. The aphasias and related disturbances. In: Baker AB, Baker LH, eds. *Clinical neurology,* vol 1. New York: Harper & Row, 1971.
9. Geschwind N, Levitsky W. Human brain: left–right asymmetries in temporal speech region. *Science* 1968;161:186–187.
10. Geschwind N. Aphasia. *N Engl J Med* 1971;284:654–656.
11. Geschwind N. Language and the brain. *Sci Am* 1972;226:76–83.
12. Geschwind N. Focal disturbances of higher nervous function. In: Beeson P, McDermott W, eds. *Textbook of medicine.* Philadelphia: WB Saunders, 1971;99–102.

ADDITIONAL READING

Benson DF, Geschwind N. Cerebral dominance and its disturbances. *Pediatr Clin North Am* 1968;15:750–769.
Benson DF, Geschwind N. Developmental Gerstmann syndrome. *Neurology* 1970;20:293.
Benson DF, Sheremata WA, Bouchard R, Segarra JM, Price DL, Geschwind N. Conduction aphasia: a clinicopathological study. *Arch Neurol* 1973;28:339–346.
Chedru F, Geschwind N. Writing disturbances in acute confusional states. *Neuropsychologia* 1972;10:343–353.
Damasio AR, Geschwind N. The neural basis of language. In: Cowan WM, Shooter EM, Stevens CF, Thompson RF, eds. *Annual review of neuroscience.* Palo Alto, CA: Annual Reviews, 1984;127–147.
Galaburda AM, Geschwind N. The human language areas and cerebral asymmetries. *Rev Med Suisse Romande* 1980;100:119–128.
Geschwind N. Carl Wernicke, the Breslau school, and the history of aphasia. In: Carterette EC, ed. *Brain function,* vol 3: *Speech, language, and communication.* Berkeley, CA: University of California Press, 1963;1–16.
Geschwind N. The development of the brain and the evolution of language. In: Stuart CIJM, ed. *Monograph series on languages and linguistics,* vol 17. Washington, DC: Georgetown University Press, 1964;155–169.
Geschwind N. The paradoxical position of Kurt Goldstein in the history of aphasia. *Cortex* 1964;1:214–224.
Geschwind N. Il problema del linguaggio in rapporto allosviluppo filogenetico del cervello. *Sistema Nervoso* 1965;6:411.

Geschwind N. Non-aphasic disorders of speech. *Int J Neurol* 1965;4:207–214.
Geschwind N. The test of time. VIII: Aphasia. *Boston Med Q* 1965;16:129–130.
Geschwind N. Wernicke's contribution to the study of aphasia. *Cortex* 1967;3:449–463.
Geschwind N. The varieties of naming errors. *Cortex* 1967;3:97–112.
Geschwind N. The neural basis of language. In: Salzinger K, Salzinger S, eds. *Research in verbal behavior and some neurological implications.* New York: Academic Press, 1967;423–427.
Geschwind N. Neurological foundations of language. In: Mykelbust HR, ed. *Progress in learning disabilities,* vol 1. New York: Grune & Stratton, 1967;182–198.
Geschwind N. Problems in the anatomical understanding of the aphasias. In: Benton AL, ed. *Contributions to clinical neuropsychology.* Chicago: Aldine, 1969;107–128.
Geschwind N. Anatomy and the higher functions of the brain. In: *Boston studies in the philosophy of science.* RS Cohen, MW Wartosky eds., Dordrect, Holland: D. Reidel, 1969;4:98–136.
Geschwind N. The work and influence of Wernicke. In: *Boston studies in the philosophy of science.* RS Cohen, MW Wartosky, eds., Dordrect, Holland: D. Reidel, 1969;4:1–33.
Geschwind N. Clinical syndromes of the cortical connections. In: Williams D, ed. *Modern trends in neurology.* London: Butterworths, 1970;29–40.
Geschwind N. Language disturbances in cerebrovascular disease. In: Benton A, ed. *Behavioral changes in cerebrovascular disease.* New York: Harper & Row, 1970;29–36.
Geschwind N. Disturbances of language, perception and memory. In: Keefer CS, Wilkins RW, eds. *Medicine: essentials of clinical practice.* Boston: Little, Brown, 1970;973–980.
Geschwind N. The organization of language and the brain. *Science* 1970;170:940–944.
Geschwind N. Review of "Traumatic Aphasia" by A. R. Luria. *Language* 1972;48:755–763.
Geschwind N. Disorders of higher cortical function in children. *Clin Proc Children's Hosp Natl Med Center* 1972;28:261–272.
Geschwind N. The brain and language. In: Miller GA, ed. *Communication, language and meaning.* New York: Basic Books, 1973;61–72.
Geschwind N. Language and cerebral dominance. In: Tower DB, ed. *The nervous system,* vol 2. New York: Raven Press, 1975;433–439.
Geschwind N. Anatomical foundations of language and dominance. In: Ludlow CL, Doran-Quine ME, eds. *The neurological bases of language disorders in children: methods and directions for research.* Washington, DC: US Government Printing Office, 1979;145–157.
Geschwind N. L'aphasie de Broca: le phenix neurologique. *Rev Neurol* 1980;136:585–589.
Geschwind N. Some comments on the neurology of language. In: Caplan D, ed. *Biological studies of mental processes.* Cambridge, MA: MIT Press, 1980;301–319.
Geschwind N. Language and communication in the elderly: an overview. In: Obler LK, Albert ML, eds. *Language and communication in the elderly.* Lexington, MA: DC Heath and Co., 1980;205–209.
Geschwind N. Linguistic distinctions in aphasia. *Contemp Psychol* 1981;26:833–834.
Geschwind N. Aphasia. Part 1: Examination of the aphasic patient. *Neurology and neurosurgery update series.* 1982;3(6).
Geschwind N. Aphasia. Part 2: Diagnosis, prognosis, and treatment. *Neurology and neurosurgery update series.* 1982;3(7).
Geschwind N. Focal disturbances of higher nervous function. In: Wyngaarden JB, Smith LH, eds. *Textbook of medicine.* Philadelphia: WB Saunders, 1982;1935–1940.
Geschwind N. Biological foundations of language and hemispheric dominance. In: Studdert-Kennedy M, ed. *Psychobiology of language.* Cambridge, MA: MIT Press, 1983;62–68.
Geschwind N, Howes D. Quantitative studies of aphasic language. In: Rioch D, Weinstein E, eds. *Disorders of communication: proceedings of Association for Research in Nervous and Mental Diseases,* vol 42. Baltimore: Williams & Wilkins, 1964;229–244.
Geschwind N, Quadfasel FA, Segarra JM. Isolation of the speech area. *Neuropsychologia* 1968;6:327–340.
Goodglass H, Geschwind N. Language disorders (aphasia). In: Carterette EC, Friedman MP, eds. *Handbook of perception,* vol 7. New York: Academic Press, 1976;390–428.
Heilman KM, Coyle JM, Gonyea EF, Geschwind N. Apraxia and agraphia in a left-hander. *Brain* 1973;96:21–28.
Heilman KM, Gonyea EF, Geschwind N. Apraxia and agraphia in a right-hander. *Cortex* 1974;10:284–288.
Heilman KM, Pandya DN, Karol EA, Geschwind N. Auditory inattention. *Arch Neurol* 1971;24:323–325.
Heilman KM, Safran A, Geschwind N. Closed head trauma and aphasia. *J Neurol Neurosurg Psychiatry* 1971;34:265–269.
Judd T, Gardner H, Geschwind N. Alexia without agraphia in a composer. *Brain* 1983;106:435–457.
Naeser MA, Alexander MP, Helm-Estabrook N, Levine HL, Laughlin SA, Geschwind N. Aphasia with predominantly subcortical lesion sites. *Arch Neurol* 1982;39:2–14.
Sherwin I, Geschwind N. Language-induced epilepsy. *Arch Neurol* 1967;16:25–31.
Sparks R, Geschwind N. Dichotic listening in man after section of neocortical commissures. *Cortex* 1968;4:3–16.
Strub R, Geschwind N. Gerstmann syndrome without aphasia. *Cortex* 1974;10:378–387.

14
Evolving Concepts of Anomia: Geschwind's Role

Martin L. Albert and Harold Goodglass

Aphasia Research Center, Boston Department of Veteran Affairs Medical Center, Department of Neurology, Boston, Massachusetts 02130.

Geschwind's work in the area of anomia began at a period when this disorder had the status of only a clinically described symptom; the classical theorists of the 19th century had made little effort to deal with it in terms of causative mechanism. Geschwind's writings on the neurology of naming, and its pathology in aphasia, constitute a modest body of work; only one paper has the word *naming* in its title. Thus, in comparison with apraxia, the principle of disconnection syndromes and the case reports that contained illustrative instances of disconnection syndromes, and Geschwind's work on cerebral dominance, the concept of naming and its disorders occupied little of his published output. Nevertheless, his views had an impact on both the neurological theory of naming and the differentiation of its clinical forms. In this chapter, we will sketch the state of the concept of anomia up to the 1950s and review Geschwind's contribution to the topic. Then we will summarize the work on anomia in the dozen years since his death, touching on Geschwind's influence on contemporary thinking.

ANOMIA IN THE 1950S

Impaired word retrieval was described as part of the core of aphasic symptomatology from the earliest documented case descriptions. It was customary to refer to the loss of word retrieval as *verbal amnesia*. The first use of the term *amnesia* in connection with aphasia appears to be by Gesner in 1770; he used the term *Sprachamnesie* (1). Marc Dax, the first person to report cerebral dominance for language, referred in his manuscript (published in 1865 by his son) to his curiosity about the loss of memory for words, which impelled him to embark on the accumulation of a series of such cases (2). Lordat, who wrote an extensive introspective analysis of his own aphasia, used the term *verbal amnesia* to refer specifically to the failure of word retrieval (3). Broca himself distinguished between *aphémie*, denoting the loss of articulatory output, and *amnésie verbale*, or impaired memory for words with preserved motor speech skills.

It is not clear whether references to verbal amnesia by Broca and others referred to pure word retrieval difficulty (today's *anomic aphasia*) or whether it included all the fluent forms of aphasia that featured impaired word retrieval in their symptomatology. What does emerge from this usage is a readiness to deal with word retrieval failure purely phenomenologically, assuming it to be some form of memory failure.

With the appearance of Wernicke's monograph *Der aphasische Symptomenkomplex* (4) in 1874, the rudiments of a mechanism for normal naming and its pathology made their appearance. The posterior portion of the first temporal convolution (Wernicke's area) was postulated to be a storehouse for the auditory images of the words acquired during a speaker's lifetime. The concepts to which the words referred were distributed in other parts of the brain, so connections between Wernicke's area and the conceptual system were vital for the auditory word images to be endowed with meaning. When these connections were impaired (in transcortical sensory aphasia), the patient might hear and repeat the recognized word-sounds without understanding them. The same store of auditory word images was the basis for word production in naming. Because of the assumption that the memory of word images was based on an auditory trace, impaired word retrieval was referred to in the classic German literature as a sensory aphasic feature. This assumption fit perfectly well with the impaired word retrieval of patients with the sensory aphasia of Wernicke but did not explain the dissociation of word retrieval from word comprehension in patients with pure anomia. Indeed, the anatomic association model of Wernicke and Lichtheim made no provision for anomic aphasia.

It was Pitres who first called attention to the pure disorder of word retrieval that today we call anomia (5). Pitres, however, did little more than describe the clinical presentation of the disorder and to resurrect the concept of verbal amnesia as an explanation.

Although Wernicke's notion of a storehouse of auditory verbal word representations remained unchallenged from the viewpoint of anatomic theorists, Kurt Goldstein (6), who represented the noetic or psychological school, provided a totally different emphasis. Goldstein regarded the act of naming as dependent on the capacity to appreciate that the association between an object and its name is arbitrary and abstract. The loss of *abstract behavior* left a person unable to conceive of the name as a label in this sense and hence unable to provide a name as a deliberate act. *Amnestic aphasia* was Goldstein's term for the syndrome of impaired word retrieval caused by an impairment of abstract behavior. Patients with amnestic behavior occasionally accessed the names of concepts, but by Goldstein's analysis, their naming was *concrete*. By this term he meant that the word became available as an automatic association within a situational context but could not be retrieved for a voluntary act of naming. Goldstein allowed that name retrieval could be impaired as part of the impairment of the *instrumentalities of speech,* without invoking a loss of abstract behavior. However, the instrumentalities of speech are not differentiated. In particular, Goldstein does not make provision for a selective disorder of naming in any context except that of amnestic aphasia.

Goldstein's strong position on the nature of amnestic aphasia encountered opposition from a number of authors [e.g., Lotmar (7) and von Kuenberg (8)], who described word-retrieval difficulty in patients with normal ability to deal with concepts on an abstract level. The approach of Henry Head (9), another member of the noetic school, shared with Goldstein a predilection for discussing word-retrieval failure on a psychologic level. Yet their accounts differed in terminology and in the details of the psychological mechanisms that they invoked.

Although Head proposed a fourfold typology of aphasias, he attributed them all to a single underlying deficit—a "loss of symbolic formulation and expression." *Nominal aphasia* was his term for the subtype in which the ability to retrieve the names of concepts of all types was interfered with, although motor articulatory and syntactical aspects remained unaffected. As with his other subtypes of aphasia, Head ascribed no other specialized mechanism to the impairment of naming except to indicate that it was one of the manifestations of the symbolic incapacity.

Thus, by 1950, the neurology of naming disorders could be quickly summarized as being expressed in terms of either the loss of access to a localized storehouse of word images or the loss of a broad symbolic capacity. The psychological analysis of the normal process of acquiring and using a naming vocabulary was somewhat more sophisticated but far different from its character in the current era of cognitive neuropsychology.

GESCHWIND'S ANATOMY OF NAMING

Rooted in clinical neurology, fascinated by rare and unexplained cases of neurobehavioral syndromes that could serve as a window on the brain, and steeped in contemporary neuroanatomy and neurophysiology, Geschwind used phenomena of aphasia after brain damage to generate a neuroanatomic model of language. Arguing backward and forward between the damaged brain and the normal brain, he also developed a neuroanatomic model of aphasia. For the purpose of this chapter, we will focus on his models of normal naming and pathological naming.

One of Geschwind's signal contributions to contemporary behavioral neurology was his reassertion of the role of neural connections and disconnections as fundamental to the neurology of language, an emphasis already asserted by Wernicke at the end of the 19th century. In 1965 in his seminal work "Disconnexion Syndromes in Animals and Man" (10), Geschwind exposed the foundation of his neuroanatomic model of naming disorders: precisely localized lesions within the left hemispheric zone of language could produce different varieties of anomia by disconnection of two or more centers, which therefore could not adequately communicate with each other to produce the desired effect. Three years before that publication, Geschwind and Kaplan had already described, by clinical analysis with special attention to psycholinguistic and neuropsychologic issues, a "human cerebral deconnection syndrome" (11). They demonstrated a unilateral tactile anomia by showing that the interruption of pathways through the corpus callosum could prevent tactile information received by the right hemisphere from crossing into the language areas of the left hemisphere.

The immediate appeal of Geschwind's anatomic model of language is its simplicity and logical clarity. He proposed a relatively hard-wired, serial system for information transfer. According to this schema, auditory input works its way through the brainstem to Heschl's gyrus. Language-related sounds then move into the posterior two thirds of the superior temporal gyrus of the left hemisphere of right-handers (Wernicke's area). For a person to fully comprehend word meaning, signals stored in Wernicke's area must be connected to associations, including those that are kinesthetic, visual, and somesthetic, stored in the appropriate motor or sensory association cortices. Signals from each of these association areas, as well as from Wernicke's area, converge in the posterior temporal/inferior parietal regions (the angular and supramarginal gyri) as "cross-modal, cortico-cortical connections." One distinctive feature of the human brain, for Geschwind, was the highly developed "tertiary association cortex" of the angular and supramarginal gyri, which facilitated the cross-connectivity of these distant association areas, thereby serving as the basis of naming and language comprehension (i.e., the understanding of word meanings by means of cross-modal corticocortical connections). Using this model, one could already predict, as we will discuss, different forms of anomia resulting from precisely located lesions within Wernicke's area or the angular gyrus, or disconnecting distant association areas from the angular gyrus region.

For words to be spoken, Broca's area, located at the foot of the third left frontal convolution, must be activated. Language-related signals are transferred from Wernicke's area, along the arcuate fasciculus, through (under) the angular and supramarginal gyri, along the superior longitudinal fasciculus, to Broca's area. From Broca's area, the signals for word production would pass to the regions of the motor cortex controlling the muscles of the glossopharyngeal apparatus. Again, one could predict the specific forms of output anomias that would result from lesions along this sequential pathway of information transmission.

Geschwind's anatomy of the normal naming process, then, would work with, for example, visual confrontation naming as follows: the seen object activates visual association cortex that transmits signals through the angular gyrus–supramarginal gyrus area to Wernicke's area, where the signals representing the name of the object are activated. As the signals pass through the angular gyrus–supramarginal gyrus area, they are cross-connected with distant motor and sensory association cortices. These are the "cross-modal, non-limbic, cortico-cortical connections" that drape the signals with additional meaning, providing the distinctively human cognitive aspect of language. From Wernicke's area, the signals representing the name of the object are transmitted along the arcuate fasciculus subcortical to the angular and supramarginal gyri, through the superior longitudinal fasciculus to Broca's area in the premotor frontal lobe. There, the signals sent forward from Wernicke's area are transformed into patterns of motor signals that are sent to the motor cortex, which controls the muscles necessary for speaking the desired name.

By today's standards, this serial-processing model of visual input to spoken-name output seems quaint. At the time, however, it served as a powerful motor, creating and driving enthusiasm for the newly emerging field of behavioral neurology, just before the explosion of facts and knowledge in neuroscience and cognitive science from the mid 1970s to the present.

GESCHWIND'S VARIETIES OF ANOMIA

Except for the group of anomias that he called *nonaphasic misnaming*, Geschwind (12,13) understood anomia to result from disconnections at one or another point along the previously described serial transmission pathway. With regard to nonaphasic misnaming, Geschwind was at pains to emphasize that a clinician, when confronted with such a disorder, "may mistakenly assume the presence of disease of the classical speech regions in the left hemisphere and thus be led to an incorrect localization with resultant errors in investigation and management."

Nonaphasic misnaming is found in acute diffuse disorders of the brain, such as encephalitides, diseases causing rapidly increasing intracranial pressure, toxic or metabolic encephalopathies, head injury, and withdrawal syndromes. Depending on the form of misnaming, an examiner may mistakenly believe that the patient is aphasic. A key to diagnosis is the frequent presence of reduction of level of consciousness and impaired attentional state. Characteristically, the errors tend to propagate. Thus, the patient being asked where he is may say, "In a bus," and then may say that the examining physician is the driver, that those around him are passengers, and that the bed he is in is used by the driver for resting.

Additional clues to the clinical diagnosis of nonaphasic misnaming are that spontaneous speech is usually, but not invariably, normal despite gross errors in naming, whereas aphasic anomia is typically accompanied by word-finding pauses, paraphasias, and empty phrases. In some instances, nonaphasic misnaming may seem bizarre, unrelated to the target word by sound or meaning.

Aphasic errors of naming, for Geschwind, fell into two major categories: classical anomias and disconnection anomias. The classical anomias are characterized by difficulty in naming on confrontation, although the patient will often accept the correct name when it is provided by the examiner. The patient with classical anomia will typically show by one means or another that he or she recognizes the object, thus ruling out that failure to name is a result of a failure of perception. For example, the patient may produce a closely related name, a related paraphasia, or a circumlocutory description. Or the patient may indicate how the object is used or may employ the correct action verb for an object. Almost invariably, when confrontation naming is impaired as part of an aphasic syndrome, the patient's spoken language output is impaired in other ways as well (such as circumlocutions, empty words or phrases, word-finding pauses).

The anatomic basis of classical anomia, according to Geschwind's model, is a lesion in the angular gyrus area of the left temporoparietal region. Lesions in this vital crossroad of cortical connectivity produce anomia that is general, affecting all modalities and all types of stimuli.

Contrasted with classical anomia are the disconnection anomias, which Geschwind argued are "best characterized as an inability to match a stimulus to its spoken name, i.e., the patient can neither produce the name when presented with the stimulus nor choose the correct stimulus when given a name." We have already referred to the case of unilateral tactile anomia. The original case of Geschwind and Kaplan was a patient with a proven infarction of the corpus callosum sparing the splenium. He had no difficulty naming objects on visual confrontation. His spontaneous speech was normal, but when he was blindfolded, he was unable to name objects placed in his left hand. Tactile naming of items placed in his right hand was normal.

A second example of disconnection anomia provided by Geschwind was the problem a patient with pure alexia had in naming colors (14). The patient had a right hemianopia; he could not read (but could write), and he could not name colors correctly. He also failed to select the correct color name from a list of names offered by the examiner. In addition, he failed to select a named color from a group of colors presented to him. He had what Geschwind called a "two-way naming deficit." This patient had an infarction in his left visual cortex and the splenium of the corpus callosum, sparing the rest of his corpus callosum.

The unilateral tactile anomia was interpreted as the result of a disconnection of the somesthetic cortex in the right hemisphere from the language area in the left hemisphere. The two-way color-naming defect was interpreted as being the result of a disconnection of an intact right hemispheric visual cortex from the undamaged language area in his left hemisphere.

Clinical distinctions can be drawn between classical and disconnection anomias. Classical anomias are multimodal, but disconnection anomias are delimited. In the disconnection anomias, one finds no other evidence of aphasia in spontaneous speech. In the disconnection anomias, few if any paraphasias are observed, in contrast with their abundance in classical anomia.

In his explanation of mechanisms underlying these two different varieties of aphasic anomia, Geschwind appealed to the serial processing model of language previously summarized. For the disconnection anomias, a lesion, by disconnecting the zone of language in the left hemisphere from some given sensory region, prevents the matching of a sensory stimulus to a speech stimulus. In classical anomia, the lesion is located in the midst of a complex sequential processing system that receives sensory information and finds the appropriate word to match it. This system uses information from all modalities and is, for Geschwind, most likely to be in the angular gyrus and supramarginal gyrus area of the left hemisphere, because this is the region involved in the formation of associations among the various sensory modalities.

CONTEMPORARY APPROACHES TO NAMING AND ITS DISORDERS

In the 12 years since Geschwind's death, investigations of normal and disordered naming have moved forward on many fronts. These include cognitively guided experimental studies aimed at developing models of the word retrieval process that would be compatible with observations from pathology. Some of these models have taken the form of computer simulations, in which a computer model is tested to see if it can be made to duplicate a clinically observed error pattern. During this period, too, there has been an explosion of case studies of patients with forms of anomia that selectively affect a particular input modality (e.g., optic aphasia) or a particular semantic category, such as animals or manipulable implements. Cases of these types have been seen as a challenge to models of the cognitive architecture that attempt to relate sensory input, semantic memory, and access to word phonology. Accounts that emphasize anatomic disconnections have competed with accounts proposing functional disconnection or accounts evoking theories of representation in neural networks. Concurrently, improvements in functional imaging techniques have led to demonstrations of focal changes in metabolism or cerebral blood flow that appear to distinguish between different picture-naming tasks.

The mechanism of picture naming most widely accepted among cognitive psychologists is, like Geschwind's, a serial stage model but one that does not make any assumptions about the brain structures that mediate processing stages or the connections between them. In the clearest exposition of this model (15), we begin with the assumption that the visual processing system has performed its function of recognizing the visual stimulus as familiar and activating the memory of its core semantic features. The first truly linguistic step in Levelt's model is the selection of a *lemma,* a construct that contains the uniquely specified meaning of a word, including its syntactic properties, but still without phonology. The selection of a lemma may entail competition between candidates in the same semantic neighborhood. On rare occasions, this competition may result in the choice of a lemma that is related to, but not an accurate label for, the target. The choice of a lemma marks the termination of the first stage—one in which semantic selection is dominant. The selection of the lemma permits the second, or phonologic, stage of word retrieval to be realized. This model holds that the phonology, or sound pattern, of the word can be activated only after the selection of a lemma. Like virtually all contemporary cognitive models, this one assumes the existence of a phonologic lexicon, or store of word forms. The actual realization of each word's phonology proceeds from left to right, syllable after syllable.

Much of the research by Levelt and his co-workers has been devoted to confirming the two-stage model in which semantic processing is completed before the determination of word phonology can begin. One approach (16) has been to expose a picture to be named, followed at a specified short interval by the subject's hearing a spoken stimulus that is to be judged as being a word or not a word. This technique, called *lexical decision,* has come into wide use as a probe of the length of the interval between a priming stimulus (in this case, the picture to be named) and the stimulus to be judged before the effect of priming becomes apparent. Stimuli related to the prime are identified as real words more quickly than those that are unrelated. Levelt and his collaborators used words related in meaning, related in sound, and unrelated to the priming picture interspersed among nonwords. They reported observing semantic priming effects at a short interval (70 milliseconds) after the picture, whereas facilitation of phonologically related stimuli appeared only after longer intervals.

Notwithstanding the appeal of the model of Levelt and colleagues, other investigators have objected to the separation of semantic from phonologic aspects of the naming process. Distributed-processing computer models offer alternatives in which interaction between phonologic and semantic aspects of a word in process influences the outcome (17). Other versions of distributed-processing models dispense entirely with the concept of a "lexical store." In such models, the phonologic representations of words are reactivated on each occasion of use on the basis of appropriate semantic or visual stimulation. They do not exist as a stored list but as latent patterns distributed in primary motor and sensory cortices (18,19).

The essential property of distributed-processing models is that multiple aspects of a complex process, such as lexical retrieval, engage a distributed network of neural activity and interactively provide information, reinforcement, and inhibition to each other. This approach contrasts with the stepwise, multistage model that Geschwind (20) described or that is represented by Levelt's cognitive model.

Optic aphasia, first described by Freund in 1889 (21) and later in many case reports (22–24), refers to the phenomenon whereby a patient cannot name objects or pictures on visual presentation but can do so by touch, by hearing the sounds that are characteristic of the objects, or in response to definitions. Optic aphasia differs from visual agnosia in that the patient can demonstrate knowledge of the identity of objects by pantomiming their use or selecting them by multiple choice when they are named by the examiner. Freund considered optic aphasia to be the result of a disconnection between the visual system of the right hemisphere and the language area on the left. Optic aphasia has stirred some controversy in contemporary cognitive neuropsychology, with some observers (22) arguing that it is evidence for a visually based semantic system that is autonomous but disconnected from the verbal semantic system. In this model, the name would be available via the verbal semantic system.

Others, such as Riddoch and Humphreys (23), question the basis for inferring a complete semantic representation in a disconnected visual system. They argue that correct pantomime may reflect the shape characteristics of the object or its picture and need not indicate complete identification of the object. In support of Lhermitte and Beauvois' view (22), Coslett and Saffran (24) found that their patient could select a picture semantically related to the target from a multiple choice among other pictures. In rebuttal, however, Hillis and Caramazza (25) have recently demonstrated that a patient who could select a picture from other unrelated ones performed at chance levels when the selection had to be made from objects of the same category. Although the indication is that preserved sense-modality-specific semantic representations may exist in cases of disconnection of a sensory association system from language, such representations are not complete.

Sense-modality-specific naming disorders may be understood in terms of anatomic disconnection, but dissociations based on semantic category present a much more intractable theoretical problem. Geschwind and Fusillo (26) observed such a category-specific disconnection in their patient with pure word-blindness, who had a two-way aphasia for color names. Geschwind attempted to deal with the following challenge: If the patient had an interhemispheric disconnection lesion that affected written words, why did it not also affect the naming of objects and why did it affect colors? Geschwind suggested that the vulnerability of colors is that, like letters of the alphabet, they are purely visual concepts and can communicate with the left hemisphere only via the splenial portion of the corpus callosum. Objects, however, have tactile and other dimensions of sensory experience that make it possible for their representation in the right hemisphere to find interhemispheric pathways through other, nonvisual parts of the corpus callosum.

But a wider range of semantic-category-specific dissociations appeared in the literature within a few years after Geschwind and Fusillo's paper. In 1966, Goodglass et al. (27) described a number of category-specific phenomena that were fairly common in aphasia—selective impairment in understanding body part names, contrasting with selective preservation of the ability to name alphabet letters. In 1973, Yamadori and Albert (28) described a fluent aphasic patient who had a selective word comprehension impairment for objects, such as furniture and parts of the room, but not for other categories of words, such as manipulable implements. In 1984, Warrington and Shallice (29) published a report of four postherpetic patients whose ability to both name and comprehend the names of naturally occurring (e.g., animate) objects was impaired but who had no difficulty with man-made ones. The general dichotomy between animate objects (impaired) and artifacts (spared) has subsequently been documented in a great many cases, chiefly of post-herpetic patients. In a few cases, the deficiency has been confined to narrower categories of animacy, such as fruits and vegetables (30) or animals (31).

Case studies of a number of these patients suggest that they are most deficient in dealing with the visually related properties of the objects that they are trying to identify. It has been suggested (32) that identification of animals is particularly dependent on visual experience because their unique identity is determined only by their visual properties. Moreover, in the case of four-legged animals, the visual distinctions are arbitrary features of the particular species. In contrast, man-made implements usually have a unique form dictated by their function.

The common anatomic site of pathology shared by most patients with category-specific naming problems is the inferior/medial temporal lobe, either bilaterally or on the left side alone—the site of predilection for herpetic lesions. It is probably not coincidental that primate research has revealed this region to be a critical part of the primate object identification system (33). There is some supporting evidence for the role of the inferior temporal lobe from metabolic studies of the active brain by positron emission tomographic (PET) scan.

As the technology of functional imaging of cognitive and linguistic brain activity with PET became practical, it was natural that the name *retrieval process* should become a focus of attention. In a report emanating from the imaging center at Washington University (34), word retrieval appears to be most associated with increased metabolism in the dorsolateral, lateral, and inferior prefrontal cortices. That is, a different picture of the neural circuitry for object naming emerges from studies of brain activation as compared to the picture that was inferred from the cerebral lesions that resulted in aphasic anomia (and that motivated Geschwind's view of the process) (35). The angular gyrus and Wernicke's area do not figure in the PET-based naming observations. Obviously, the PET-based observations do not nullify the clinicoanatomic correlations emerging from a century of lesion data, but the two sources of information clearly need to be reconciled in an overall functional/anatomic model.

According to Tranel et al. (18), there is consistency between lesion data and functional imaging data as to the anatomy of category-specific naming disorders. Consistent with most other observations of anomia for animate objects, the investigators' patients had lesions in the anterior portion of the inferior temporal lobe. The same site was activated in normal subjects when they were required to name animate objects during PET scan activation.

CONCLUSION

The course of contemporary investigations of naming disorders in aphasia reveals that Geschwind's rigorous anatomic connectionism continues to play a significant role in the understanding of important neurolinguistic phenomena. In particular, the concept of disconnection anomia is unchallenged as a way of understanding optic aphasia and the unilateral tactile and visual anomias of callosal syndromes. However, the focus of interest in contemporary research has shifted to the nature of the partial processing that may be retained in the capacity of the isolated right hemisphere system. Geschwind's anatomic account of classical anomia has had little support from functional imaging techniques, whereas the phenomenon of category-specific anomia appears to lie outside the scope of Geschwind's circuit from vision to articulation of object names. However, this phenomenon does not so much negate the principle of an anatomic pathway for naming, as it raises the question of whether multiple, simultaneously active pathways are brought into play.

REFERENCES

1. Gesner JAP. *Samlung von Beobachtungen aus der Arzneygelahrheit und Naturkunde.* Nördlingen, Germany, 1770.
2. Dax M. Lésions de là moitié gauche de l'encéphale coincidant avec l'oubli des signes de là pensée. *Gazette Hedomodaire Medecine Chir* 1865;33:259.
3. Lordat J. *Analyse de là parole pour servir à là théorie de divers cas d'alalie et de paralalie.* Montpellier, France, 1843.
4. Wernicke C. *Der aphasische Symptomenkomplex.* Breslau, Poland: M Cohn and Weigert, 1874.
5. Pitres A. L'aphasie amnésique et ses variétés cliniques. *Progr Med (Paris)* 1898;28:17–23.
6. Goldstein K. *Language and language disturbances.* New York: Grune & Stratton, 1948.
7. Lotmar F. Zur Kenntniss der erschwerten Wortfindung und ihrer Bedeutig für das Denken des Aphasischen. *Arch Neurol Psychiatr* 1919;5.
8. von Kuenberg M. Ueber das Erfassen einfacher Beziehungen an anschaulichem Material bei Hirngeschädigten, insbesondere bei Aphasischen. *Z Gesamte Neurol Psychiatr* 1923;85.
9. Head H. *Aphasia and kindred disorders of speech.* Cambridge, MA: Cambridge University Press, 1926.
10. Geschwind N. Disconnexion syndromes in animals and man (2 parts). *Brain* 1965;88:237–294, 585–644.
11. Geschwind N, Kaplan E. A human cerebral deconnection syndrome. *Neurology* 1962;12:675–685.
12. Geschwind N. Non-aphasic disorders of speech. *Int J Neurol* 1964;4:207–214.
13. Geschwind N. The varieties of naming errors. *Cortex* 1967;3:97–112.
14. Geschwind N, Fusillo M. Color-naming deficits in association with alexia. *Arch Neurol* 1966;15:137–146.
15. Levelt WJM. *Speaking: from intention to articulation.* Cambridge, MA: MIT Press, 1989.
16. Levelt WJM, Schriefers H, Vorberg D, Meyer AS, Pechman T, Haringa J. The time course of lexical access in speech production. *Psychol Rev* 1991;98:122–142.
17. Dell GS, Reich PH. Stages in sentence production: an analysis of speech error data. *J Verbal Learning Verbal Behav* 1981;20:611–629.
18. Tranel D, Damasio H, Damasio AR. On the neurology of naming. In: Goodglass H, Wingfield A, eds. Anomia. San Diego, CA: Academic Press. 1996 *(in press)*
19. Goodglass H. *Understanding aphasia.* San Diego, CA: Academic Press, 1993.
20. Geschwind N. Problems in the anatomical understanding of the aphasias. In: Benton AL, ed. *Contributions to clinical neuropsychology.* Aldine Press, 1969.
21. Freund CS. Ueber optische Aphasie und Seelenblindheit. *Arch Psychiatr Nerven Krankh* 1884;20:276–297, 371–416.
22. Lhermitte F, Beauvois MF. A visual-speech disconnexion syndrome: report of a case of optic aphasia, agnosic alexia, and color agnosia. *Brain* 1973;96:695–714.
23. Riddoch MJ, Humphreys GW. Visual optic processes in optic aphasia: a case of semantic access agnosia. *Cognit Neuropsychol* 1987;4:131–185.

24. Coslett HB, Saffran EM. Optic aphasia and the right hemisphere: a replication and extension. *Brain Lang* 1992; 43:148–161.
25. Hillis A, Caramazza A. Cognitive and neural mechanisms underlying visual and semantic processing: implications from "optic aphasia." *J Cognit Neurosci* 1995;7:457–478.
26. Geschwind N, Fusillo M. Color-naming defects in association with alexia. *Arch Neurol* 1966;15:137–146.
27. Goodglass H, Klein B, Carey P, Jones KJ. Specific semantic word categories in aphasia. *Cortex* 1966;2:74–86.
28. Yamadori A, Albert ML. Word category aphasia. *Cortex* 1973;9:83–89.
29. Warrington EK, Shallice T. Category-specific semantic impairments. *Brain* 1984;107:828–856.
30. Hart J, Berndt RS, Caramazza A. Category-specific naming deficit following cerebral infarct. *Nature* 1985;316: 4339–4440.
31. Hart J, Gordon B. Neural subsystems for semantic knowledge. *Nature* 1992;359:60–64.
32. Warrington EK, McCarthy R. Categories of knowledge: further fractionations and an attempted integration. *Brain* 1987;110:1273–1296.
33. Ungerleiter LG, Mishkin M. Two cortical visual systems. In: Ingle DJ, Goodale MA, Massfield RJW, eds. *Analysis of visual behavior.* Cambridge, MA: MIT Press, 1982;549–586.
34. Petersen SE, Fox PT, Posner MI, Mintun M, Raichle ME. Positron emission tomographic studies of the cortical anatomy of single-word processing. *Nature* 1988;331:585–589.
35. Bachman D, Albert ML. Cerebral organization of language. In: Peters A, Jones E, eds. *Cerebral cortex: normal and altered states of function.* New York: Plenum, 1991.

15
Anatomy of Developmental Dyslexia: Geschwind's Last Legacy

Albert M. Galaburda

Department of Neurology, Beth Israel Hospital, Boston, Massachusetts 02215.

It is hard to pin to a single philosophical conviction a man as complex as Norman Geschwind, but it would be fair to state that he had a strong phrenologic bent. By phrenology, I specifically mean the belief in at least two principles of brain organization: (a) localization of function, and (b) the concept that bigger is better. The former, of course, has been one of the central concerns of neurologists, neurophysiologists, and neuropsychologists since the time of Gall, Broca, and Wernicke and has evolved accordingly during our own century. I believe that, for Geschwind, localization implied that circumscribed areas of cortex processed information locally and were capable of informing or being informed by other areas of cortex, where other processing took place—in short, a traditional and, today, old-fashioned view of localization of function (1).

The second component of phrenology, that bigger is better, tended to be trivialized in the phrenologic exercises of the last century, whereby palpation of the cranium was used to determine a person's mental and moral characteristics. Geschwind never told me that he believed in the validity of these attempts, but he often spoke in terms suggesting that he believed that more cortex devoted to a particular function equaled better performance. Thus, both aspects of phrenology served as lenses through which Norman Geschwind attempted to understand the neurologic underpinnings of behavior in general and developmental dyslexia, the focus of this chapter, in particular.

Norman Geschwind was interested in language and aphasia, about which he wrote extensively. He took as his subjects of study patients with acquired disorders of language, mostly arising from stroke but also occasionally from other forms of brain injury—infection, degeneration, developmental anomaly, and neoplasm. His main tenets about language and the brain were that the brain contained, in the left hemisphere in most people, a handful of specialized regions with phylogenetic and ontogenetic histories, and that these regions were responsible for processing various aspects of language (production, comprehension, repetition, naming, reading, and writing) and communicated with each other via long axonal connections (2–7). Injury to one of these centers was accompanied by loss of function in that center; likewise, injury to the connecting fiber bundles led to disconnection syndromes, whereby the symptoms could be explained not on the basis of processing itself but rather on that of loss of transfer of information from one center to another (3–4,8–11).

Geschwind's work in developmental dyslexia was less well specified and much less detailed about mechanisms, although not so about etiologies (see the following discussion). Although he recognized and often spoke about the effects of brain plasticity on the clinical consequences of acquired brain injury (he believed that plasticity was bad for acquired injury), he was, I believe, somewhat uncomfortable with clinical entities such as developmental disorders, in which plasticity might have played a huge role. He often cited with befuddlement the Kennard principle [after Margaret Kennard (12)], which claimed that it is better to acquire a brain lesion early than late in life, and he was rather fond of the work of Gerald Schneider (13) that pointed out experimental examples to the contrary.

In fact, Geschwind preferred to stay away from considerations of plasticity and instead to treat developmental disorders as special cases of acquired disorders. Therefore, his approach to this area was mainly phrenologic. It was this approach that launched his inquiries into the nature of dyslexia. The hypothesis he expressed first was the following: The human brain contains language areas (phrenologic principle 1). In most people, the language areas are obviously asymmetrical anatomically [see, for instance, his seminal paper with Walter Levitsky (14), which explains why the left hemisphere is affected more often than the right in acquired disorders of language). The left hemisphere language areas (in most people) are larger (phrenologic principle 2) in order to support the left hemisphere's superiority for language. A handful of people show right-sided anatomic superiority, and this group is simply the mirror image of the former, larger group, without pathological implications. Still a third group fails to show any asymmetry or may become asymmetrical on the opposite side for "the wrong reasons" (see the following discussion), and persons in this group must be considered anomalous anatomically and functionally. The mildest case of "pathology" in this third group is represented by many left-handers (he preferred the appellation non-right-handers), but anomalies of language development, such as dyslexia, may also be present. Whereas in most non-right-handers, the size of the two symmetrical plana can be relatively large, in persons with developmental dyslexia, the plana must be symmetrical and small (15). This first hypothesis of Geschwind on the anatomy of dyslexia was in keeping with his belief in phrenologic principle 2. My task, after the end of my residency in neurology under his mentorship and at the beginning of my own research career, was to look into this possibility. The year was 1978.

It was, therefore, not until the late 1970s that Geschwind was able to pursue his first hypothesis on the anatomy of developmental dyslexia. Just before that time, the brain of a young man with that diagnosis had come to be part of the collection of serially sectioned human brains held by Dr. Thomas L. Kemper, chief of neuropathology at the Harvard Neurological Unit of Boston City Hospital, of which Geschwind was director. This collection was an offshoot of the famous Yakovlev Collection, then and now held at the Armed Forces Institute of Pathology in Washington, D.C. This was truly a rare specimen. Throughout the history of this disorder, beginning in the late 19th century with the work of Pringle Morgan (16) and James Hinshelwood (17), there had been controversy about the brain basis of dyslexia. Yet, review of the literature failed to show that any brain had actually been studied until the case report by Drake (18). That study had been carried out using standard neuropathological approaches, which, although they produced pathological findings, could not address the questions of interest to Geschwind: namely, are the language areas small on both sides, and specifically, is Wernicke's area small on both sides?

Why Wernicke's area specifically? Geschwind held to the notion that the organization of language in the brain was focused in Wernicke's area, which he felt brokered all linguistic activities, including reading. [More recently, it has been shown by positron emission tomography studies that this idea is not accurate in all instances (19). This emphasis was in contrast to the more traditional view, championed by Hinshelwood in Glasgow at the turn of the century after the work of Déjérine in Paris, that reading was the business of the occipital and parietal lobes, and that dyslexia reflected abnormal development of those areas.

Geschwind argued that, anatomically, Wernicke's area was an elusive concept. He emphasized in his teachings that Wernicke's area was the area that, when damaged, could lead to Wernicke's aphasia. It was not, however, a specific anatomic site, because some patients had more extensive damage than others, some patients had lesions that were relatively distant from the posterior superior region of the temporal lobe, and moreover some patients had extensive damage in that region of the temporal lobe with no aphasia whatsoever. Nonetheless, Wernicke's area was to be found in the caudal end of the superior temporal gyrus in most brains, and this is where Geschwind thought the secret of dyslexia lay. This belief, plus the discovery that a natural landmark located in this region of the temporal lobe was usually asymmetrical on the left side (14), led Geschwind to suggest focusing on the planum temporale.

Brooke Seckel was a senior Neurology resident when I was a first-year resident. He was a colorful young man with many interests, and it fell on his shoulders to begin to study the dyslexic brain. Thus, he began the reconstruction of the planum temporale from the serial sections. But he soon decided to pursue a career in microvascular surgery instead and ceased his dyslexia research. Geschwind picked me to continue Seckel's work, and so I did. At that time, I had been working with the architectonicist Friedrich Sanides, on leave from his post in West Germany, and had become familiar with the superior temporal gyrus and the architectonic areas that it comprises (20,21). So, naturally, I took a peek at the familiar areas before plunging into the tedious task of reconstructing the planum temporale. It was then that I found the cortical malformation that triggered a line of research that has lasted over a decade.

The anomaly was unfamiliar to me, and so I asked Tom Kemper to help in its characterization and classification, which he did in his usual scholarly fashion (22). It turned out to be an instance of micropolygyria within the planum temporale on the left side. The anomaly was only the most striking of a collection of malformations that included ectopic collections of neurons and glia in the molecular layer, which we termed *ectopias,* and myelinated glial scars, both affecting the cortex mainly of the perisylvian region, and often more so on the left side. Later we discovered that these malformations were related to one another etiologically but represented instances of varying severity (23).

Contrary to Geschwind's predictions, the plana were not small. They were relatively large and bilaterally symmetrical. This finding also became an area of further study. Among other things, it threw doubt on the phrenologic notion that size related directly to quality (24); instead it began to orient the research program toward the demonstration that differences in asymmetry indicated differences in the organization of neural networks, which could reflect early injury leading to alterations in the numbers and types of neurons and connections (for a review, see ref. 25). The conclusion from the line of research that was pursued throughout the 1980s could only be that the size of the plana, their degree of symmetry or asymmetry, and the side of the brain involved did not, in and of themselves, determine normal or abnormal processing. Rather, understanding the exact nature of the circuits instantiated in these structures, and their relationships to task demands, was probably more useful in predicting the adaptability of a brain substrate for a specific behavior. Dyslexia, therefore, was not turning out to be simply the result of an atrophic language area.

In the last years of his life, Geschwind focused his attention on etiology of dyslexia rather than mechanisms. Other than mentioning atrophic language areas, he did not specify further mechanisms underlying poor reading performance. He was content with imagining that atrophy of language areas would lead to weakness proportional to the level of difficulty of the language task. Thus, spoken language would be least affected because it is easier than reading and most people have the opportunity of a great deal of practice. Reading, on the other hand, is more difficult because it requires cultural input and most people do not get nearly as much practice in reading as they do in speaking.

The prediction that persons with dyslexia have two small plana gave way to a different anatomic hypothesis after the presentation, in 1982 (26), of the first data in support of what came to be known as the Geschwind hypothesis or the Geschwind-Behan hypothesis (27), also sometimes called the Geschwind-Behan-Galaburda model (28,29). By 1982, my colleagues and I had seen several brains from developmental dyslexics that exhibited two sizable plana, but I do not recall Geschwind's ever citing this finding as a reason for looking for a different anatomic hypothesis. It is quite striking, furthermore, that another cardinal finding in the brain of dyslexics, the minor cortical malformations we have referred to as *ectopias* in our writings (see the following discussion), never seemed to play a role in Geschwind's subsequent considerations on the anatomy of dyslexia. Instead, the latest concept Geschwind developed on the anatomy of dyslexia emerged *de novo* from the Geschwind hypothesis and not as a phoenix resurrected from the ashes of the older hypothesis.

THE GESCHWIND HYPOTHESIS

The Geschwind hypothesis may be summarized as a program of research to help explain why certain traits having to do with handedness or other aspects of cerebral lateralization, immunologic disorders, learning disabilities, or other disorders may co-occur. The common denominator, but not the sole factor, is sex steroids acting on the brain and immune system during development; these effects introduce variations according to sex, sex hormone levels, and sex hormone sensitivity into cerebral lateralization, immunology, and learning and related disorders. The Geschwind hypothesis is based strongly on clinical observations made by Geschwind himself and on a detailed survey of the medical literature. Some of the original observations, such as the relationship between learning and immune disorders, have largely stood the test of time (30), whereas others, such as the relationship between handedness and immune disorders, and handedness and learning disorders, have remained at best tenuous (30).

It is not possible here, nor is it the purpose of this review, to discuss more thoroughly the literature that was triggered by the original publication of the Geschwind hypothesis, other than to focus on the issues of anatomy and developmental dyslexia. There were several aspects to Geschwind's thinking on this topic. First, he was interested in the mechanisms by which the planum temporale would become symmetrical during development. His interest gave rise to the so-called testosterone hypothesis (a restricted interpretation of the Geschwind hypothesis, because the latter deals with other effects in addition to the effects of sex steroids), which has been extensively reviewed elsewhere (31–34), but which can be summarized as follows. The planum is naturally asymmetrical on the left side. This asymmetry is ostensibly due to a universally inherited gene or set of genes. The expression of the genetic effect, however, can be altered by the activity of (mainly male) sex hormones, which produce a shift away from the standard pattern of asymmetry. Partial hormonal effect leads to great symmetry, whereas full effect leads to reverse asymmetry. Because part of the hypothesis states that, with the shift away from the standard, left-side-larger pattern of asymmetry, there is accompanying increased non-right-handedness and left-handedness, this hypothesis has sometimes been called the left-shift hypothesis. This hypothesis is in contrast to the one proposed by Marian Annett (35–37), which states that the neutral case is symmetrical, producing random-handedness, and that there may be a single or double dose of "right-shift" gene that produces greater right-handedness. This gene is not universally present, and the variation in the population is the result of the presence or absence of only one or two right-shift alleles.

The left-shift hypothesis makes important and testable predictions about the size of the planum temporale. For instance, testosterone activity predicts that the larger the right planum, the smaller the left planum. The reason for this prediction is that implicit in the hypothesis is the notion that the testosterone effect is on storage rather than on independent production of neural material in one or the other hemisphere. Therefore, the two plana should comprise the same amount of neural tissue. Thus, in some cases (those with the standard pattern) most of the tissue is on the left side; in other cases (the symmetrical ones) the tissue is divided about equally between the two hemispheres; and in still other cases (the rightwardly asymmetrical ones) most of the tissue is on the right side. In effect, the hypothesis does not predict a great deal of variability in the total amount of planum tissue, left plus right, in the population (other than that which would be explained by variations in total brain size). As it turns out, the total amount of planum tissue does vary greatly, as my colleagues and I learned when we examined the photographs used to carry out the famous study by Geschwind and Levitsky (14). We also found that the total amount of neural tissue varies independently of total brain size and is a function of the coefficient of asymmetry (24). The data showed that symmetrical plana were uniformly large, similar in size to the left planum in the standard case. That state could not have been achieved by a simple shift of planum tissue toward the right hemisphere and away from the left.

Another prediction of the left-shift hypothesis might have been that, because the amount of total neural tissue does not vary with the pattern of asymmetry, the number of neurons and connections in the tissue, though perhaps not their pattern, remains unchanged, too. Instead, studies showed that the size of a particular cortical area is a function mainly of the number of neurons in that area (38), which means that symmetrical cortical areas contain more neurons than asymmetrical ones. Additional studies showed that the number and patterns of callosal connections differ greatly between asymmetrical and symmetrical cortical areas (39), which again indicates that storage differences would not adequately characterize differences between dyslexic and nondyslexic brains. So, two predictions made by Norman Geschwind about the planum temporale in dyslexic brains—that the two plana are small (early hypothesis) and that the two plana are of medium size (left-shift hypothesis)—have not been corroborated by the data. However, one important prediction was indeed found to hold true: the finding that in developmental dyslexia there is greater symmetry of the planum temporale. That finding has indeed been confirmed in many brains studied either at postmortem or using imaging techniques in living dyslexic subjects (40–42). Together with the data on size, neuron numbers, and connections, this finding began to point the way to current research on the anatomy of developmental dyslexia.

ANATOMY OF DEVELOPMENTAL DYSLEXIA: STATE OF THE FIELD

The biological basis of developmental dyslexia may be attributed to genetic influences on the fetus even before anatomic characteristics of the disorder become visible during mid gestation. We can only surmise, from our knowledge of how these anatomic features develop, that they become manifest at that time. We cannot witness their actual appearance for the simple reason that dyslexia cannot be diagnosed until after birth, and substantially after birth at that. Nonetheless, we have learned a great deal about these anatomic characteristics and can state categorically that the anatomy of dyslexia precedes any significant cultural experience, even the beginning of language development, which may indeed be slightly before birth. As mentioned earlier, developmental dyslexia has two important anatomic features: symmetry of the planum temporale and minor cerebrocortical malformations termed *ectopias*. We have learned from developmental studies in normal brains that symmetry or asymmetry of the planum is visible by the 31st week of gestation (43), and there is no compelling reason not to believe that the process of the planum becoming asymmetrical takes place following a comparable schedule in dyslexic brains. The ectopias are probably traceable to an even earlier period, perhaps as early as the 16th week of gestation, when neuronal migration to the cerebral neocortex is thought to begin.

It is not possible to say with certainty which of the two neuroanatomic characteristics is more important to the development of the dyslexic behavioral trait. However, it may be a moot point because the two features affect each other during development. In fact, current anatomic research on developmental dyslexia emphasizes that changes at one site propagate to alter the development of structures or systems at other sites. This is the strong element of plasticity that distinguishes thinking in this field from the type of thinking usually associated with the understanding of acquired disorders of language—localization of function and pathology. Thus, my colleagues and I have shown, in the mouse, that the presence of ectopias changes the nature of brain asymmetry (44). Although, as we have learned, there is a strongly negative correlation between the coefficient of asymmetry and the total amount of neural tissue attributed to the planum on both sides, this relationship breaks down in the presence of ectopias. We are able to state, therefore, that cerebral lateralization is not simply shifted or reconfigured in developmental dyslexia but, instead, damaged. This finding helps to explain the fact that lack of asymmetry in the planum temporale or reversal of asymmetry is seldom associated with developmental dyslexia, being instead a normal variant. On the other hand, if non-right-handedness is a common consequence of any deviation from the standard pattern of leftward asymmetry, either for normal or pathological reasons, it may follow that non-right-handedness may be more common among dyslexics, as some studies have shown (45,46).

ECTOPIAS

Ectopias consist of collections of neurons and glia in the molecular neocortical layer, usually associated with visible distortion of the underlying laminar architecture. They are variable in number and location in the dyslexic brains we have studied at postmortem. All brains appear to have at least some ectopias in the inferior premotor and prefrontal region, corresponding roughly to architectonic areas (Brodmann) 45, 46, and 47. The presence of ectopias in other perisylvian cortex is less predictable, but in some cases (of a total of nine) they have been found on the superior temporal gyrus and parietal operculum and inferior parietal lobule. They may be more numerous in the left hemisphere. In human specimens (the ectopias have been modeled in experimental animals, as discussed later), the distortion of the lamination subjacent to the ectopia gives the impression of fiber bundles reaching or leaving (or both) the ectopia. In a couple of instances, there has been focal microgyria, which is a more severe cortical anomaly, often with ectopias at its edges. We have shown experimentally that, indeed, the pathogenesis, if not the severity, of these two malformations is shared (23).

Neocortical ectopias are frequently found in the developmental neuropathology laboratory and reflect a common outcome of subtle brain injury during critical developmental stages. My colleague Gordon Sherman has studied a model of neocortical ectopia presented by the New Zealand Black autoimmune mouse [also other strains; (47–49)], in which these ectopias, as well as autoimmunity, spontaneously develop (50). My colleague Glenn Rosen has furthered a rat model, begun by the Czechoslovakian researchers Dvorák, Feit, and Juránková (51,52), whereby microgyria and ectopias can be induced by a freezing injury at birth or shortly thereafter (53,54). Using these models, we have made several interesting observations about the nature of neocortical ectopias. First, the ectopias are more broadly disturbing to the architecture of neurons and connections than first suspected. For instance, the composition of neuronal types in the cortex subjacent and adjacent to the ectopia is altered (55–57). The malformations contain abnormal connections, even across the corpus callosum and to the subcortex (55,56,58,59). The ectopias and related malformations arise soon after the beginning of neuronal migration to the neocortex and cannot be induced after migration arrest (60,61). This fact helps to date the malformation in the dyslexic brain to somewhere between the 16th and 24th weeks of gestation, probably closer to the former date. A measure of developmental arrest is evident in the experimental malformations, whereby radial glial fiber immunocytochemical markers remain in the tissue well beyond their usual time of disappearance, ostensibly for the life of the animal (62). The development of the malformations can be relatively inhibited by the use of neuroprotective agents (63). The ectopias are associated with unique behavioral changes in the affected animals (64), which can be ameliorated by early environmental enrichment (65).

PROPAGATION OF CHANGES

More recently, the anatomic characteristics of the ectopias have been studied in light of a new hypothesis of the brain basis of dyslexia. Paula Tallal and her colleagues, for more than 20 years, have made the claim that dyslexia results from disturbed perception of rapidly changing sounds (66–68). This hypothesis is in apparent conflict with the leading hypothesis in the field, which maintains that dyslexia results from abnormal phonologic processing (69–73). In fact, the dispute should have to do with ontogenesis, rather than mechanism. The fundamental question is whether the perceptual problem represents the first event, which triggers abnormal phonologic development in higher centers, or whether anomalies occur first in regions processing phonology, which then propagate to centers closer to the input and modify the development of perceptual capacities there. Tallal would seem to claim that perceptual problems occur first, but she agrees that the significant outcome is abnormal phonologic processing. The other camp does not address this issue and simply dismisses the effect of perceptual input anomalies. We have begun to use the anatomic models to answer this question at the level of brain structure, in order to argue back to the development of functional dyslexic traits such as phonologic capacity. Paula Tallal's work and independent thinking by my colleague Margaret Livingstone led to a study in which dyslexic persons showed anomalies in the early phases of the visual evoked potential elicited by rapidly changing checkerboard patterns, particularly at low contrasts (74). We interpreted this finding to mean that the magnocellular pathway of the visual system (75) was abnormal in this population. There were also psychophysical studies implicating abnormal fast processing in the visual system (76–78). Together, these results implicated abnormal fast processing in more than one modality and suggested multimodal cortices as possible starting points in the abnormal development.

Again, we began with observations in the human brain and generated hypotheses to be tested in the autoimmune mice and the neonatal rat model. A subsequent anatomic study found smaller neurons in the magnocellular layers of the lateral geniculate nucleus of dyslexic brains than in the brains of normal controls (74). Tallal's own work suggested that we look at the medial geniculate nucleus, because her work implicated auditory pathways. Here, too, we found relatively too many small neurons and too few large neurons in the left medial geniculate nucleus (79). This finding was evidence that the abnormal anatomy of dyslexia concerns not only cortical areas commonly associated with high-level language processing, including phonologic processing, but also regions much closer to the sensory (visual, auditory) input. What could not be determined from these observations was whether the thalamic changes preceded or were a consequence of the cortical changes. A third possibility was that changes occurred at many levels in the systems at the same time. Evidence for the last hypothesis, albeit inconsistent among the brain specimens studied at autopsy, was the finding in some brains of migrational anomalies in the thalamic relay nuclei themselves (74,80), in addition to the changes in neuronal size. The experimentally induced malformation model in the rat was chosen to look at this question further.

Glenn Rosen and Paula Tallal's postdoctoral fellow Holly Fitch first looked at temporal auditory processing capacity in rats with induced cerebrocortical malformations and found that animals with neonatal lesions were worse at processing rapid sound transitions than their littermates without induced malformation (81), a finding reminiscent of those of Tallal's original study in language-impaired children. Interestingly, the induced microgyri were in the frontal cortex in areas homologous to those in the dyslexic brain receiving the bulk of ectopias, but the behavioral findings could be demonstrated in auditory function. This finding indicated that developmental frontal cortical malformations might propagate anatomic and functional changes along connectional pathways toward areas closer to sensory inputs. If so, that could explain why cortical changes arising very early in development could still be the first event that led to the disarray of brain centers processing sounds at much lower levels in the thalamus. In this case, therefore, the perceptual anomalies seen by Tallal, and demonstrated electrophysiologically, psychophysically, and anatomically in the visual system as well, could be the result rather than the cause of processing anomalies in cognitive brain areas.

Anatomic confirmation of this hypothesis has only begun to emerge. Changes in cell size in the sensory thalamus present in both the rats with induced cortical malformations in the frontal lobe and in New Zealand Black mice with spontaneous cortical malformations in sensorimotor cortex (82,83). The mechanism of top-down propagation of anatomic changes during development is probably one that plays a role in the distortion of systems involved in the learning of the native language, a prerequisite for efficiently learning to read. This propagation is probably quite active and may involve all areas connectionally related to the area with the original anomaly. On the other hand, if the pathway for propagation is cortical connectivity, this would lead to sparing of cortical and subcortical areas as well, thus explaining the specificity of the learning disorder. Ongoing research aims at testing these possibilities in greater detail and at finding the agent responsible for the initial event; that is, the cause of the minor cortical malformations. Preliminary indications that this agent may have been passed transplacentally from the mother have not stood up to testing. Studies using autoimmune mice and involving ova transfer experiments, whereby susceptible embryos have been raised in normal uteruses and vice versa, have not demonstrated a maternal effect on the malformations (84). Breeding studies, on the other hand, have demonstrated genetic effects (85). The objective of present work in this area is to discover the gene responsible for the cortical malformation in affected animals.

CONCLUSION

Geschwind made several predictions about dyslexia and brain asymmetry. Although some have not stood the test of experimental research, it is clear that he asked the right questions and stimulated research in the right direction, and among many of us. This fact, more than the answers themselves, constitutes the best legacy of Norman Geschwind and his work. Eleven years after his untimely death, papers continue to be published in which the authors claim that Geschwind was or was not right about something or other (e.g., refs. 28,86). I anticipate and hope that this reaction will continue for many years to come.

REFERENCES

1. Damasio AR, Damasio H, Tranel D, Brandt JP. Neural regionalization of knowledge access: preliminary evidence. *Cold Spring Harbor Symp Quant Biol* 1990;55:1039–1047.
2. Damasio AR, Geschwind N. The neural basis of language. *Ann Rev Neurosci* 1984;7:127–147.
3. Geschwind N. Disconnexion syndromes in animals and man. I. *Brain* 1965;88:237–294.
4. Geschwind N. Disconnexion syndromes in animals and man. II. *Brain* 1965;88:585–644.
5. Geschwind N. The organization of language and the brain. *Science* 1970;170:940–944.
6. Geschwind N. Language and the brain. *Sci Am* 1972;226:76–83.
7. Goodglass H, Geschwind N. Language disorders (aphasia). In: Carterette EC, Friedman MP, eds. *Handbook of perception.* New York: Academic Press, 1968;390–428.
8. Geschwind N. The clinical syndromes of the cortical connections. In: Benton, A, ed. *Behavioral changes in cerebrovascular disease.* 1970;29–40.
9. Geschwind N, Kaplan E. A human cerebral deconnection syndrome. *Neurology* 1962;12:675–685.
10. Geschwind N, Quadfasel FA, Segarra JM. Isolation of the speech area. *Neuropsychologia* 1968;6:327–340.
11. Mesulam MM, Geschwind N. On the possible role of neocortex and its limbic connections in the process of attention and schizophrenia: clinical cases of inattention in man and experimental anatomy in monkey. *J Psychiatr Res* 1978;14:249–259.
12. Kennard MA. Age and other factors in motor recovery from precentral lesions in monkeys. *Am J Physiol* 1936;115:138–146.
13. Schneider GF. Is it really better to have your brain lesion early? A revision of the "Kennard principle." *Neuropsychologia* 1979;17:557–583.
14. Geschwind N, Levitsky W. Human brain: left-right asymmetries in temporal speech region. *Science* 1968;161:186–187.
15. Geschwind N. Disorders of higher cortical functions in children. *Clin Proc Child Hosp Washington* 1972;28:261–272.
16. Morgan WP. A case of congenital word-blindness. 1896;23:357–377.
17. Hinshelwood J. *Congenital word-blindness.* London, England: Lewis, 1917.
18. Drake WE. Clinical and pathological findings in a child with a developmental learning disability. *J Learning Disabil* 1968;1:9–25.
19. Petersen S, Fox P, Snyder A, Raichle M. Activation of extrastriate and frontal cortical areas by visual words and word-like stimuli. *Science* 1990;249(31):983–986, 1041–1042.
20. Galaburda AM, Sanides F. Cytoarchitectonic organization of the human auditory cortex. *J Comp Neurol* 1980;190:597–610.
21. Galaburda AM, Sanides F, Geschwind N. Human brain: cytoarchitectonic left-right asymmetries in the temporal speech region. *Arch Neurol* 1978;35:812–817.
22. Galaburda AM, Kemper TL. Cytoarchitectonic abnormalities in developmental dyslexia: a case study. *Ann Neurol* 1979;6:94–100.
23. Rosen GD, Galaburda AM. Neocortical dysplasia, microgyria, and porencephaly: common etiologies? *Soc Neurosci Abstr* 1995;21:1712.
24. Galaburda AM, Corsiglia J, Rosen GD, Sherman GF. Planum temporale asymmetry: reappraisal since Geschwind and Levitsky. *Neuropsychologia* 1987;25:853–868.

25. Galaburda AM. Developmental dyslexia and animal studies: at the interface between cognition and neurology. *Cognitia* 1994;50:133–149.
26. Geschwind N, Behan PO. Left-handedness: association with immune disease, migraine, and developmental disorder. *Proc Natl Acad Sci USA* 1982;79:5097–5100.
27. Hugdahl K, Ellerstsen B, Waaler PE, Klove H. Left and right-handed dyslexic boys: an empirical test of some assumptions of the Geschwind-Behan hypothesis. *Neuropsychologia* 1989;27(2):223–231.
28. Kaplan BJ, Crawford SG. The GBG model: is there more to consider than handedness? *Brain Cogn* 1994;26(2): 291–299.
29. Previc FH. Assessing the legacy of the GBG model. *Brain Cogn* 1994;26(2):174–180.
30. Tonnessen FE, Lokken A, Hoien T, Lundberg I. Dyslexia, left-handedness, and immune disorders. *Arch Neurol* 1993;50(4):411–416.
31. Geschwind N, Galaburda AM. Cerebral lateralization: biological mechanisms, associations, and pathology. I. A hypothesis and a program for research. *Arch Neurol* 1985;42:428–459.
32. Geschwind N, Galaburda AM. Cerebral lateralization: biological mechanisms, associations, and pathology. II. A hypothesis and a program for research. *Arch Neurol* 1985;42:521–552.
33. Geschwind N, Galaburda AM. Cerebral lateralization: biological mechanisms, associations, and pathology. III. A hypothesis and a program for research. *Arch Neurol* 1985;42:634–654.
34. Geschwind N, Galaburda AM. *Cerebral lateralization: biological mechanisms, associations, and pathology.* Cambridge, MA: MIT Press/Bradford Books, 1987.
35. Annett M. *A single gene explanation of right and left handedness and brainedness.* Coventry, England: Lanchester Polytechnic, 1978.
36. Annett M. The right shift theory of handedness and developmental language problems. *Bull Orton Soc* 1981;31: 103–121.
37. Annett M. Handedness as a continuous variable with dextral shift: sex, generation, and family handedness in subgroups of left and right-handers. *Behav Genet* 1994;24(1):1–63.
38. Galaburda AM, Aboitiz F, Rosen GD, Sherman GF. Histological asymmetry in the primary visual cortex of the rat: implications for mechanisms of cerebral asymmetry. *Cortex* 1986;22:151–160.
39. Rosen GD, Galaburda AM, Sherman GF. Neocortical symmetry and asymmetry in the rat: different patterns of callosal connections. *Soc Neurosci Abstr* 1987;13:44.
40. Steinmetz H, Galaburda A. Planum temporale asymmetry: in vivo morphometry affords a new perspective for neuro-behavioral research. *Reading Writing* 1991;3:331–343.
41. Leonard CM, Voeller KKS, Lombardino LJ, Morris MK, Hynd GW, Alexander AW, Anderson HG, Garafalakis M, Honeyman JC, Mao JT, Agee OF, Staab EV. Anomolous cerebral structure in dyslexia revealed with magnetic resonance imaging. *Arch Neurol* 1993;50(5):461–469.
42. Hynd G, Semrud-Clikeman M, Lorys A, Novey E, Eliopulos R. Brain morphology in developmental dyslexia and attention deficit disorder/hyperactivity. *Arch Neurol* 1990;47:919–926.
43. Chi JG, Dooling EC, Gilles FH. Gyral development of the human brain. *Ann Neurol* 1977;1:86–93.
44. Rosen GD, Sherman GF, Mehler C, Emsbo K, Galaburda AM. The effect of developmental neuropathology on neocortical asymmetry in New Zealand Black mice. *Int J Neurosci* 1989;45:247–254.
45. Eglinton E, Annett M. Handedness and dyslexia: a meta-analysis. *Percept Motor Skills* 1994;79(3, pt 2): 1611–1616.
46. Richardson AJ. Dyslexia, handedness and syndromes of psychosis-proneness. *Int J Psychophysiol* 1994;18(3): 251–263.
47. Denenberg VH, Sherman GF, Morrison L, Schrott LM, Waters NS, Rosen GD, Behan PO, Galaburda AM. Behavior, ectopias and immunity in BD/DB reciprocal crosses. *Brain Res* 1992;571:323–329.
48. Schrott LM, Morrison L, Wimer R, Wimer C, Behan PO, Denenberg VH. Autoimmunity and avoidance learning in NXRF recombinant inbred strains. *Brain Behav Immun* 1994;8:100–110.
49. Schrott LM, Waters NS, Boehm GW, et al. Behavior, cortical ectopias, and autoimmunity in BXSB-Yaa and BXSB-Yaa+ mice. *Brain Behav Immun* 1993;7(3):205–223.
50. Sherman GF, Rosen GD, Galaburda AM. Neocortical anomalies in autoimmune mice: a model for the developmental neuropathology seen in the dyslexic brain. *Drug Dev Res* 1988;15:307–314.
51. Dvorák K, Feit J. Migration of neuroblasts through partial necrosis of the cerebral cortex in newborn rats: contribution to the problems of morphological development and developmental period of cerebral microgyria. *Acta Neuropathol (Berlin)* 1977;38:203–212.
52. Dvorák K, Feit J, Juránková Z. Experimentally induced focal microgyria and status verrucosus deformis in rats: pathogenesis and interrelation histological and autoradiographical study. *Acta Neuropathol (Berlin)* 1978;44: 121–129.
53. Humphreys P, Rosen GD, Sherman GF, Galaburda AM. Freezing lesions of the newborn rat brain: a model for cerebrocortical microdysgenesis. *Soc Neurosci Abstr* 1989;15:1120.
54. Rosen GD, Sherman GF, Richman JM, Stone LV, Galaburda AM. Induction of molecular layer ectopias by puncture wounds in newborn rats and mice. *Dev Brain Res* 1992;67(2):285–291.
55. Rosen GD, Galaburda AM, Sherman GF. Cerebrocortical microdysgenesis with anomalous callosal connections: a case study in the rat. *Int J Neurosci* 1989;47:237–247.
56. Sherman GF, Stone JS, Press DM, Rosen GD, Galaburda AM. Abnormal architecture and connections disclosed by neurofilament staining in the cerebral cortex of autoimmune mice. *Brain Res* 1990;529:202–207.

57. Sherman GF, Stone JS, Rosen GD, Galaburda AM. Neocortical VIP neurons are increased in the hemisphere containing focal cerebrocortical microdysgenesis in New Zealand Black mice. *Brain Res* 1990;532:232–236.
58. Jenner AR, Galaburda AM, Sherman GF. Connectivity of cortical ectopias in autoimmune mice. *Soc Neurosci Abstr* 1995;21:1712.
59. Rosen GD, Humphreys P, Sherman GF, Galaburda AM. Connectional anomalies associated with freezing lesions to the neocortex of the newborn rat. *Soc Neurosci Abstr* 1989;15:1120.
60. Rosen GD, Press DM, Sherman GF, Galaburda AM. The development of induced cerebrocortical microgyria in the rat. *J Neuropathol Exp Neurol* 1992;51(6):601–611.
61. Sherman GF, Stone LV, Walthour NR, et al. Birthdates of neurons in neocortical ectopias of New Zealand Black mice. *Soc Neurosci Abstr* 1992;18:1446A.
62. Rosen GD, Sherman GF, Galaburda AM. Radial glia in the neocortex of adult rats: effects of neonatal brain injury. *Dev Brain Res* 1994;82(1–2):127–135.
63. Rosen GD, Sigel EA, Sherman GF, Galaburda AM. The neuroprotective effects of MK-801 on the induction of microgyria by freezing injury to the newborn rat neocortex. *Neuroscience* 1995;69:107–114.
64. Rosen GD, Sigel EA, Sherman GF, Galaburda AM. The neuroprotective effects of MK-801 and GM1 ganglioside on injury to the newborn rat cortex. *Soc Neurosci Abstr* 1993;19:1657.
65. Schrott LM, Denenberg VH, Sherman GF, Waters NS, Rosen GD, Galaburda AM. Environmental enrichment, neocortical ectopias, and behavior in the autoimmune NZB mouse. *Dev Brain Res* 1992;67(1):85–93.
66. Tallal P. Auditory perception, phonics and reading disabilities in children. *J Acoust Soc Am* 1977;62:S100.
67. Tallal P, Piercy M. Defects of non-verbal auditory perception in children with developmental aphasia. *Nature* 1973;241:468–469.
68. Tallal P, Piercy M. Developmental aphasia: the perception of brief vowels and extended stop consonants. *Neuropsychologia* 1975;13:69–74.
69. Alegria J. Phonetic analysis of speech and memory codes in beginning readers. *Mem Cognit* 1982;10:451–456.
70. Bradley L, Bryant P. Visual memory and phonological skills in reading and spelling backwardness. *Psychol Res* 1981;43(2):193–199.
71. Bradley VA, Thomson ME. Residual ability to use grapheme-phoneme conversion rules in phonological dyslexia. *Brain Lang* 1984;22:292–302.
72. Liberman IY, Shankweiler D. Phonology and the problems of learning to read and write. *RASE* 1985;6:8–17.
73. Morais J, Luytens M, Alegria J. Segmentation abilities of dyslexics and normal readers. *Percept Motor Skills* 1984;58:221–222.
74. Livingstone MS, Rosen GD, Drislane FW, Galaburda AM. Physiological and anatomical evidence for a magnocellular defect in developmental dyslexia. *Proc Natl Acad Sci USA* 1991;88:7943–7947.
75. Livingstone MS, Hubel DH. Psychophysical evidence for separate channels for the perception of form, color, movement, and depth. *J Neurosci* 1987;7(11):3416–3468.
76. Lovegrove W, Garzia R, Nicholson S. Experimental evidence for a transient system deficit in specific reading disability. *J Am Optom Assoc* 1990;2(2):137–146.
77. Lovegrove WJ. Is the question of the role of visual deficits as a cause of reading disabilities a closed one? Comments on Hulme. *Cognit Neuropsychol* 1991;8(6):435–441.
78. Slaghuis WL, Lovegrove, WJ, Davidson JA. Visual and language processing deficits are concurrent in dyslexia. *Cortex* 1993;29(4):601–615.
79. Galaburda AM, Menard MT, Rosen GD. Evidence for aberrant auditory anatomy in developmental dyslexia. *Proc Natl Acad Sci USA* 1994;91(17):8010–8013.
80. Galaburda AM, Eidelberg D. Symmetry and asymmetry in the human posterior thalamus. II. Thalamic lesions in a case of developmental dyslexia. *Arch Neurol* 1982;39:333–336.
81. Fitch RH, Tallal P, Brown C, Galaburda AM, Rosen GD. Induced microgyria and auditory temporal processing in rats: a model for language impairment? *Cereb Cortex* 1994;4(3):260–270.
82. Herman AE, Fitch RH, Galaburda AM, Rosen GD. Induced microgyria and its effects on cell size, cell number, and cell packing density in the medial geniculate nucleus. *Soc Neurosci Abstr* 1995;21:1711.
83. Sherman GF, Stone LV, Galaburda AM. Neuronal area is increased in the ventrobasal complex in autoimmune NZB mice with cortical ectopias. *Soc Neurosci Abstr* 1995;21:1712.
84. Denenberg VH, Mobraaten LE, Sherman GF, et al. Effects of the autoimmune uterine/maternal environment upon cortical ectopias, behavior and autoimmunity. *Brain Res* 1991;563(1,2):114–122.
85. Sherman GF, Stone LV, Denenberg VH, Beier DR. A genetic analysis of neocortical ectopias in New Zealand Black mice. *Neuroreport* 1994;5:721–724.
86. McManus IC, Bryden MP. Geschwind's theory of cerebral lateralization: developing a formal, causal model. *Psychol Bull* 1991;110(2):237–253.

*Behavioral Neurology and
the Legacy of Norman Geschwind,*
edited by S. C. Schachter and O. Devinsky,
Lippincott-Raven Publishers, Philadelphia © 1997.

16
Stuttering

David B. Rosenfield

Stuttering Center Speech Motor Control Laboratory, Department of Neurology, Baylor College of Medicine, Houston, Texas 77030.

I have long been interested in speech motor output, stuttering in particular. Norman Geschwind's interest in neurobehavior and language, including speech, greatly influenced our laboratory as well as my own personal development. In this chapter, I hope to convey why and how Norman Geschwind held meaning in my own life and to honor him accordingly.

I first met Norman Geschwind while I was a house officer at the University of Iowa. My interest in neurology had been catalyzed during the neurology rotation of my medical internship, when I also had the pleasure of interacting with Arthur Benton. He later introduced me to Norman when he was a Visiting Professor at the University of Iowa. Norman and I discussed (in Arthur Benton's office and later that evening in his home) the imperatives of handedness and why some people were left-handed.

I completed 1 year of my Neurology residency at Iowa and spent the next 2 years as a Neurology resident at Duke University, training under Stanley H. Appel. An elective with Marcel Kinsbourne consolidated my interest in disorders of language and neurobehavior. I was fortunate to spend the next 3 years as a Fellow at the Boston Aphasia Unit, working under D. Frank Benson and Harold Goodglass. That period came to include 1½ years, part-time, at the Massachusetts Institute of Technology (MIT), where the Sloan Foundation had encouraged Morris Halle, Noam Chomsky, and Salvador Luria to establish an institute to investigate the biological basis of language. Morris Halle, chairman of linguistics, was kind enough to select me for neurologic input.

Norman, Frank, or Harold easily could have preempted my taking on a simultaneous fellowship position in linguistics, but none of them did. Indeed, they were all supportive. One of my contributions to the field may be that, while a Fellow at MIT, I helped establish a lectureship, asking Norman to be our first lecturer. Although the audience was dissimilar to that of the Aphasia Unit, his talk was extremely well received, including by linguists.

During the preceding 7 years (1970–1977: internship, residency, fellowship), many changes had occurred in my own personal realm. But whatever degree of growth I had achieved paled in comparison with the effects on me of the numerous personal and professional interactions I later had with Norman (including telephone conversations, Winter Conferences in Brain Research, the American Neurological Association, the American Academy of Neurology, and being invited guest speaker at the Harvard Neurobehavior Course). What struck me then, and now looking back, was Norman's open-mindedness, especially concerning why human beings stutter, and the ease with which he listened to evolving ideas and thoughts, all the while offering constructive critical comments and support.

I frequently spoke to Norman, asking him his thoughts on Orton and Travis's theory that disrupted cerebral laterality for language caused stuttering [reviewed in Rosenfield, 1984 (1)]. He thought that the idea had merit. We had many discussions about handedness, including ones about his ongoing investigations with Steve Schachter. Norman believed that most studies of handedness were fraught with error because strong and mild preferences were not always considered. As we further discussed handedness, he commented that computerized literature searches were often inadequate, partly because important information was sometimes buried in papers and, therefore, did not show up in computerized searches. Thus, when I visited him in his home during his sabbatical, I was not surprised to see a number of references on handedness that I had scarcely heard of stacked on his dining room table (functioning as his desk). The references concerned the crossover between left-handedness and immunity, a concept that Norman helped discover and promulgate.

I also remember sitting with Norman at one of the Winter Conferences in Brain Research (Steamboat Springs, Colorado, 1982), held at a time when our laboratory was investigating whether stapedius reflex abnormalities could cause stuttering. I told Norman that I questioned whether the "real definition" of cerebral dominance was the brain's ability to override intrinsic laryngeal reflex mechanisms, thereby producing normal phonation. I questioned whether stapedius reflex abnormalities interfered with normal speech production in stutterers. We discussed prephonatory and phonatory tuning, during which sensory stimuli might prompt vocal fold adduction, this reflex needing to be overridden by cerebral dominance for language (a concept that I have long since abandoned) (2).

I eagerly discussed speech acoustics, jitter, shimmer, formants, and theories of sound production, and I hailed the new technology of speech acoustics, proud of my mastery of heretofore foreign ideas. Norman listened, found some of the concepts cogent, looked at me directly, and said, "Never forget, you are a behavioral neurologist. Relate everything to behavior." He went on to discuss the reasons why doing so was important, not the least of which was the clinical constraint that observed behavior placed on any theory. He contended that we, as behavioral neurologists, had much to add, providing a clinical filter on many theories of function. Those words remain in my memory, highlighting the necessity of relating theories of laryngeal function and articulator neuromotor control to clinical observations.

Geschwind loved behavioral neurology. We all know many people who hate their job, but Norman loved his. He had long been committed to behavioral neurology, commenting that the American Academy of Neurology, in its early years, would give neurobehavior only a Saturday morning position and that, sometimes, he bolstered attendance by packing the audience with members of his family. Behavioral neurology has certainly expanded considerably since then, both in the eyes of the Academy and among our neurologist peers. The field of neurobehavior has grown, encompassing investigations on language, movement disorders, dementia, and other areas of behavior compromise, including dysfluency and other speech disorders.

Our laboratory studies aberrations in speech motor control, especially dysfluency. Further, we sponsor a consumer-oriented speech organization, which publishes a newsletter called *Speech News*. We have a mailing list of over 5,000 stutterers, we investigate stuttering clinically and from the perspectives of acoustics and speech science, and we are currently participating in studies in animal modeling. It is within this context that I discuss stuttering and Norman Geschwind.

WHY DO PEOPLE STUTTER?

Stuttering has been with us throughout time; it is referred to in all languages and occurs in all cultures. When I told Norman about my interest in stuttering, he said that he knew little about it but was struck with its rarity in women. His observation was correct: most studies indicate that stuttering is 3 to 4 times more common in men (3). Any theory of stuttering must explain this fact.

The prevalence of stuttering among adults is slightly greater than 1% (3). Porfert and Rosenfield (4), in the most recent investigation of this topic, studied students who were registering at the University of Massachusetts. The prevalence of stuttering among that sociologically skewed population was slightly greater than 2%. One can conservatively conclude, using the world birth rate of over 200 births per minute and the lower prevalence figure for stuttering among adults of 1%, that a person destined to stutter as an adult enters the world every 30 seconds.

References to stutterers appear on Mesopotamian clay tablets, in Egyptian hieroglyphics, and in Chinese poems thousands of years old. The Koran refers to Moses as a stutterer (1). The Old Testament also states that Moses stuttered, but some Hebrew scholars interpret the words to mean "heavy of mouth." Virginia Congressman Frank Wolf underscored these facts in a conversation with me a few years ago. He also commented that there were five members of Congress, including himself, who stuttered. Indeed, Congressman Wolf, who actively participated in establishing the Institute of Hearing and Speech within the National Institutes of Health (NIH), sponsored the institute's commitment to stuttering, which is mentioned in the organization's charter. Although funding for research on stuttering is limited, investigations in this field continue.

One could argue that a period of stuttering is universal in childhood, whether that period lasts only a few hours, several days or months, or years. At issue is not only whether one stutters but whether everyone has the capacity to develop motor skills that will enable them to overcome their stuttering. Depending on how stuttering is defined, 4% to 5% of children aged 4 to 5 stutter. Approximately 80% of these children stop stuttering by adulthood. Children who do not cease stuttering by late adolescence are very likely to continue to be stutterers throughout adulthood. As noted, the prevalence of stuttering among adult men is significantly greater than among women. It may be that once the association cortex is fully myelinated, which occurs near the end of the second decade, one's motor pattern is set and stuttering has become "hardwired" (3).

The dysfluencies of stutterers occur primarily at the beginnings of sentences and phrases, not randomly in their speech. Thus stutterers say, "Wh-Wh-Wh-Where is the hospital?" and never "Where is the hospital-l-l-l?" (1,3). Any theory of stuttering must address this finding.

Altering what a stutterer hears can alter what the person produces, promoting fluency. Specifically, hearing loud, broadband noise while they are speaking renders most stutterers fluent. This is a striking observation: altering input (i.e., hearing) alters output (i.e., speech). This phenomenon was first noted by a stutterer while he was standing next to a waterfall, talking to a friend. He realized that when he did not hear what he was saying, he was able to speak fluently. This observation later inspired the development of auditory masking devices, which are frequently used by speech/language pathologists to demonstrate to stutterers the kinesthetic feeling of fluent speech, as well as the development of therapeutic auditory masking devices to be worn by stutterers during ongoing speech (2,3).

Are the effects of auditory masking on stuttering akin to the phenomenon of "deaf speech," in which abnormal speech output sometimes develops in formerly normal-speaking adults after total loss of hearing? These persons do not produce abnormal speech, such as slurred words, altered enunciation, and abnormal modulation of volume, immediately after they lose their hearing, but later, over time. Some type of orchestrated system must exist in the brain such that when hearing loss compromises sensory input (auditory) to the brain, motor output (speech) is significantly compromised, although not immediately (1–3).

A test called the DAF (delayed auditory feedback) can render stutterers fluent and fluent people dysfluent. Sometimes used by the Armed Forces to detect malingerers on the battlefield who claim hearing loss due to loud explosions, the DAF produces markedly dysfluent speech in fluent persons when they hear their speech output 250 milliseconds after its production. Curiously, stutterers are often fluent in DAF paradigms, possibly because of the sing-song nature of their output. Again, altering auditory input alters speech motor output (2).

Familiarity as well as repetition improves motor performance, not only in tasks of athletic prowess but also in speech. Reading the same passage repeatedly and choral reading are both moderately effective in decreasing dysfluent production in stutterers. Increased fluency from the practice effect of repeatedly reading a passage, referred to as adaptation, occurs only if the stutterer actually voices the sounds. If the stutterer lip-reads or whispers the sounds and does not engage the laryngeal sound system in producing actual phonated sounds, fluency is not enhanced. The practice of the motor system must involve employing the components to make sounds, not merely using the components for other tasks, such as whispering or lipreading (3,5–7).

WHAT IS SPEECH?

A stutterer's problem lies within the domain of speech, not language. Stutterers are not aphasic. They know what they want to say but cannot always say it. Any theory of stuttering must address the problem of speech motor output, even though stuttering may occur because of problems related to hearing, behavior, or language. Stuttering itself is compromised speech output, which is, *a priori,* motor output. Although speech is motor output and differs from language, it does not exist without language. Thus, "Wha- ti- -s -t?" is understood by most people to mean "What time is it?" because of top-down cognitive processing, in which the "rules" of the language supply the missing sounds.

Acquired compromise of language can render someone aphasic, compromising the domains of comprehension, word choice, or syntax. Many persons who are aphasic, especially those who are nonfluent, have accompanying dysarthria. However, a compromised speech motor control system can render a person dysarthric, dysfluent, or dysphonic but need not extend into the realm of grammar or semantics.

Expanding technology within the field of speech acoustics has permitted increasing characterization of human speech. Most of the studies done to date have been related to speech perception rather than speech output. Studies of vowel perception have prompted new conceptions of vowels as articulatory, acoustic, and perceptual events. Fundamental frequencies that emanate from the vocal folds at the laryngeal-level sound source and the subsequent peaks of resonant frequencies, termed *formants,* can be measured so that the relationship of the various sound waves that compose vowels can be mathematically described.

The simple target model of vowel perception initially characterized vowels from an articulatory perspective as static vocal tract shapes and from an acoustic perspective as points in a first and second formant vowel space. Subsequent theories represented vowels as target zones in perceptual spaces whose dimensions are perceived as ratios between formants. These elaborated target models evolved because they could explain the various modes of vowel production (e.g., children's speech and dysarthric speech are dissimilar to the speech of normal adults but still comprehensible). Later, dynamic specification models evolved, emphasizing the importance of formant trajectory patterns in specifying vowel identity (8).

The preceding discussion emphasizes a major problem in analyzing speech and, therefore, stuttering. What is the stutterer actually producing while uttering dysfluencies? How descriptive need one be in analyzing the disrupted output? Most of what the stutterer produces is fluent. Any theory of stuttering must explain not only why stutterers stutter but why they do not stutter all the time or on all words.

Why do fluent persons occasionally stutter? Their stuttering, too, occurs at the beginning of sentences and phrases. A theory is needed to explain why stutterers stutter and why the majority of their output is fluent, as well as why fluent persons are sometimes dysfluent. What are the measures and models that characterize this system (3,9)?

In certain instances, stutterers never stutter. The moderate fluency-evoking power of choral reading, adaptation, and loud, broadband, masking noise has already been discussed. The fluency-evoking potency of singing is immense. Stutterers never stutter when they sing. A 10-year-old stutterer might be terrified to give a book report in front of his class because he stutters, but he might be just as embarrassed to sing in front of the class even though he is fluent when he sings. Why do stutterers not stutter when they sing?

When a person sings, subglottic pressure (i.e., the pressure beneath the vocal folds) is higher than during normal speech. One's pitch is higher when singing than during normal speech. Further, the prevalence of voiced sounds (e.g., /z/, /b/, /d/, /g/) increases during singing, whereas the prevalence of voiceless sounds (e.g., /s/, /p/, /t/, /k/) decreases. Some people are good speakers but poor singers and vice versa. Singing and speaking are perceptually, as well as physiologically, dissimilar (1,3,9,10).

Any theory of stuttering must address its prevalence in males; the fact that many children who stutter do not stutter in adulthood, so that the prevalence of stuttering among adults is slightly more than 1%; the location of stuttered dysfluencies at the beginnings of words and phrases; the fluency-evoking power of singing; and the fact that psychiatry-oriented therapies do not cure stuttering. I frequently pondered these issues during my fellowship at the Aphasia Unit. Unfortunately, because I did not then recognize my interest in speech motor control, I did not initiate any discussions with experts in acoustics or speech science while in Boston. Had I done so, I might have more fully enjoyed studying language and linguistics. Elliot Ross, a behavioral neurologist who had trained under Norman, had recently moved to Dallas. Elliot and I were good friends and we frequently spoke about Texas. After my fellowship, I left Boston and moved to Houston to join Stanley Appel in a new department he was establishing at the Baylor College of Medicine/The Methodist Hospital.

Norman continued to interact with me in a professional manner and did not act as though he thought I had abandoned my research. In fact, I continued to do research as well as see patients. As the laboratory grew, I returned to seeing some patients but focused on our research efforts. I valued Norman's counsel not only on scientific matters but also on dealing with the frustrations of academe.

I later (1981) stopped seeing patients and spent more time on establishing the Stuttering Center Speech Motor Control Laboratory. Norman was very supportive of my efforts. He was enthusiastic and inspiring. Throughout this period, he stressed the importance of my relating everything that I was doing to neurobehavior: the speech motor control system does not exist in a vacuum; it is intricately tied into language and behavior. How does one model this connection?

Norman was interested in obtaining a research grant from the NIH on the biology of language, and we were to be the sector that investigated stuttering. We were able to contact stutterers in any geographical area deemed important for the project. We were very excited about working with Norman on the grant, because he was one of very few people who could have enlisted the cooperation of many centers around the globe to study the biology of language. His untimely death prompted abandonment of that grant proposal.

Norman visited us the year before his death and had dinner with the Appels, the Nudelmans, and me. It was then that I learned that he had worked with two of Harvey's heroes in cybernetics and modeling, Norbert Wiener and Warren McCulloch. I had had no idea that Norman had worked with mathematicians and modelers in cybernetics. Harvey and I had frequently argued about whether some concepts, particularly in motor control, could be explained only mathematically, necessitating calculus equations. Norman contended that this was true and discussed calculus. Norman Geschwind knew calculus! Not only was I amazed that he knew calculus, that he had personally interacted with Wiener and McCulloch, and that he was familiar with their theories of cybernetics, but, when I ordered a fine, single-malt scotch on the rocks and Stanley Appel jokingly belittled my mixing such a good scotch with ice, Norman politely and with a friendly smile ordered a glass of scotch, setting a separate glass of water on the side. He also knew about scotch!

Earlier that day, I had vented with Norman some of my frustrations. While showing him my original set of Broca's anatomy books (which I considered giving him then but decided to do so at a future time—and later regretted my decision), I told him that I felt totally overwhelmed by the incredible academic workload. Risking being too familiar while simultaneously recognizing his status as a chaired professor at Harvard, I asked him whether he ever felt inundated by his workload. He replied that if one felt at pace with one's workload, then one probably wasn't doing enough work. If someone else had made that remark, I would have considered the person hyperactive, academically egocentric, wrong, or any combination thereof. However, Norman loved what he was doing, he seemed to have thought about everything, and in some ways he was laid back. He was so human that, in the same breath that he discussed the workload in academic medicine, he stated that he was astounded by a colleague of his who had spent an inordinate amount of time battling the Boston phone company, making a big moral issue out of a dispute over less than 30 dollars.

Norman and I frequently discussed the Aphasia Unit, including the training of residents and Fellows. When I was a Fellow at the Unit, we had no computed tomography or magnetic resonance imaging scanners, which sometimes made it necessary to decide where a lesion was by vote but, always, while paying careful attention to the details of the patient's history and the physical examination. Similarly, I asked myself where the lesion was in stutterers.

In 1972, the *New England Journal of Medicine* published a letter of mine in which I described the first known case of a formerly fluent person being rendered dysfluent, without aphasia, after cerebral compromise (11). I had seen the patient while at the University of Iowa and had presented her to Dr. Arthur Benton, a leading neuropsychologist in the university's department of Neurology. The description of that patient has become a model for describing patients who have become dysfluent after cerebral compromise.

We have since carried out many studies on acquired stuttering, as have others. Acquired stutterers have dysfluencies throughout their sentences and fail to respond to adaptation, broadband noise, or deliberate slowing of speech (which helps most routine developmental stutterers). Also, unlike developmental stutterers, they seldom appear anxious about their speech (12).

Carefully listening to the speech of a developmental stutterer reveals that the stutterer does not correctly produce the sounds in those of the target word that he is dysfluently repeating. Thus, a developmental stutterer may say "ba-ba-ba-believe," uttering the incorrect sound at the beginning of the dysfluent output. In contrast, an acquired stutterer will usually say "be-be-be-believe," employing the appropriate sound at the beginning of the dysfluent output. The developmental stutterer fails to reach the target even after trying various maneuvers. The acquired stutterer does reach the target the first time and then keeps repeating the target sound. Indeed, it is in this context that one might query a psychogenic component (e.g., if the acquired stutterer has already reacted to the intended target, why does he keep repeating it?)

One can well argue that the main problem in developmental stuttering is not the stuttering itself but some other problem, to which stuttering is a response. One can easily make a stutterer stop stuttering—have the person stop talking. A stutterer can "wait out" the dysfluency until becoming able to produce the target sound or try to struggle through the dysfluency in sundry ways. Sometimes, the stutterer opts for repeating the sound; at other times the person holds the sound, waiting for resolution; and sometimes the person circumlocutes, substituting a more readily produced synonym for the target word (e.g., "guh-guh-guh—see you later," as opposed to "good-bye").

Many stutterers' corrective strategies are learned and, unfortunately, inappropriate and counterproductive to the production of normal speech. Norman and I once discussed this problem, comparing it to downhill skiing. When skiing, one is supposed to lean down the mountain for balance, although it may feel more natural to lean uphill, into the mountain. However, leaning uphill is more likely to cause a fall. So it is with stuttering. Contracting the articulator muscles with excessive force in an attempt to get a word out is not as effective at producing the intended sound as less rigorous muscle contraction (this is a major principle in speech therapy).

On one occasion, Mitchell Brin, Nagalapura S. Viswanath, Celia Stewart, and I, as well as other colleagues, sought to answer the question, Is stuttering a movement disorder? My perspective is that stuttering is not one of the clinically recognized movement disorders but, rather, a disorder of movement. One might regard a tremor as an underdamping of an oscillation system, and a dystonia as an overdamping of that system (13,14). If so, a person could have dystonic tremors and, at different times, more dystonia or more tremor. The problem might be the same in terms of damage to the oscillation system but, depending on the degree of anxiety and neurochemical changes in the physiological milieu, underdamping might sometimes occur, producing tremor, or overdamping, producing dystonia.

This perspective leads into the question of whether the nosology used in movement disorders is as productive as it might be in a physiological sense. Perhaps the current nosology too closely follows the hierarchy of current clinical diagnoses and the efficacy of particular medications. Dystonia and tremor might be far more similar than we think, especially if they are viewed respectively as an overdamping and underdamping of the same system.

One can model stuttering as a disorder of motor movement, interacting with language as well as behavior. Further, stuttering might not be the actual problem itself but, rather, a response to an underlying problem. During dysfluent output, the stutterer is trying to reach the target word fluently. In attempting to do so, the stutterer can engage in many different maneuvers. He or she can hold the sound (e.g., aaaaaaangry) or repeat the initial sound several times (ah-ah-ah-angry). The stutterer can also engage in facial distortion and obvious struggling behaviors, producing classic "secondary characteristics" of stuttering.

The speech/language pathologist is usually able to teach the stutterer not to produce these secondary characteristics and to employ various speech therapy techniques instead, such as gentle-onset speech and slowed speech. These techniques are used to manage the stutterer's compromised speech-motor output in a way that is similar to the way physical therapy techniques are used to replace abnormal maneuvers in a patient stricken with a gait disorder.

When they speak, stutterers are doing something inappropriate that keeps them from reaching the target. Using this premise and recognizing that one of the core features of developmental stuttering is repetition of parts of words (fragments), followed by fluent production (resolution) of the target words, Viswanath and Neel (15) studied a group of adult stutterers. The investigators discussed the articulatory implications of their acoustic data for each of the two fragment types (those with vowels and those without) within the framework of speech as an act designed to achieve contextually conditioned acoustic goals. A more recent study found similar articulatory patterns for the different fragments in child stutterers (16).

Is there a part of the brain that, when compromised, makes a person dysfluent? I erroneously used to argue that just as one's eyeball can be too long, producing myopia, or too short, producing hyperopia, and just as one's gain and phase of a motor system (e.g., synchrony of amplitude and frequency in a sensorimotor feedback loop) might be better than average (good athlete) or below average (poor athlete), some people must lack appropriate control of their speech motor system. I presumed that these people were stutterers. However, the search for this lesion(s) has failed to produce fluent persons who, after sustaining brain damage, developed dysfluency similar to that in developmental stutterers. True, some of these persons became dysfluent after brain lesions, but their dysfluency, as noted earlier, is different from that of developmental stutterers. In effect, we have accumulated data demonstrating that developmental stuttering is not due to a singular brain lesion or to multiple lesions.

Several investigators have demonstrated that people can become acquired stutterers with lesions in either hemisphere, anteriorly or posteriorly (12). The prognosis is usually good when the lesion is unilateral and poor when it is bilateral. However, none of these people stutter the way developmental stutterers do. Thus, in the search for a lesion that produces developmental stuttering, we have identified people who stutter, but they are different from developmental stutterers. Could it be that developmental stuttering is not due to a lesion? Could it be that one can have a problem in brain function without any lesion?

Norman stressed neurobehavior. Can a person exhibit an abnormal neurobehavior without having any "lesion," focal or otherwise? The ringing of a public address system serves as an analogy. When it rings, where is the lesion? A public address system has a microphone, an amplifier, and a loudspeaker. The system can ring for different reasons at different times, even though all components are working normally; that is, the system can ring without anything being broken. In one instance the system might ring because the microphone is too sensitive; in another because the microphone is too close to the amplifier; in another because the gain of the amplifier is too high; and in yet another because the loudspeaker volume is too high. If various public address systems across the nation were analyzed, in one study the sensitivity of the microphone might be found responsible for the ringing in 40% of the systems, the gain of the amplifier in 30%, and the loudspeaker volume in another 30%. In a different study, completely different percentages might be obtained. If one then prepared a detailed "case report" on the ringing of a single public address system, one might find that in the morning the microphone was too close to the amplifier, in the afternoon the gain of the amplifier was too high, and the following day the loudspeaker volume was too high. The point is that the public address system can become unstable (e.g., ring) at different times for different reasons. Why should the brain be any different? Both have inputs and outputs, and both are intricately tied into feedback control systems (17–20). The ringing is not caused by a single component within the system but, rather, by the interaction of various components within that system. To understand the ringing, one need not know how each component of the system actually works, only how to analyze the interaction of the components.

Nudelman and colleagues model stuttering as a momentary instability in a complex multiloop control system (17–20). This instability is similar to that in a public address system. The model predicts the temporal conditions under which this instability occurs in a speech sensorimotor negative feedback loop and accounts for the efficacy of fluency-evoking maneuvers and speech therapy and for the variability of speech output in stutterers. The problem with the model is that it does not state what parts of the brain are involved in the functioning of this loop. Indeed, different parts of the brain might be compromised at different times, or perhaps the connections between them (ranging from ion channels, to voltage gating mechanisms, to anything that involves time) are compromised.

This model might be a somewhat novel concept in behavioral neurology. Can a cognitive/cerebral deficit exist without a focal lesion? Yes, indeed. One could argue that in someone who is addicted to power, money, drugs, or reading, a particular sector (or sectors) in the brain promotes the addiction. This line of reasoning need not imply that there is a focal point of abnormality. Our laboratory investigates such concepts. I believe that Norman's open-mindedness helped me to expand my thinking about neurological disease, such that we can contemplate ideas such as these.

I once told Norman that I thought people should view stuttering in much the same way they view migraine—as a disease. He had written a review of the play *Wings* for the *New England Journal of Medicine* several years earlier. That prompted me to write a review of the movie *A Fish Called Wanda,* a caper comedy embodying various styles of British humor in which a stutterer named Ken (played by Michael Palin) does funny things (21). Never mind the fact that Ken stuttered when real stutterers do not (he stuttered on every sound, not just those at the beginnings of sentences and phrases). I deplored the fact that this movie belittled a stutterer and made stuttering appear funny, and I was surprised that it apparently did not offend the audience's sensibilities. In my review, I stated that such a film probably would not have been made if stuttering were regarded as a bona fide disease. I also raised the question whether such a movie would have been made if the affliction were breast cancer. The *Journal* editors and I corresponded back and forth for some time about this point, and ultimately they decided to condense the review into a letter. That decision reminded me, again, about my talks with Norman about whether stuttering is a significant disease, warranting such discussions. Norman's view was that a disease was something that was infectious, plain and simple. I pointed out that stuttering was almost a stepchild of medicine, without true disease status. Surely no one would make a movie poking fun at someone with Alzheimer's disease, prostate cancer, or the like, but stuttering is considered fair game. Norman and I had often discussed the fact that in the field of speech, the disease is often the obvious symptom. No self-respecting physician would opt for a single treatment for back pain, arguing that all back pain patients should have an operation, or that everyone with chest discomfort warrants open heart surgery. Rather, the physician should try to classify the symptom before treating it. But no bona fide nosology for stuttering exists. Only recently has there been one for spasmodic dysphonia, and there is none for voice abuse or poor diction. Until we are able to relate the signs of stuttering to the symptoms and classify stuttering as a disease, we will have difficulty unraveling this disturbance. Indeed, stuttering is a syndrome, and different people can stutter for different reasons.

The corpus of investigations on stuttering is expanding. The reader is referred to several texts for further discussion (3,22–24). Recently, positron emission tomography scans of the brains of stutterers suggest that they lack normal left hemisphere dominance for language, have exaggerated disruption in their right cerebral motor control areas, and have inappropriate auditory feedback to their left auditory cortex during ongoing speech. These preliminary findings are in keeping with the theory that many regions of the brain are involved in stuttering, perhaps different ones at different times in different people [analogous to the public address system ringing (25,26)].

A number of new texts have been published on stuttering, new journals have been created that discuss dysfluency, and the International Fluency Association, an organization dedicated to disseminating information about stuttering and its treatment and to promoting related research, has been established. Researchers in our laboratory are excited about their work in analyzing patterns of output in stutterers' disrupted speech fragments and our recent entry into the fields of genetics and functional neuroimaging. We are beginning to study phonatory disruption in birds as a model of human dysfluency. This enterprise is truly multidisciplinary, reflecting Norman's emphasis on being open-minded and Stanley Appel's prompt that we need an animal model.

Numerous advances are being made in the field of stuttering. As investigations into dysfluency expand into other areas, I often think of Norman, smiling, moving his hands in and out of his coat pockets, not being afraid of new ideas or expanding technologies, and listening intently, always having intelligent things to say. He would have welcomed the current technologies, would have related them to neurobehavior, and would be pleased to see so many of his students and colleagues continuing to do research (he once told me that a scientist can be judged only by the students whom he or she trains). I respected Norman Geschwind a great deal. We all miss him.

ACKNOWLEDGMENT

This work was supported by the M. R. Bauer Foundation and the Benjamin-Gideon-Jeremiah-Abigail-Rebekah-Maida Lowin Medical Research Foundation.

REFERENCES

1. Rosenfield DB. Stuttering. *CRC Critical Rev Clin Neurobiol* 1984;1:117–139.
2. Rosenfield DB, Jerger J. Stuttering and auditory function. In: Curlee RF, Perkins WH, eds. *Nature and treatment of stuttering: new directions.* San Diego, CA: College Hill Press, 1984;73–87.
3. Bloodstein O. *A handbook on stuttering.* Chicago, IL: National Easter Seal Society, 1987.
4. Porfert AR, Rosenfield DB. Prevalence of stuttering. *J Neurol Neurosurg Psychiatry* 1978;41:954–956.
5. Wingate ME. Sound and pattern in "artificial" fluency. *J Speech Hear Res* 1969;12:677–686.
6. Adams MR, Ramig P. Vocal characteristics of normal speakers in stutterers during choral reading. *J Speech Hear Res* 1980;2:457–469.
7. Brenner NC, Perkins WH, Soderberg GA. The effect of rehearsal on frequency of stuttering. *J Speech Hear Res* 1972;15:483–486.

8. Strange WJ. Evolving theories of vowel perception. *J Acoust Soc Am* 1989;85:2081–2087.
9. Van Riper C. *The treatment of stuttering.* Englewood Cliffs, NJ: Prentice-Hall, 1973.
10. Borden GJ, Harris KS, Raphael LJ. *Speech science primer: physiology, acoustics and perception of speech,* 3d ed. Baltimore, MD: Williams & Wilkins, 1994.
11. Rosenfield DB. Stuttering in cerebral ischemia. *N Engl J Med* 1972;287:991.
12. Rosenfield DB, Viswanath NS, Callis-Landrum L, DiDanato R, Nudelman HB. Patients with acquired dysfluencies: what they tell us about developmental stuttering. In: Peters HFM, Hulstijn W, Starkweather CW, eds. *Speech motor control in stuttering.* New York: Elsevier, 1991;277–284.
13. Stein RB, Oguztöreli MN. Reflex involvement in the generation and control of tremor and clonus. In: Desmedt JE, ed. *Physiological tremor, pathological tremors and clonus,* vol 5: *Progress in clinical neurophysiology.* Basel, Switzerland: Karger, 1978;28–50.
14. Stein RB, Oguztöreli MN. Tremor and other oscillations in neuromuscular systems. *Biol Cybern* 1976;22:147–157.
15. Viswanath NS, Neel AT. Part-word repetitions by persons who stutter: fragment types and their articulatory processes. *J Speech Hear Res* 1995;38:740–750.
16. Joullian AL, Viswanath NS, Rosenfield DB. *Motor processes underlying incipient and chronic stuttering.* Poster presentation at the 120th annual meeting of the American Neurological Association; October 22–25, 1995; Washington, D.C.
17. Nudelman HB, Herbrich KE, Hoyt B, Rosenfield DB. Dynamic characteristics of vocal frequency functioning in stutterers and non-stutterers. In: Peters H, Hulstijn W, eds. *Speech motor dynamics in stuttering.* New York: Springer-Verlag, 1987;161–169.
18. Nudelman HB, Hoyt B, Herbrich KE, Rosenfield DB. A neuroscience model of stuttering. *J Fluency Disord* 1989;14:399–427.
19. Nudelman HB, Herbrich KE, Hoyt BD, Rosenfield DB. A neuroscience approach to stuttering. In: Peters HFM, Hulstijn W, Starkweather CW. *Speech motor control in stuttering.* New York: Elsevier, 1991;157–162.
20. Nudelman HB, Herbrich KE, Hoyt BD, Rosenfield DB. Phonatory response times of stutterers and fluent speakers to frequency-modulated tones. *J Acoust Soc Am* 1992;92:1882–1888.
21. Rosenfield DB. Stuttering. *N Engl J Med* 1989;320:1630–1631.
22. Herman FM P, Hulstijn W, Starkweather CW. *Speech-motor control in stuttering.* Amsterdam, the Netherlands: Excerpta Medica, 1991.
23. Bloodstein O. *Stuttering: the search for cause and cure.* Boston, MA: Allyn and Bacon, 1993.
24. Starkweather CW, Herman FM P. *Stuttering: proceedings of the First World Congress on Fluency Disorders.* University Press Nijmegen, Nijmegen, the Netherlands, August 8–11, 1995.
25. Fox PT, Ingham RI, Ingham IC, Downs H, Hersch T, Lancaster IL. *Supplementary motor and premotor overactivity in stuttering: a pet study of stuttering and induced fluency.* Presented at the 25th Annual Meeting of the Society for Neuroscience; San Diego, CA, November 11–16, 1995.
26. Ludlow CL, Braun A. Advances in stuttering research using positron emission tomography brain imaging. Panel discussion at the American Speech-Language Hearing Association; Orlando, FL; December 7–10, 1995.

Other Disorders
of Higher Cortical Function

17

Disconnexion Syndromes

Orrin Devinsky

Department of Neurology, NYU School of Medicine, Hospital for Joint Diseases, New York, New York 10003.

Norman Geschwind's career could never be duplicated today. He became the chairman of Neurology at Boston University School of Medicine at age 40 (in 1966), and at age 42, the James Jackson Putnam Professor of Neurology at Harvard Medical School. He had no major funding from the National Institutes of Health. He had neither discovered nor utilized any new technology. He had neither discovered nor cured any disorder. By age 42 years, he had published a dozen papers and a dozen chapters on topics ranging from muscle disease to aphasia. Among the papers was a long, two-part treatise, "Disconnexion Syndromes in Animals and Man" (DSAM), published in *Brain* (1,2). DSAM synthesized case reports from nearly a century before, together with more recent observations, into a document that swayed contemporary neurological thought on behavior back towards a conceptual framework of anatomy, pathways, and localization. The DSAM paper launched Geschwind's career.

"Disconnexion Syndromes in Animals and Man" remains Norman Geschwind's most powerful and persisting influence in neurology. The DSAM papers resurrected the late 19th and early 20th century German and French literature buried by neglect and misinterpretation. More importantly, it united the forgotten masters with the recent anatomic, physiological, and clinical data. Geschwind rediscovered that neuronal masses and fiber pathways are essential to deciphering the mechanisms of behavior. The anatomic and mechanistic model of behavioral analysis was not new and was still being applied to help understand isolated problems. In DSAM, Geschwind applied this model to many normal functions and pathological states, covering a diverse range of topics. The synthetic originality and scope of this manuscript helped forge the modern field of behavioral neurology.

CHANCE FAVORS THE PREPARED MIND BUT ONE MUST SPIN THAT LITTLE WHEEL—NORMAN GESCHWIND

In 1961, Edith Kaplan evaluated a 41-year-old policeman who had a left frontal resection for a glioblastoma. Postoperatively, he developed a marked grasp reflex in the right hand, but not the left. For Kaplan, this case provided an opportunity to test the assertions made by Bouman and Grunbaum that the grasp reflex caused characteristic mechanical defects in writing (3). Kaplan found that the man could write normally with his right hand but aphasically with his left hand. She was astonished to find aphasic writing restricted to the left hand. She could have told a thousand neurologists about this case, and it would have remained merely one of those curiosities that do not conform to the pigeon-holes of current knowledge, but she told Norman Geschwind. She related this case history to Geschwind a week after he had read Déjérine's description of callosal syndromes in man (3). The timing was fortuitous, but Pasteur was right, chance does favor the prepared mind.

Déjérine described several callosal syndromes, including alexia (pure word-blindness) without agraphia, which Geschwind summarized in 1962 (4). In 1891, Déjérine described a 63-year-old man who developed the sudden onset of inability to read and write, and a right hemianopia, but no other neurological deficits (5). Postmortem revealed a lesion of the angular gyrus and underlying white matter. Déjérine reasoned that the lesion destroyed a "visual memory center for words," impairing reading and writing abilities. A year later, in a more detailed paper, Déjérine (6) reported a patient who suddenly developed inability to read letters, words, or musical notation, and a right hemianopia. The man could copy words accurately but could not transcribe print to script. He could write in script to dictation or spontaneously, but could not read what he had written. He could read tactilely, with his fingers tracing over the outline of letters. Naming of low-frequency, complex words was intact. Intelligence was intact. Despite the alexia, he remained successful at business and gambling at cards. Ten days before he died, he developed agraphia. Postmortem revealed an infarct of the left occipital lobe and splenium of the corpus callosum. The occipital lobe was old—shrunken and yellow and adherent to the meninges. There was an additional fresh infarct of the angular gyrus that caused agraphia shortly before death. Déjérine postulated that the splenial lesion disconnected visual input in the preserved left visual field from the visual memory center for words (left angular gyrus). The ability to write demonstrated that the "visual word center" was intact. Ability to read tactilely demonstrated that the pathway from somesthetic cortex to angular gyrus was intact.

Déjérine's 1892 description of the classic disconnection syndrome, alexia without agraphia, well recognized by English authorities such as Bastian (7), was lost to the English-speaking neurological community after World War I. Geschwind revived the syndrome (1,2,4). It provided him with the background to recognize a disconnection syndrome in a man with alexia associated with a color-naming defect, who was similar to Déjérine's patient both clinically and neuropathologically. In this man's brain, disconnection of visual input from the angular gyrus prevented the language cortex from receiving the data to be named. Geschwind reported his original observations regarding the defect in a paper published with Fusillo (8). Geschwind later described, together with Judd and Gardner, alexia and agraphia in a composer (9).

Geschwind and Kaplan presented two cases to the Boston Society of Neurology and Psychiatry on December 14, 1961 (10,11). The first patient had alexia without agraphia from a lesion of the left visual cortex and splenium. The second patient was Edith Kaplan's policeman, described previously, who had a left frontal resection. In a brief report of the meeting, published in *The New England Journal of Medicine* (10), Geschwind and Kaplan anonymously reported that callosal syndromes were well known before 1940. In the early 1940s, Akelaitis' studies (12–14) of patients after callosal section for intractable epilepsy appeared to refute previously well-documented cliniconeuropathological cases of callosal syndromes. However, Gazzaniga and coworkers demonstrated dramatic results after callosal sections using new examination techniques (15).

In 1961, Geschwind met Oliver Zangwill at a meeting on dyslexia in Baltimore. "He listened patiently to the exposition of my ideas on the significance of the cortico-cortico connections for the higher functions. A short time later, while on a trip to Boston, he suggested to me that I should prepare an extended account of these ideas" (3). The result was the two-part opus, DSAM (1,2).

HISTORICAL BACKGROUND

The roots for Geschwind's disconnection syndromes, as well as his major contributions in aphasia, lie in late 19th century Germany and France. Wernicke's life and contributions were a source of great interest to Geschwind (16–18). Wernicke wrote "The Symptom Complex of Aphasia: A Psychological Study on an Anatomical Basis" in 1874, at age 26 years (19). He began this monograph with a tribute to his teacher: "Meynert's theory of the connections of the brain contains the foundations of a precise physiology of the central nervous system. It provides only a broad, general outline, to be sure, but one of such brilliant inner truth that it can even now be applied without hesitation to individual cases.

The present case is an attempt to make practical use of Meynert's neuroanatomical teachings in an area in which fundamental principles of this kind are badly needed but up to now have scarcely been applied—the normal speech process and the disturbances of this process, which are known as aphasia."

In the introduction to this classic work on fluent aphasia with paraphasia from posterosuperior temporal lesions, Wernicke added, "The surface of the brain is a mosaic of very simple elements of this kind, which are characterized by their anatomical connections with the periphery of the body. Everything beyond these elementary functions, such as the linking of different sense impressions to form a concept, thought, and consciousness, is a function of the fiber tracts that connect different cortical regions with each other, i.e., a function of the association systems, to use Meynert's terminology."

Geschwind's DSAM revived Meynert's attention to anatomy and corticocortical connections. In turn, Meynert and Wernicke relied on Burdach (19), Flechsig (20), and others anatomists, who carefully mapped the association bundles that made up much of the cerebral white matter and their patterns of myelination. Wernicke's 1874 monograph established that posterosuperior temporal lesions caused an aphasic syndrome with fluent speech and paraphasia. However, Meynert previously identified the adjacent temporal cortex (Heschl's gyrus) as the termination for the auditory pathways, and he determined that lesions in the posterosuperior temporal gyrus cause an aphasia distinct from the disorder following destruction of Broca's area (18). Wernicke created a new approach to behavioral analysis, postulating conduction aphasia *(Leitungsaphasie)* from lesions disconnecting Wernicke's and Broca's aphasia. Wernicke predicted that patients with conduction aphasia would have fluent speech with paraphasias, strongly resembling the speech in patients with posterior superior temporal lesions. However, conduction aphasics would recognize their language errors, as they had normal comprehension. Wernicke did not predict impaired repetition with conduction aphasia. Lichteim (21) correctly identified repetition defect as a cardinal feature of conduction aphasia, and reported a case with this finding. Wernicke predicted that the lesion in conduction aphasia would lie in the insula. Subsequent clinicopathological cases confirmed Wernicke's clinical prediction of fluent paraphasic speech with preserved comprehension, but von Monakow's studies (22) identified the lesion in the inferior parietal region, disrupting the arcuate (superior longitudinal) fasciculus, not in the insula. More than a century later, the insula region, as well as the inferior parietal region, would find support in neuroimaging studies (23).

The transcortical aphasias stood in bold contrast to conduction aphasia. The former were summarized by Goldstein in his early and later writings (24,25). The term *transcortical aphasia* was coined by Wernicke; it was later used to describe patients with preserved repetition but impaired spontaneous speech (transcortical motor aphasia), impaired comprehension (transcortical sensory aphasia), or both (mixed transcortical aphasia) (26). Geschwind and colleagues' description (26) of a man whose speech cortex was isolated after carbon monoxide poisoning helped reestablish the existence of the transcortical aphasias. Geschwind recognized the role of the neocortical language areas, as well as that of the white matter tracts that connect them. His rediscovery of disconnection syndromes brought two aphasic syndromes back to clinical neurology: conduction aphasia (1,2,27) and the transcortical aphasias (1,2,24).

The integration of Meynert's anatomic approach with Wernicke's psychological (behavioral) studies led to a productive period in European neurology. Broca's localization of the motor speech area was supplemented by attention to connections and associations of different cortical areas. Lesions of these fiber bundles caused specific deficits, such as alexia without agraphia (6). At the turn of the century, Liepmann, Wernicke's disciple, reported the first neuropathological study of a unilateral lesion causing pure word deafness (28). This disconnection syndrome resulted from a lesion isolating Wernicke's area from auditory inputs of both hemispheres.

Apraxia, like aphasia, was lucidly identified through brilliant clinicopathological correlations by early German neurologists. However, in post–World War I England and France, apraxia was rarely mentioned in its original forms. Rather, the term was loosely and incorrectly applied to a variety of other motor disorders such as constructional tasks, gait, speech, and clumsiness (16). For Liepmann, *apraxia* was conceptually more than a *motor asymbolia* (Meynert's term). Recognizing the brilliant analysis of the Regierungsrat case with *apraxia*, Geschwind fully credited Liepmann with showing that the patient's inability to perform learned movements was explained by a series of disconnecting lesions (29). The patient died 2 years later and neuropathology confirmed the predicted lesion sites (30). The following year (1907), Liepmann and Maas published the case of Ochs, in whom apraxia resulted from a callosal lesion (31). These authors, as well as Geschwind, applied Flechsig's rule to their interpretations: primary receptive areas have no direct neocortical connections except with immediately adjacent sensory association areas (20). Leipmann and Maas later reported apraxia from a callosal lesion (31). Geschwind and Kaplan's subsequent description of a similar patient with apraxia from a callosal (and left frontal) lesion (11) was a major impetus to DSAM.

DISCONNEXION SYNDROMES IN ANIMALS AND MAN

Geschwind's two-part opus, "Disconnexion Syndromes in Animals and Man," revisited the data of Wernicke, Déjérine, Liepmann, Jackson, Flechsig, Foix, Lissauer, Bonhoeffer, and Maas. The clinical and pathological information was clear and well documented. The intrahemispheric and callosal disconnection syndromes were reconfirmed by neurologists and accurately summarized by authorities such as Kinnier Wilson (32) over the next 30 years, but these syndromes were relegated to oblivion. Holistic neurologists such as Head (33), Marie (34), von Monakow (35), and Goldstein (24,25) confirmed cases of disconnection syndromes. Yet they denied the value of localization—tossing out the overzealous microlocalization of Kleist (36) together with the accurate localizations described by Wernicke, Déjérine, and Liepmann. Karl Lashley's holistic Gestalt psychology viewed the cerebral cortex as an equipotential mass (37). Henry Head (33), in his influential monographic "Aphasia and Kindred Disorders of Speech," concluded that the contributions of those such as Wernicke were based on faulted theories and were of no consequence. As Déjérine and Liepmann exited academia, Akelaitis reported that callosal lesions in epilepsy patients caused no deficits (12–14), thus hammering nails into the coffin of disconnection syndromes. Norman Geschwind removed the nails with DSAM. With his marvelous mind, he simultaneously looked backward and forward, while attending fully to the cases that lay in front of him.

Geschwind's DSAM integrated the historical data with more recent observations in neuroanatomy (38–45), neurophysiology (46–51), animal neurobehavioral studies (52–60), and clinical neurology and neuropsychology (15,61–65). The style of DSAM was distinctly Geschwind:

long (as were his conversations and rounds!)
informal and personal (frequent references to what he thought, whom he agreed and disagreed with)
highlighted anatomy
highlighted mechanisms
synthetic
far-reaching (from the historical roots of neurology to philosophical implications).

The outline of DSAM is summarized below:

Part I
  Introduction
    Acknowledgments
  I. Anatomic background: Flechsig's rule
    Connexions of the visual association areas
  II. Agnosias in animals
    Removals of temporal neocortex: the visual–limbic disconnexion syndrome
    The effects of the extent of the lesion
    Nonlimbic associations
    "Motor" learning
    Objections to the theory
    Negative experiments
    Other reward systems
    Lesions of somesthetic association areas
    The auditory system
    The problem of mirror foci
    Disconnection from the limbic system in man
  III. Disconnexion syndromes in man
    The anatomic basis of language
    Pure word-blindness without agraphia
    Pure word-deafness
    Lesions of Wernicke's area
    Tactile aphasia
  Summary

Part II
  Introduction
  IV. The agnosias
    The problem of confabulatory response
    Inability to identify colors
    Classical visual agnosia
    The lesions of classical visual agnosia
    The handling of objects
    The conditions for confabulatory responses
    The problem of right parietal dominance
    Visual imagery
  V. The mechanisms of the apraxias
    Disconnexion from the speech area

Extension of the theory of the apraxias
The apraxias of the supramarginal gyrus region
Facial apraxia
Whole body movements
Other bilateral movements
The problem of "motor" versus "cognitive" learning
VI. Other aphasic disturbances
Conduction aphasia
The case of Bonhoeffer
Echolalia
VII. Possible objections and pitfalls
The results of Akelaitis and his coworkers
VIII. Philosophical implications
The whole man
The unity of consciousness
The value of introspection
Language and thought
Summary
Bibliography

Any of these sections is a rich source for discussion. I will first consider the role of the association cortex and nonlimbic connections as postulated by Geschwind, and its later revisions, and I will then briefly review his contribution to the apraxias.

THE ASSOCIATION AREAS

The most significant difference between the brain of man and the higher ape—the expansion of the association cortex in the former—formed a cornerstone of Geschwind's theory of anatomic mechanisms underlying behavior. Flechsig's rule (20)—primary receptive areas connect only to adjacent unimodal association cortex—was critical to DSAM. For Geschwind, the term *disconnexion syndrome* applied to lesions of the associational pathways. The unimodal sensory association cortices project to higher order, polymodal association cortices—"the association area of association areas." Geschwind stressed that unlike the brain of other primates, the human brain is well endowed with connections between different cortical associational areas. Man could link visual and tactile, or visual and auditory inputs without using limbic structures as the connection. If animals are shown a picture of a cross, they are unable to match it to a cross presented tactilely to their hand when blindfolded. A young child can make this cross-modal association quite easily. The implications of this wiring were profound—it served, as Meynert said, as the foundation for human language and thought. It is *"only in man that associations between two nonlimbic stimuli are readily formed and it is this ability which underlies the learning of names of objects"* (66). In Geschwind's lectures on the origins of human language, he cogently argued that naming ability is the basis of language. If you were trapped on a desert island with a man who spoke another language, you would start to communicate by naming objects—from yourself to food (Geschwind, personal communication).

Geschwind brought clinical meaning to the cytoarchitectural and functional divisions of the brain—primary motor and sensory, unimodal motor and sensory association cortex, and heteromodal cortex. Like many new theories and perspectives, these ideas can help obscure one picture while illuminating another. Geschwind's formulation of information flow in the brain was partly correct—from primary sensory cortex (e.g., striate cortex; area 17), to unimodal association cortex (e.g., visual association cortex; areas 18 and 19), to higher-order association cortex (e.g., angular gyrus; area 39). Like Hubel and Wiesel's discovery of simple, complex, and hypercomplex cells in the primate visual cortex (67), Geschwind also postulated a hierarchical, serial progression of information flow and data analysis.

This serial model of visual analysis is correct but incomplete. Additional concepts must also be considered—two visual processing systems, parallel processing, data flowing from "higher" to "lower" centers (i.e., feedback), the nonreplicated role of "lower" centers for detailed analysis, and neuronal synchrony. The nonhierarchical, parallel model of visual processing by the brain was only recently conceptualized (68). Cases supporting this model were reported more than a century ago, but as Geschwind stressed many times for the aphasias, apraxias, and agnosias, they were not accepted because they lacked a theoretical framework.

Independent extracalcarine visual areas mediating color and motion perception were postulated in the late 19th century and supported by clinical and neuropathologic data (69–74). However, neurological authorities, such as Henschen (75), von Monakow (35), and Holmes (76,77), emphatically dismissed evidence for color or motion areas as inconclusive, but most importantly, inconsistent with their views. The concept of separate centers for motion and color vision and the existence of patients with isolated loss of motion (akinetopsia) and color (achromatopsia) vision vanquished from neurology for more than 50 years.

The theoretical structure to accept the clinical data was built by anatomic and physiological studies of visual cortex in monkeys, demonstrating that multiple visual association areas (V3 to V5) contain independent but different retinal representations (68,78–81). Each of these areas is smaller than V1 and contains cells with receptive fields larger than in V1. The multiple representations of the visual world do not neatly fit into the hierarchical model of serial processing. Rather than being redundant, these areas are specialized and receive different inputs from V1 and V2. The connections between V3, V4, and V5 strongly support a primarily parallel—not serial—communication network.

The presence of parallel outputs is a consistent feature of cortical connectivity (82). Cortical areas parcel different output signals to different areas, serving as segregators undertaking multiple operations (68). Cortical connections are usually between areas with similar functions. Thus, portions of V1 and V2 that segregate color input from other inputs have strong connections to V4, the cortical color vision area in the fusiform gyrus. Parallel processing occurs in other cortical areas, such as prefrontal cortex and limbic system (83,84).

Parallel processing can be applied to concepts of "bottom-up" and "top-down" analysis of visual input. Bottom-up analysis refers to the construction of a visual object or spatial scene by integrating many tiny bits of raw data. Thus, the hierarchical analysis with increasing size of neuronal receptive field and complexity of neuronal responsiveness is a bottom-up process. In contrast, top-down processing refers to the influence of other cognitive domains, such as attention, other senses, or emotion, on visual analysis. For example, if we wander through a game park where someone was recently killed by a lion, it is likely that we would more vigorously scan the visual field to detect a lion and might "see" a lion's tail where there is only a patch of sand-colored plants blowing in the wind.

Feedback Connections and the Role of V1 and V2. The hierarchical model of visual processing conceptualizes visual input travelling down a one-way avenue towards a more complex and integrated visual image. However, there are robust connections from association to primary visual cortices. Whereas the forward connections from V1 and V2 are modality specific, the feedback connections from V3 to V5 to V1 to V2 are diffuse (85). Thus, for example, the feedback from cortical units in V4 are not limited to cells in V1 and V2 that project to V4; it also includes cells in V1 and V2 that project to V3 and V5. These feedback fibers may contribute to several functions (68), such as the following:

1. They may provide access to the detailed visual field map. Benefits of selective motion or color recognition are balanced by losses in topographical detail.

2. They may access data in V1, "zooming in" for a "precise focus" on an area of interest.

3. They may aid in the linking and activating of one visual modality from another. For example, when a moving structure is recognized by V5, direct and indirect (via V1 and V2) connections to V3 activate the form-selective cells that permit recognition of the moving structure's shape. The visual image can be integrated by pathways joining form, color, and motion.

Neuronal Synchrony and Integration of the Visual Image. How is the visual image integrated by the brain? The multiple specialized cortical visual areas "see" different aspects of the world—orientation, depth, form, motion, and color. These areas do not provide convergent input to a "visual integration center" that "sees the whole picture." They are connected in parallel with each other and reciprocally with V1 and V2. When two specialized visual areas project to a common cortical area, their inputs are largely distinct. Local circuits could integrate these inputs, but then we are left with multiple local circuits in separate areas.

Neuronal synchrony may provide the solution to integration. Synchrony in neuronal populations depends on neuronal groups interconnected by mutually excitatory and inhibitory synaptic connections (86) and has been demonstrated in multiple cortical and limbic areas (87–90). With a continuous stimulus, cells in different visual areas and hemispheres can synchronize their responses to stimuli sharing particular features, such as the same orientation or direction of motion (91,92). With visual experience, cells in the visual cortex may become functionally linked with other cells sharing certain properties. As certain cells become synchronously activated over time, they may form repertoires, or groups, and their connections may selectively compete for space on other cells (93). The stability of groups is increased if the probability of their firing in synchrony is high.

Synthesis of the visual image may depend on activity in nonspecialized (V1 and V2) and specialized (V3 to V6) visual areas being both simultaneous and in temporal synchrony (68). *Perceptual awareness (consciousness)* of visual input may rely on synchronously linked activity in multiple areas.

THE APRAXIAS

Geschwind first visited the apraxias in DSAM, but he continued to provide original insights and reviews throughout his career (4,11,15,16, see chapter 22). He helped non-German neurologists revisit apraxia, emphasizing that apraxia is common, especially in patients with acute dominant hemisphere frontal strokes, although it was considered very rare. The error is made because most apraxic patients can correctly manipulate familiar objects in their environment, but they fail with specific testing. In other patients, apraxia is missed because it is present only transiently, during the early stage of the disorder. Geschwind stressed that apraxias are disorders characterized by impaired execution of a learned movement in response to a stimulus that would normally elicit the movement in the setting of intact sensation, strength, attention and cooperation (4). He recognized four principal apraxic deficits:

failure to produce a correct movement in response to a verbal command
failure to correctly imitate a movement performed by the examiner
failure to correctly perform a movement in response to seeing an object
failure to handle and use an object correctly.

Geschwind's analysis and teaching about apraxia reveals the fundamentals of his style: (a) a passion for the history of an idea, even when it has been discarded; (b) looking at what others are looking at and seeing something new; (c) appreciating the value of detailed clinical and pathological case study; (d) synthesis of observations, from daily life*, to novels, to current science; and (e) a love of talking about his thoughts and soliciting comments and criticisms.

EPILOGUE

As a first year medical student, Geschwind granted my unreasonable request for a weekly tutorial with him. I would read, and then meet with him to discuss my attempt to comprehend some aspect of behavioral neurology. My understanding of neurophysiology, neuroanatomy, and neurology was meager. I struggled for some time to fully follow his orations.

After several months, I came to one of those Friday sessions to disagree with Geschwind. He had asked me to read about right parietal lesions, the syndrome of left-sided neglect, and the associated confabulatory responses. In part II of his disconnection paper, Geschwind seemed to stretch the disconnexion theory too far. "The right hemisphere is probably always at a disadvantage in relation to the left, since the pathway from any part of it to the speech area is probably at least one neuron longer than the pathway from the corresponding part of the left hemisphere" (7). Geschwind then went on to note that Jackson (94), Mullan and Penfield (95), and others found that *déjà vu* most often resulted from right-seizure foci. "This tendency of the minor hemisphere to give rise to such illusions is not the result of emotion or memory in the minor hemisphere, but another example of the increased tendency to confabulatory response in cases of lesions of the association cortex on the right side."

I suggested that in the title of that section, "The Problem of Right Parietal Dominance," was the solution to the problem. The right parietal lobe was dominant for surveying and attending to space and the body. He opened his eyes wide, paused as I trembled inside—perhaps this would be our last session. He then launched into a 40-minute monologue, from which I could comprehend momentary bits and pieces. He circled back to the right parietal lobe, smiled, and said he thought that I was right. He had revised his ideas significantly. He liked my idea, but he broke my heart when he told me it was not new—Marsel Mesulam had already formulated it.

In his 1974 book, *Norman Geschwind: Selected Papers on Language and the Brain,* he ends the preface to DSAM with the comment that he has revised many of his ideas and plans to publish these revisions in book form. Geschwind never presented a revised

---

*He loved to cite the example of multiple motor pathways for facial expression—a volitional one arising in pyramidal pathways, and a mesial/subcortical pathway arising in cingulate, supplementary motor, amygdala, and subcortical sites that mediate smiling. A patient with a frontal motor cortex lesion would smile quite asymmetrically when asked to smile, but the smile would be perfectly symmetrical in response to a joke. In contrast, a patient with a limbic lesion might smile volitionally fairly well, but asymmetrically to a funny remark. "Only actors and politicians can fairly well reproduce a natural smile to command." (Geschwind, teaching rounds).

DSAM. The lure of a new, uncharted area—the developmental aspects of the brain and how immunity, hormonal influence, and cerebral development interact, would largely occupy Geschwind's thoughts during the next, final decade of his life.

When Geschwind studied at Harvard College and Medical School in the 1940s, academics did not consider neuroanatomy in relation to behavior. In his DSAM, Geschwind helped to make the brain's connection to behavior a fundamental tenet in the neurosciences (96). The connections between association cortices have been reconceived by Geschwind's students, creating a network approach to understanding human cognition (97–99). Ultimately, Geschwind refocused our thoughts on the clinical details—what the patient can and cannot do, a systematic approach to evaluate patients, an individual approach to see each patient, first compassionately as a human, and secondly, as an invaluable experiment of nature teaching us something if we can only be granted the curiosity, intelligence, patience, and perseverance to see what lies in front of us. Geschwind had all those qualities, in abundance. He refocused our thoughts towards a neuroanatomic model. How does the brain work this behavioral function? What are the roles of different areas? What role do the connections between different areas play? His genius shone brightly as he approached behavior—he never lost the child's fascination, he never lost his focus on mechanism and anatomy, he brought together thoughts and observations that would have never been linked in another mind. Geschwind brought topics such as the aphasias from a collection of bizarre symptom concatenations to a comprehensible group of language disorders. In DSAM, he helped create a foundation for modern behavioral neurology.

REFERENCES

1. Geschwind N. Disconnexion syndromes in animals and man. I. *Brain* 1965;88(2):237–294.
2. Geschwind N. Disconnexion syndromes in animals and man. II. *Brain* 1965;88(3):585–644.
3. Geschwind N. Preface, chapter II. *Selected works of Norman Geschwind on language and behavior.* Boston: Boston University Press, 1974.
4. Geschwind N. The anatomy of acquired disorders of reading. In: Money J, ed. *Reading disability.* Baltimore: Johns Hopkins Press, 1962;115–129.
5. Déjérine J. Sur un cas de cecite verbale avec agraphie, suivi d'autopsie. *Mem Soc Biolog* 1891;3:197–201.
6. Déjérine J. Contribution a l'etude anatomo-pathologique et clinique des differences variete verbale. *Mem Soc Biolog* 1892;4:61–90.
7. Bastian HC. *Treatise on aphasia and other speech defects.* London, 1898.
8. Geschwind N, Fusillo M. Color-naming defects in association with alexia. *Arch Neurol* 1966;15:137–146.
9. Judd T, Gardner H, Geschwind N. Alexia without agraphia in a composer. *Brain* 1983;106:435–457.
10. (Geschwind N, Kaplan E.) Random reports: human split-brain syndromes. *N Engl J Med* 1962;266:1013 (published anonymously).
11. Geschwind N, Kaplan E. A human cerebral deconnection syndrome: a preliminary report. *Neurology* 1962;12: 675–685.
12. Akelaitis AJ. Studies on the corpus callosum. The higher visual functions in each homonymous field following complete section of the corpus callosum. *Arch Neurol Psychiatry* 1941;45:788.
13. Akelaitis AJ. Studies on the corpus callosum. Study of the language-functions tactile and visual lexica and graphia unilaterally following section of the corpus collosum. *J Neuropath Exp Neurol* 1943; 226.
14. Akelaitis AJ. A study of the gnosis, praxis, and language following section of the corpus callosum and anterior commisure. *J Neurosurg* 1944;1:94.
15. Gazzaniga MS, Bogen JE, Sperry RW. *Proc Nat Acad Sci* 1962;48:1765.
16. Geschwind N. Carl Wernicke, the Breslau School and the history of aphasia. In: Carterette EC, ed. *Brain function,* vol III: *Speech, language, and communication.* Berkeley, CA: University of California Press, 1963;1–16.
17. Geschwind N. Wernicke's contribution to the study of aphasia. *Cortex* 1967;3:449–463.
18. Geschwind N. The work and influence of Wernicke. In: Cohen RS, Wartofsky MW, eds. *Boston studies in the philosophy of science,* vol IV. Dordrecht, Holland: D. Reidel, 1969;1–33.
19. Wernicke C. The symptom complex of aphasia: a psychological study on an anatomical basis. In: Cohen RS, Wartofsky MW, eds. *Boston studies in the philosophy of science,* vol IV. Dordrecht, Holland: D. Reidel, 1969; 34–97.

20. Flechsig P. Developmental (myelogenetic) localization of the cerebral cortex in the human subject. *Lancet* 1901;2:1027.
21. Lichtheim L. On aphasia. *Brain* 1885;7:433–484.
22. Wernicke C. The symptom-complex of aphasia. In: Church A, ed. *Diseases of the nervous system,* New York: Appleton, 1908:265–324.
23. Damasio H, Damasio AR. The localization of lesions in conduction aphasia. In: Kertesz A, ed. Localization in neuropsychology. Orlando, FL: Academic Press, 1983;231–243.
24. Goldstein K. Die transkortikalen Aphasien. *Jena* (pt II), 1917.
25. Goldstein K. *Language and language disturbances: aphasic symptom complexes and their significance for medicine and theory of language.* New York: Grune & Stratton, 1948.
26. Geschwind N, Quadfasel FA, Segarra JM. Isolation of the speech area. *Neuropsychologia* 1968;6:327–340.
27. Benson DF, Sheremata WA, Bouchard R, Segarra JM, Price D, Geschwind N. Conduction aphasia: a clinicopathological study. *Arch Neurol* 1973;28:339–356.
28. Liepmann H. *Ein Fall von reiner Sprachtaubheit.* Breslau, 1898.
29. Liepmann H. *Das Krankheitsbild der Apraxie ('motorischen Asymbolie').* Berlin, 1900.
30. Liepmann H, Storch E. *Mschr Psychiat Neurol* 1902;11:115.
31. Liepmann H, Maas O. *J Psychol Neurol* 1907;10:214.
32. Wilson SAK. *Brain* 1908;31:164.
33. Head H. *Aphasia and kindred disorders of speech.* Cambridge: Cambridge Univ Press, 1926.
34. Marie P, Chatelin C. Les trouble visuels dus aux lesions des voies optiques intracerebrales et de la sphere visuelle corticale dans les blessures du crane par coup de feu. *Rev Neurol (Paris)* 1915;22:882–925.
35. von Monakow C. Die Lokalisation im Grosshirm. The mechanism of vision, XVIII. Effects of destroying the visual associative areas of the monkey. *Genet Psychol Monogr* 1914;37:107–166.
36. Kleist K. *Gehirnpathologie.* Liepzig: JA Barth, 1934.
37. Lashley KS. *Brain mechanisms and intelligence.* Chicago: University of Chicago Press, 1929.
38. Aring CD. In: Bucy PC, ed. *The precentral motor cortex.* Clinical Symptomatology, Urbana, IL. 409–424.
39. Bailey P, Bonin G. *The isocortex of man.* Urbana, IL. 1951.
40. Bailey P, McCulloch WS. *The isocortex of the chimpanzee,* University of Illinois Press, Urbana, IL. 1950.
41. Kreig WJS. *Connections of the frontal cortex of the monkey.* Charles C. Thomas, Springfield, 1954.
42. NAUJA, WJH. Neural associations of the Amygdaloid complex in the monkey. Braun 85, 505–520. 1962.
43. Whitlock DG, Nauta WJH. *J Comp Neurol* 1956;106:183.
44. Meyers RE. *J Comp Neurol* 1962;118:1.
45. Nauta WJH. *Brain* 1962;85:505.
46. McCulloch WS, Garol HW. *J Neurophysiol* 1941;4:555.
47. Bailey P, von Bonnin GV, et al. Functional organization of temporal lobe of monkey *(Macaca mulatta)* and chimpanzee *(Pan satururs)*. *J Neurophysiol* 1943;6:121.
48. Bailey P, Bonnin G. *J Neurophysiol* 1943;6:129.
49. Pribram KH, Rosner BS, et al. *J Neurophysiol* 1954;17:336.
50. Kaada BR. In: *Handbook of physiology.* Washington, DC: American Physiological Society, 1960; sect 1, vol 2, p 1345.
51. Morrell F. *Epilepsia* 1960;1:538.
52. Kluver H, Bucy P. *J Psychol* 1938;5:33.
53. Bucy PC. *The precentral motor cortex.* University of Illinois Press, Urbana, IL; 1944.
54. Kennard MA. *Arch Neurol Psychiat* 1939;41:1153.
55. Bucy P, Kluver H. An anatomic investigation of the temporal lobe in monkeys. *J Comp Neurol* 1955;103: 151–252.
56. Welch K, Stuterville P. Experimental producion of unlateral neglect in monkeys. *Brain* 1958;81:341–347.
57. Weiskrantz L, Mishkin M. *Brain* 1958;81:406.
58. Wilson WA, Mishkin M. *J Comp Physiol* 1959;52:10.
59. Downer JDC. *Brain* 1959;82:251.
60. Ettlinger G, Morton HB. *Science* 1963;139:485.
61. Penfield W, Boldrey E. Cortical spread of epileptic discharge on the conditioning effect of habitual seizures and psychiatry. 1939;96.
62. Hecean H, Ajuriaguerra JD, David M. *Mschr Psychiat Neurol* 1952;123:239.
63. Bingley T. Mental symptoms in temporal lobe epilepsy and temporal lobe gliomas. *Acta Psychiat Scand* 1958 (suppl);120.
64. Segarra JM, Quadfasel FA. *Proceedings of the VII International Congress of Neurology*, vol II, 1961;377.
65. Kinsbourne M, Warrington EK. *J Neurol Neurosurg Psychiat* 1962;25:339.
66. Geschwind N. The development of the brain and the evolution of language. In: Stuart CIJM, ed. *Monograph series on languages and linguistics,* vol. 17. Washington, DC: George Washington University Press, 1964;155–169.
67. Hubel DH, Wiesel TN. Receptive fields and functional architecture in two nonstriate visual areas (18 and 19) of the cat. *J Neurophysiol* 1965;28:229–289.
68. Zeki S. *A vision of the brain.* Oxford, England: Blackwell Scientific Publications, 1993.
69. Wilbrand H. *Ophthalmiatrische Beitrage zur Diagnostik der Gehirkrankheiten.* Wiesbaden: JF Bergmann, 1884.
70. Verrey L. Hemiachromaqtopsie droite absolue. *Archs Ophtalmol* 1888;8:289–301.

71. MacKay G. A discussion on a contribution to the study of gemianopsia, with special reference to acquired colour. *Br Med J* 1888;2:1033–1037.
72. Harris W. Hemianopics, with special reference to its transient varieties. *Brain* 1897;20:308–364.
73. MacKay G, Dunlop JC. The cerebral lesions in a case of complete acquired colour-blindness. *Scot Med Surg* 1899;5:503–512.
74. Riddoch G. Dissociation of visual perception due to occipital injuries, with especial reference to appreciation of movement. *Brain* 1917;40:15–57.
75. Henschen SE. On the visual path and centre. *Brain* 1893;16:170–180.
76. Holmes G. Disturbances of vision by cerebral lesions. *Br J Ophthalmol* 1918;2:353–384.
77. Holmes G. The Ferrier Lecture: the organization of the visual cortex in man. *Proc R Soc Lond B* 1945;132: 348–361.
78. Zeki SM. Representation of central visual fields in prestriate cortex of monkey. *Brain Res* 1969;14:271–291.
79. Cragg BH. The topography of the afferent projections in the circumstiate visual cortex of the monkey studied by the Nauta method. *Vision Res* 1969;9:733–747.
80. Allman JM, Kaas JH. A representation of the visual field in the caudal third of the middle temporal gyrus of the owl monkey *(Aotus trivirgatus)*. *Brain Res* 1971;31:85–105.
81. Allman JM, Kass JH. Representation of the visual field in striate and adjoining cortex of the owl monkey *(Aotus trivirgatus)*. *Brain Res* 1971;35:89–106.
82. Zeki S, Ship S. The functional logic of cortical connections. *Nature* 1988;335:311–316.
83. Goldman-Rakic P. Modular organization of prefrontal cortex. *Trends Neurosci* 1984;7:419–429.
84. Schwartzkroin PA, Scharfman HE, Sloviter RS. Similarities in circuitry between Ammon's horn and dentate gyrus; local interactions and parallel processing. *Prog Brain Res* 1990;83:269–286.
85. Perkel DJ, Bullier J, Kennedy H. Topography of the afferent connectivity of area 17 in the macaque monkey: a double-labelling study. *J Comp Neurol* 1986;253:374–402.
86. Nunez PL. *Neocortical dynamics and human EEG rhythms.* New York: Oxford University Press, 1995.
87. Eckhorn R, Bauer R, Jordan W, et al. Coherent oscillations: a mechanism of feature linking in the visual cortex? Multiple electrode and correlation analysis in the cat. *Biol Cybern* 1988;60:121–130.
88. Gray CM, Konig P, Engel AK, Singer W. Oscillatory responses in cat visual cortex exhibit inter-columnar synchronization which reflects global stimulus properties. *Nature* 1989;338(B):334–337.
89. Engel AK, Konig P, Gray CM, Singer W. Stimulus-dependent neuronal in cat visual cortex: inter-columnar interaction as indicated by cross-correlation analysis. *Exp Neurol* 1990;6:12–29.
90. Horowitz JM. Evoked activity of single units and neural populations in the hippocampus of the cat. *Electroenceph Clin Neurophys* 1972;32:227–240.
91. Singer W. Search for coherence: a basic principle of cortical self-organization. *Concepts Neurosci* 1990;1:1–26.
92. Engel AK, König P, Kreiter AK, Singer W. Interhemispheric synchronization of oscillatory neuronal responses in cat visual cortex. *Science* 1991;252:1177–1179.
93. Edelman G. *Neural Darwinism: the theory of neuronal group selection.* New York: Basic Books, 1987.
94. Jackson JH. In: Taylor J, ed. Selected writings of John Hughlings Jackson. *Brain* 1880;3:192. (Reprinted: vol 1, 1958. New York, Basic Books.)
95. Mullan S, Penfield W. *Arch Neurol Psychiatry* 1959;81:269.
96. Absher JR, Benson DF. Disconnection syndromes: an overview of Geschwind's contributions. *Neurology* 1993;43:862–867.
97. Heilman KM, Watson RT, Valenstein E. Neglect and related disorders. In: Heilman KM, Valenstein E, eds. *Clinical Neuropsychology,* New York: Oxford University Press, 1985:243–93.
98. Damasio AR. Time-locked multiregional retroactivation: a systems-level proposal for the neural substrates of recall and recognition. *Cognition* 1989;33:25–62.
99. Mesulam M. Large-scale neurocognitive networks and distributed processing for attention, language and memory. *Ann Neurol* 1990;28:597–613.

18

Geschwind's Influence on the Study of Disorders of Attention

Edward Valenstein

Department of Neurology, University of Florida College of Medicine, Gainesville, Florida 32610–0236.

It is not surprising that Norman Geschwind's name rarely appears in the reference lists of the current burgeoning literature on the neuropsychology of attention, because his direct contributions to the study of attention were modest, especially when compared with his profound writings on, for example, disconnection syndromes, aphasia, apraxia, and agnosia. Nonetheless, in 1982, just 2 years before his death, he said in an address to the Royal Society of London that "attentional systems represent the highest level of cognitive accomplishment . . ." and that attentional disorders were a "frontier in neuropsychology" (1). Regrettably, he never had the opportunity to write more extensively on the elaborate systems that subserve attention, but he contributed to our clinical understanding of attentional deficits, and he had an important influence on research in attention.

In his address to the Royal Society, he distinguished between unilateral disorders of attention, which he thought included "a variety of conditions of various mechanisms," and global deficits of attention, in which the rules that governed the selectivity, maintenance, and appropriate shifting of attention were disrupted. I shall accordingly consider each in turn. It is important to point out, however, that Geschwind believed that "unilateral disturbances of orientation to one side of space are in some instances true disturbances of attention and the full understanding of their mechanism can be attained only by consideration of the more global disorders." Thus he used similar anatomic arguments to help explain each condition.

GESCHWIND'S INFLUENCE ON THE STUDY OF HEMISPATIAL INATTENTION (UNILATERAL NEGLECT)

Geschwind's reputation in the scientific community was established with the publication in 1965 of his landmark paper on disconnection syndromes (2). This monograph demonstrated his command of the neuroanatomic and behavioral animal literature and his ability to relate this work to the behavior of human beings with brain lesions, accomplishments that were unsurpassed by other neurologists at that time. Geschwind stressed the hierarchical nature of corticocortical connectivity, citing Flechsig's rule that primary sensory cortices have no long corticocortical connections but project only to immediately adjacent association cortices. These in turn are connected with higher-order unimodal, and then with polymodal, association cortices. The expansion of high-order polymodal association cortex in human beings was, he believed, the anatomic substrate for the development of language. Geschwind also interpreted in anatomic terms the process by which animals learn stimulus–reward associations. In the visual modality, the stimulus is elaborated in the hierarchy of occipital and inferotemporal visual association cortices, and its reward significance is established through connections with limbic areas in the anteromedial temporal lobes. He thought that the connections were likely reciprocal, providing a means by which limbic structures could affect perceptions. As we shall see, the hierarchical organization of the cerebral cortex and the relationship of limbic cortex to the highest-order association cortices were integral to the mechanisms proposed by Geschwind and his students to explain attentional disorders.

When Geschwind became director of the Harvard Neurological Unit at Boston City Hospital in 1969, he recruited Dr. Deepak N. Pandya, a physician and neuroanatomist who was investigating cortical connections in primates. Dr. Pandya continued his studies using Dr. Derek Denny-Brown's primate facility on the top floor of the Harvard Medical Building. At the Boston City Hospital, Geschwind inherited a group of residents who had been recruited by Denny-Brown. One of these residents, Dr. Kenneth Heilman, was fascinated by the neglect syndrome, in which patients appeared completely unaware of stimuli in one half of space even though there was no evidence that their brain lesions affected primary sensory pathways. Geschwind directed Heilman to the 1958 paper by Welsh and Stuteville (3) and, thereby, to previous studies by Bianchi (4) and Kennard and Ectors (5). Welsh and Stuteville had described visual, somatesthetic, and auditory neglect in monkeys after small unilateral lesions were surgically created in the frontal arcuate sulcus. Heilman had noted similar trimodal neglect in patients with right hemisphere lesions. In reviewing the literature, he found scant mention of auditory disturbances in patients with neglect, and no reference to auditory neglect in monkeys with parietal or temporal lesions. Because the predominate lesion in patients with neglect affected the right parietal lobe, he wanted to try to reproduce the neglect syndrome in animals by creating parietal lesions. Dr. Geschwind and Dr. Pandya were kind enough to allow him to use monkeys from Dr. Denny-Brown's colony.* Furthermore, in selecting the site for lesioning, they suggested that the lesion be designed to selectively destroy the regions of parietal and temporal cortex that Pandya and Kuypers (6) had previously demonstrated to be polymodal association areas (areas that receive input from the association cortices of two or more modalities). Pandya and Kuypers (6) had suggested that both the frontal arcuate cortex and the inferior parietal lobule (IPL) represented areas of polymodal convergence, that the regions were connected with each other, and that "somewhat similar unilateral neglect" had been shown to arise from lesions in either location (5,7–9). Heilman and Pandya proceeded to ablate the IPL and both banks of the superior temporal sulcus (STS) in four rhesus monkeys (Fig. 1). Three monkeys with control lesions in the anterior temporal lobe had no neglect. The experimental monkeys developed contralateral neglect to visual, tactile, and auditory stimuli (10,11).

In these early publications, there was no general formulation of the mechanisms underlying unilateral neglect. But several points were made. First, all patients with auditory inattention whose cases were described up to that time also had visual and somatesthetic hemineglect. Second, the lesions producing unilateral neglect in monkeys did not affect primary sensory pathways, and, conversely, it was known that lesions of primary pathways did not produce neglect. Third—and here the input of Geschwind and Pandya is

---

*It is sobering to consider that an experiment requiring the use of seven primates was accomplished without the investigators first having to submit to institutional review boards or their animal care committees and without their having procured additional grant support.

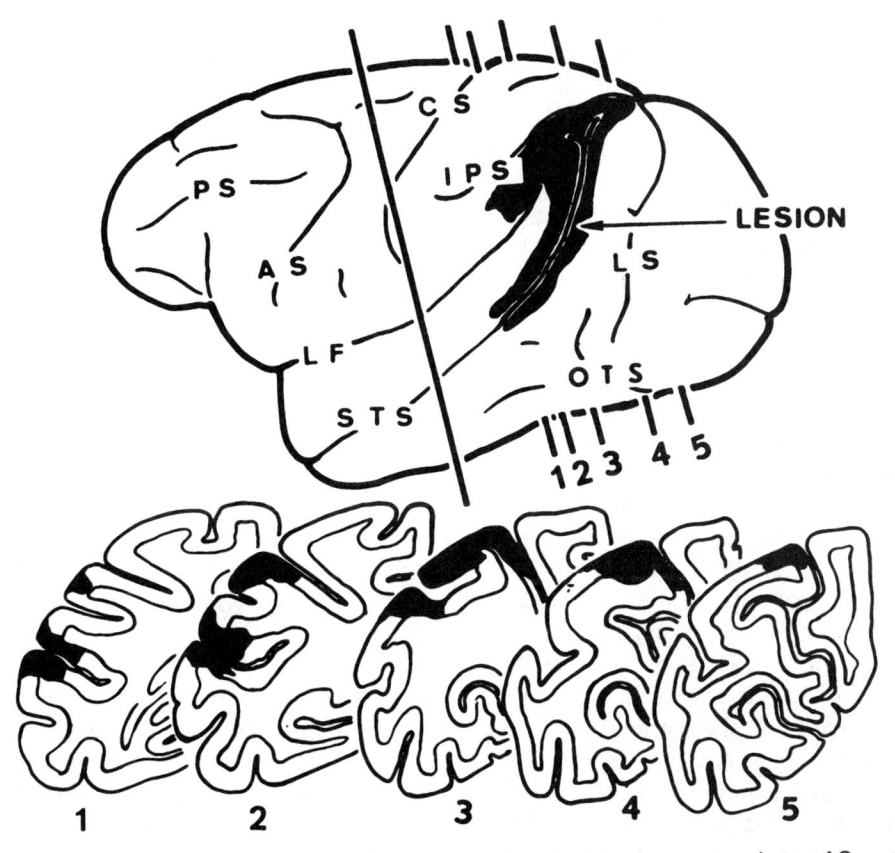

FIG. 1. The extent of the lesions causing unilateral neglect in rhesus monkeys. AS, arcuate sulcus; IPS, intraparietal sulcus; LF, lateral fissure; LS, lunate sulcus; PS, principal sulcus; STS, superior temporal sulcus; OTS, occipital temporal sulcus. (From ref. 11, with permission.)

clear—lesions that did induce neglect affected polymodal sensory association cortices: "In order to obtain auditory inattention one must ablate areas that associate the association areas of . . . different sensory modalities" (11).

The absence of a coherent formulation of the mechanisms underlying unilateral neglect was congruent with what I recall of Geschwind's clinical teaching at the time of my residency at Boston City Hospital (1968–1971). Geschwind did mention that aspects of the neglect syndrome suggested the confabulations of a left hemisphere disconnected from right hemisphere sensory association cortices, a theory detailed in his 1965 monograph on disconnection syndromes. After damage to these high-order sensory association cortices, "the left side of the body and of space is then 'lost.'" Confabulatory responses could entail "a major readjustment of all space . . . distort[ing the] . . . body image." Even in that paper, Geschwind admitted that "this is a very tentative suggestion which probably needs recasting in a clearer form. . . ." Elsewhere in this paper he suggested that denial of illness (anosognosia) might similarly reflect a disconnection from limbic influences. I recall him frequently (in 1969 and 1970) remarking, during rounds, on the emotional flatness of some patients with right hemisphere lesions and speculating very tentatively that the right hemisphere might in some way be "dominant" for emotion (see also Chapter 23). At that time, however, he did not talk about the right hemisphere playing a special role in attention.

In 1970, after completing his residency, Dr. Heilman took a position at the University of Florida in Gainesville, where he continued his study of unilateral neglect. From this point, any influence Geschwind had was indirect, because Heilman's subsequent work on neglect was independent. Using radionuclide scan localization, Heilman and Valenstein (12) demonstrated that 9 of 10 patients with trimodal neglect had right parietotemporal lesions; one had a left dorsolateral frontal lesion. The frontal localization could be explained if the neglect syndrome was in fact related to damage to polymodal association cortices. This concept was supported by the investigators' finding six additional patients with neglect induced by right frontal lobe lesions (13). Three of these lesions were dorsolateral, involving areas analogous to those damaged in Welch and Stuteville's monkeys. The fact that in the other three the lesions were medial required explanation. Pandya and Kuypers (6) had found that both periarcuate and parietotemporal association cortices projected to the cingulate gyrus. Heilman suggested that neglect resulted from an inability of sensory stimuli to "excite or alert" the animal and that pathways from multimodal sensory association cortices to limbic areas (including the cingulate gyrus) were necessary for this to occur. In turn, limbic connections with brainstem reticular systems involved in arousal might provide a mechanism by which cortically processed stimuli could alert the organism (13,14). Dr. Robert Watson, while still a neurology resident at the University of Florida, set up a primate laboratory to investigate these ideas. He found that neglect could be produced in monkeys by lesions of the cingulate gyrus (14) or mesencephalic reticular formation (15). Thus, by 1974, Heilman and his colleagues had adduced considerable evidence to suggest that unilateral neglect resulted from a disturbance in a "cortico-limbic-reticular loop," the normal function of which was to produce arousal and orienting in response to salient sensory stimuli. The inclusion of high-order association cortices in this loop provides a means by which attention can be preferentially given to meaningful stimuli. Later, Watson et al. (16) suggested that the reticular nucleus of the thalamus may function to gate sensory stimuli in response to input from the cerebral cortex.

Whereas, in monkeys, unilateral neglect appeared to be similar regardless of the hemisphere damaged, neglect in human beings was clearly more severe with lesions of the right hemisphere (17–19). During the 1970s, Heilman and his colleagues made several important observations about patients with right hemisphere disease. They demonstrated that patients with right hemisphere lesions and unilateral neglect failed to detect emotional intonation in speech (11). Minnesota Multiphasic Personality Inventory (MMPI) profiles of left- and right-hemisphere-damaged patients differed, with depression being a feature of left- but not of right-hemisphere-damaged groups (20). Patients with unilateral neglect from right hemisphere lesions also had absent or markedly attenuated electrodermal responses, even when stimulated on the normal (right) side, in contrast to left-hemisphere-damaged patients, who often demonstrated increased electrodermal responses (21). Thus, right hemisphere damage resulted in decreased emotional responsiveness and bilaterally decreased arousal. This hemispheric functional asymmetry was confirmed by studies of normal subjects: Heilman and Van den Abell analyzed reaction times (22) and electroencephalographic desynchronization (23) in normal human subjects in response to lateralized stimuli. Stimuli to the left visual field/right hemisphere were more effective in reducing reaction time of the right hand than stimuli to the right visual field, and the electroencephalogram (EEG) of the right parietal lobe showed desynchronization with stimuli to either field, whereas the EEG of the left parietal lobe showed desynchronization only to right-sided stimuli. These findings suggested that the right hemisphere monitored stimuli in either hemifield and was able to activate (reduce reaction time in) both hemispheres. This hypothesis helped to explain why unilateral neglect was more common and more severe with right than with left hemisphere lesions.

Monkeys and humans with neglect tended not to use the limbs contralateral to their lesion, even though they were not paralyzed (3,4). This lack of movement was difficult to explain entirely on the basis of sensory hypoarousal. Watson et al. (24) developed a paradigm to distinguish between motor and sensory aspects of neglect in the monkey. They suggested that monkeys be trained to respond with the limb contralateral to a stimulus. After undergoing unilateral frontal arcuate ablations, monkeys responded normally with the arm ipsilateral to the lesion when stimulated on the opposite leg. This response indicated that the animals did not neglect contralesional stimuli but failed to respond with the arm contralateral to the lesion when stimulated on the leg ipsilateral to the lesion, even though ipsilesional stimuli should have been appreciated (24). Hemiakinesia or motor neglect could not be explained on the basis of sensory inattention and was therefore a separate component of the neglect syndrome.

In summary, Heilman and colleagues suggested that unilateral neglect could result from lesions in a variety of interconnected brain areas involved in mediating attention to stimuli, preparation for action, or both. Brainstem and thalamic regions were critical for arousal. The cortical regions involved were high-order association cortices and limbic-associated (cingulate) cortices, the latter presumably involved in defining the emotional significance of stimuli. Anterior lesions might be associated with deficits of "intention." The strong tendency for severe unilateral neglect to be associated with lesions of the right hemisphere might be explained by evidence suggesting that, in normal persons, the right hemisphere can monitor stimuli delivered to either hemisphere and prepare either hemisphere for action. In contrast, the left hemisphere is more narrowly focused on contralateral stimuli and activity (25).

In the meantime, anatomic research in Dr. Pandya's laboratory provided additional information about the connectivity of the monkey parietal lobe. Working with Dr. Pandya and Dr. Gary Van Hoesen, Dr. Marek-Marsel Mesulam, a resident in Dr. Geschwind's program, used a technique of retrograde neuron labeling with horseradish peroxidase that he had perfected to restudy projections to the dorsal IPL (area 7a or PG) of the monkey. Mesulam and colleagues (26) confirmed that area PG received input principally from polymodal association cortices, including the superior temporal gyrus and periarcuate (prefrontal) cortex. They also demonstrated a major contribution from the cingulate and retrosplenial cortex. They suggested that different aspects of attention might be integrated by these three interconnected cortical areas: sensory and spatial integration in the IPL, integration of motivational significance in the cingulate gyrus, and efferent integration in the prefrontal (periarcuate) cortex. They also demonstrated anatomic connections of area PG with the intralaminar thalamus and with the basal forebrain, locus ceruleus, and raphe nuclei, areas that might modulate activity in area PG according to the organism's level of arousal. In 1981, Mesulam elegantly restated these ideas in a very influential paper (27). Like Heilman and colleagues, he explained unilateral neglect as a deficit in attention with contributions from sensory, motor, limbic, and reticular pathways, in which the right hemisphere played a special role. Mesulam used the computer analogy of networks to explain why lesions in different regions could have similar (but not identical) effects.

Evidence from anatomic studies (cited earlier in this chapter) and physiologic (28,29) studies in primates supported the importance of the IPL in spatial attention. In humans, unilateral neglect is most commonly associated with lesions of the right IPL (30). Although it is tempting to consider these lines of evidence mutually reinforcing (27,31,32), two difficulties arise. First, the IPLs in human beings and monkeys may not be homologous areas (Fig. 2). Even though in both humans and monkeys the intraparietal sulcus (IPS) separates the superior parietal lobule (SPL) and the IPL, in humans

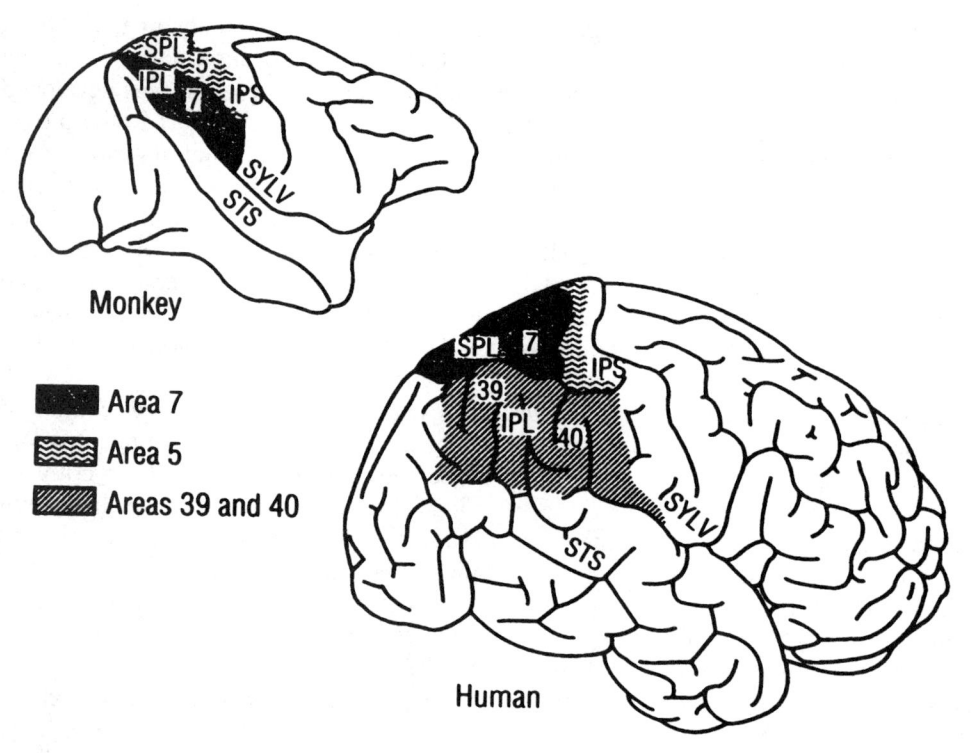

FIG. 2. Comparison of the monkey and human parietal lobes, demonstrating displacement of areas 5 and 7 above the intraparietal sulcus (IPS) in humans. SPL, superior parietal lobule; IPL, inferior parietal lobule; STS, superior temporal sulcus; SYLV, sylvian fissure. (From ref. 41, with permission.)

Brodmann's area 7 is above the IPS and, therefore, part of the SPL, whereas in monkeys Brodmann's area 7 occupies the IPL. It is variously argued that the cortex below the IPS in humans, areas 39 and 40, has no homolog in the monkey (33), is homologous with area 7 (areas 7a and 7b of the Vogts or areas PG and PF of von Bonin and Bailey) (34), or is homologous in part with cortex within the monkey's STS (13,35,36). Second, although lesions restricted to area 7 in the monkey have produced misreaching (37,38), they have not been associated with severe unilateral neglect. Lesions causing neglect in monkeys that have involved the IPL have also involved STS cortex. Monkeys with bilateral lesions of the STS show striking inattention to visual, auditory, and somesthetic stimuli (39), and animals with unilateral lesions (40) have difficulty orienting to contralateral visual, somatosensory, and auditory stimuli. We therefore compared monkeys with lesions restricted to either the IPL or STS (41). Four of 5 STS lesions were associated with unilateral neglect. In striking contrast, 0 of 6 IPL lesions was associated with unilateral neglect.

Why might damage to the STS be more likely to cause neglect than damage to the IPL? Ungerleider and Mishkin (42) proposed that the visual projections from primary visual cortex (V1) divide into two major parallel pathways, a dorsal pathway projecting to parietal cortex subserving localization of objects in space, and a ventral pathway to inferotemporal visual association cortex subserving object identification. Watson and colleagues (41) argued that IPL (area 7a), a convergence area for the dorsal pathway, would have little direct input from the ventral object identification pathway, whereas areas in the STS have input from both pathways, in addition to having connections with dorsolateral prefrontal cortex, cingulate cortex, and reticular pathways. Most corticocortical connections are reciprocated; thus the STS, after responding to convergent inputs on the nature and position of a visual stimulus, as modified by limbic input on its biologic significance, may, by means of reciprocal cortical connections, modify the responsiveness of lower-order visual cortical areas to this stimulus. Similar pathways in somatosensory and auditory systems may exist, again with convergence in the STS. Thus, damage to the STS may induce trimodal neglect. In addition, stimulation of the STS in the monkey can increase brainstem reticular activity (43), providing a means by which the STS can influence arousal. Damage to the STS may thus make it more difficult for an animal to enhance cortical activity in response to a biologically significant stimulus. Watson et al. (41) pointed out that patients with unilateral neglect act as if they are unaware of the stimuli.

Geschwind argued that cortex in the human STS and IPL represents an expansion of polysensory cortical regions in the monkey (2). In the human left hemisphere, these cortical areas are important for language. "It is tempting to speculate . . . that the same regions in the right hemisphere are indispensable for the complex integrative processes required for the effective execution of selective attention" (44). Geschwind believed that hemisphere dominance patterns for attention were established before specialization for language. Whereas hemispheric language dominance is quite variable in left-handers, it is a common clinical impression that both left- and right-handers show more severe unilateral neglect with right hemisphere lesions. Geschwind believed that "there is a group of right-hemisphere functions that are closely linked precisely because they all relate to functions of monitoring the environment and making decisions as to shifting on the basis of the importance of the monitored stimuli for survival of the self or of the species. The importance of the right hemisphere for attention and emotion, and for the configuration of space, appear to be possibly related to this function. Furthermore, it appears likely to me that this form of cerebral dominance first appeared in the animal kingdom with right-sided localization many millions of years ago." Geschwind, however, appeared to consider some spatial deficits as being unrelated to the core attentional mechanisms, whereas "the great predominance of inattention to the left side of space and of the body can be accounted for only by a theory that takes into account the dominance relations of . . . more global attentional systems. . . ." The clinical deficit associated with failure of these more global attentional disturbances was not hemispatial neglect but the acute confusional syndrome.

GLOBAL ATTENTIONAL DISTURBANCES

Acute confusional states most commonly result not from focal brain lesions but rather from systemic metabolic disturbances. It may seem curious that a neurologist who was deeply involved in explaining behavior in terms of anatomy should choose to investigate disorders that most commonly had no obvious neuroanatomic correlate. In part, Geschwind's clinical interest in these disorders arose from the need to avoid mistaking symptoms such as nonaphasic misnaming and the agraphia associated with confusional states from similar disorders that predicted focal brain pathology. In part, he was fascinated by the complex symptomatology that these disorders presented. Finally, he demonstrated that, upon occasion, these more global defects in attention could result from focal lesions in specific brain regions.

I recall, from my residency, Geschwind's vivid descriptions of the behavior of patients with the acute confusional state. He was particularly intrigued by the syndrome of nonaphasic misnaming that had been described by Edwin Weinstein in the 1950s and 1960s

(45,46). Geschwind believed that Weinstein's important observations were in danger of being forgotten. Nonaphasic misnaming was usually associated with "paramnesia." Patients with this syndrome often appear disoriented, even when their responses indicate that they should have sufficient knowledge to provide the correct response. Thus, for example, one of Dr. Weinstein's patients said she was in the "Mount Cyanide Rest Home," instead of the Mt. Sinai Hospital. Other patients might correctly name the hospital but place it closer to their home and, when pressed, state that there are two hospitals, one of which is in their neighborhood. The tendency to create a neighborhood instance of the hospital was an example of what Weinstein called "reduplicative paramnesia." Capgras syndrome is a particularly striking form of reduplicative paramnesia: patients with this syndrome claim that familiar persons are not actually the people they appear to be, but strangers who are otherwise identical (47). More commonly, patients make naming errors that have a tendency to propagate to other aspects of their environment: thus, patients who state that they are at home might misname objects in their hospital room to correspond to objects at home, however improbable—for example, calling an intravenous pole a Christmas tree—and the patient who responded that he was in a bus "may then say that the examining physician is the driver, that those around him are passengers and that the bed he is in is used by the driver for resting" (48). Geschwind added to these observations that such patients often were agraphic, even though they had no other language deficits. Chédru and Geschwind (49,50) described agraphia in 30 of 31 patients with an acute confusional state. The agraphia consisted of motor impairments, spatial disorders, and reluctance to write, as well as syntactical, spelling, and other linguistic disorders. Some patients had occasional word-finding difficulty and made a few errors in reading, but the agraphia was an isolated disturbance in many patients and the most striking linguistic abnormality in all. Patients performed poorly on tests of temporospatial orientation and attention but normally on tests of spontaneous speech, comprehension, oral spelling, and praxis (50). Chédru and Geschwind speculated that writing, a late-acquired skill not as overlearned as speaking or reading, is more "fragile" and thus more likely to be disrupted by general disturbances in attention.

In his address to the Royal Society of London in 1982, Geschwind placed the acute confusional syndrome within the broader context of confusional states (1). Confusional states are disorders of attention. Geschwind, while disclaiming any attempt to address the problem of attention systematically, listed five important components of normal attention: selectivity, coherence, distractibility, universality, and sensitivity. Selectivity refers to the ability to select from all available stimuli those that are to be attended. Selective attention must be maintained long enough to enable appropriate thought or action. Geschwind called this persistence of attention coherence. Of course, focused attention must be interrupted if a more important event takes place. The necessity of monitoring the internal and external environment continually while maintaining focused attention, and of maintaining an optimal balance between these aspects of attention "confers the utmost complexity on the system." There must be rules for distractibility that take into account the state of the animal and the nature of the distracting event, such as its novelty and biological significance. Universality indicates that the monitoring system must "register as many unattended stimuli as possible, both externally and internally." Finally, the rules governing shifts of attention must reflect sensitivity to the state of the organism. A hungry animal will attend to food differently from a satiated one.

Geschwind goes on to describe the clinical characteristics of confusional states, among which he includes paramnesias, propagation of error, inattention to environmental stimuli, and isolated agraphia, mentioned previously, plus a tendency to use occupational jargon, lack of concern about or denial of illness, and the making of seemingly witty or amusing remarks through random juxtaposition of ideas and phrases. But the cardinal feature of confusional states is the loss of coherence of thought. I can do no better than to abstract from one of Geschwind's articulate consultations. This quote will, I hope, convey to readers who have not experienced clinical rounds with Geschwind the nature of his clinical teaching. In this neurological consultation, dated January 16, 1979, Geschwind describes a physician who had suffered a right hemisphere stroke 3 months earlier. The patient had uncharacteristic emotional outbursts after the stroke, which had subsided. He was left with a left hemiparesis and left visual neglect. Dr. Geschwind examined the patient in the patient's room at home.

> He looked quite alert and awake and carried on a very good conversation. When he was pressed by me, he nearly always performed quite normally. Thus I was able to get him to identify the day of the week, the month, the year. He knew who I was instantly, although he had last seen me over a year before. He recalled in great detail the circumstances of the visit to me. He was able to disentangle, with some effort, the story of his original admission to the hospital. On the other hand, he denied knowledge of the precise episodes in which he had shown unusual rage. He was also able to copy a cube, do calculations, identify right and left, and identify fingers. There was no aphasia. Indeed, what was striking was a mental state that seemed to be remarkably normal.
>
> There were, however, certain clues that what we were dealing with here was not really a loss of memory or language, but rather a confusional state in the strict sense, or a delirium as some might prefer to call it, although of mild degree. He would thus, from time to time, amalgamate certain data that should not have gone together. Thus, having perfectly correctly identified where he was and why I was seeing him, he then proceeded to say that the room was not the real room in Cambridge, but was a reconstruction made by his wife so that he would be in familiar surroundings wherever he went. He would, at times, quite unexpectedly speak of having traveled great distances on the previous day. He seemed a bit surprised when I pointed out that these interpretations were not fully accurate. A further clue that he was in a confusional state was found when he was asked to write. He wrote a perfectly correct description of the weather, but the second line was written over almost entirely over the first one.
>
> In brief, the major difficulty in his mental state is not that of diminution of consciousness in the usual sense, nor of memory disorder or loss of intellectual function in the usual sense, but rather the inability to maintain a coherent stream of thought or action. This type of disorder is, of course, very familiar in the aged after almost any type of event and most of the time the major insult lies outside of the central nervous system. It can occur, however, with lesions in the central nervous system and for reasons that I will not detail here, particularly lesions in the right hemisphere, which he has, of course, suffered.

CONFUSIONAL STATES AFTER FOCAL RIGHT HEMISPHERE LESIONS

Geschwind's association of acute confusional states with focal right hemisphere lesions had some precedent in the clinical literature. Elements of the acute confusional state were known to be common in patients with unilateral neglect (51). In 1963, Boudin and colleagues (52) reported on nine patients with putative right hemisphere lesions whose clinical presentation was dominated by acute confusion. Only two had pathological localization, both to the right temporal lobe. Neither of these two patients had focal neurological signs, but clinical details were sparse. Juillet and colleagues (53) reported four additional cases the following year, but the provided clinical details indicated either that the confusional states were part of a more extensive right hemisphere syndrome including visuospatial dysfunction (two cases), or that there were additional lesions outside the right temporal lobe. In the 1970s, when computed tomography (CT) scanning had just become available, Mesulam and colleagues (44) described three patients with lesions involving, respectively, parietotemporal, parieto-occipital, and inferior frontal cortex. These patients were inattentive, could not maintain a coherent stream of thought, and had cognitive deficits similar to those described by Chédru and Geschwind (50) in patients with acute confusional states from nonfocal disorders. Elementary signs suggestive of a lateralized hemisphere lesion were mild or absent. The authors stated that before the era of CT scanning, such disorders would probably have been misdiagnosed as metabolic encephalopathy. The authors predicted that with the advent of routine neuroimaging, this presentation of focal right hemisphere pathology would come to be recognized as typical and perhaps not uncommon.

Geschwind believed that right hemisphere dominance for attention could account for global attentional deficits after focal right hemisphere lesions. Although the right hemisphere's superiority in certain spatial tasks was considered in part the basis of right hemisphere attentional dominance, the absence of obvious hemispatial neglect in patients presenting with acute confusional states from right hemisphere lesions was difficult to explain. Evidence that the right hemisphere is able to attend to stimuli in either hemispace, whereas the left hemisphere attends only to stimuli in the contralateral (right) hemispace (22,23,54), would help to explain global attentional disorders in patients with hemispatial neglect from right hemisphere lesions (25,51,55), but it would not explain the absence of hemispatial neglect in right-hemisphere-damaged patients presenting with the acute confusional state, because left hemisphere attentional mechanisms should bias attention toward the right (23,56). If right hemisphere attentional dominance is not dependent entirely on right hemisphere mechanisms for spatial attention, it is possible that a lesion could spare these spatial mechanisms and yet impair attention globally.

Subsequent clinical studies have not entirely resolved these issues. Mullally and colleagues (57) assessed the frequency of focal lesions among 60 patients with acute confusional state on a neurology in-patient consultation service. The etiology in 24 patients was systemic. The remaining 36 patients had focal lesions consistent with pathology on the basis of either definite CT findings (26 patients) or definite clinical signs alone (10 patients). Thirteen had lesions in the right parietal lobe, 4 had right temporal lesions, and 2 had changes in the left occipital lobe. These data were published only in abstract form; no information was provided concerning neglect in the confused patients with right hemisphere lesions. Dunne et al. (55) retrospectively assessed the incidence of confusional states or acute dementia in 661 patients with acute stroke. Of 592 noncomatose patients, 44% were disoriented or confused on admission. After patients with a history of stroke or psychiatric disease, with active toxic or metabolic disorders that might impair attention, or with aphasia or obvious hemineglect were excluded, there remained only 15 patients who had acute-onset confusion or dementia. Nine had acute confusion lasting from 1 week to 3 months, and seven had acute onset dementia that did not resolve. Of the nine patients presenting with acute confusional states, eight had right middle cerebral artery (MCA) lesions, of whom five had visual or somatosensory inattention and one without inattention had mild hemiparesis. Only two of these patients had no elementary neurologic findings.

Other studies addressed the occurrence of acute confusional states in patients with right MCA territory infarctions. Schmidley and Messing (58) found only two such patients among 46 with right MCA infarctions. Caplan and colleagues (59) reviewed the records of ten patients identified as having infarctions in the territory of the inferior division of the right MCA. Three had severe agitated delirium at onset, two had intermittent agitation and mood swings, two were restless and had difficulty cooperating for tests, and one was inappropriately unconcerned and jocular. Nine of these ten patients had either visual field defects or visual neglect; the remaining patient was too agitated to be tested. The presence of agitation correlated with lesions involving the superior and middle temporal gyri; the patients without agitation had more superior (parietal) lesions. The authors suggested that temporal lesions might have been better situated to disrupt corticolimbic pathways regulating emotion. Mori and Yamadori (60) studied 41 consecutive patients with acute right MCA strokes. Of these, 25 had an acute confusional state, as defined by poor performance on the minimental status examination and the assessment of clinicians, and six had an acute agitated delirium. Patients with acute confusion without agitation had large lesions that most often included frontal cortex and basal ganglia. Agitated delirium was associated with involvement of the inferior division of the MCA.

The studies just cited suggest that an acute confusional state is a frequent accompaniment of stroke, but that other neurological abnormalities, such as unilateral neglect, are obvious in the vast majority of such patients. In a small number, the localizing neurological findings are more subtle, and very infrequently they are absent entirely, so that the patient presents in a fashion that is perhaps indistinguishable from one with metabolic encephalopathy. Finally, among patients with right hemisphere stroke and confusion, agitation may correlate with temporal rather than parietal lesions.

OTHER LESIONS ASSOCIATED WITH THE ACUTE CONFUSIONAL STATE

Clearly, lesions affecting right hemisphere high-order association cortex are not the only focal lesions to be associated with the acute confusional state. Elements of confusional behavior may also be seen in patients with acute frontal lobe, basal forebrain, and diencephalic lesions. Large lesions in either hemisphere are commonly associated with altered arousal and attention. Interruption of pathways involved in selective attention and arousal, diaschisis, severe acute cognitive deficits, and secondary metabolic dysfunction (61,62) are among the possible mechanisms. Discrete lesions affecting inferotemporal cortex may also cause agitation and confusion (63,64). Mesulam et al. (44) suggested that lesions in these cases involved heteromodal convergence pathways in inferotemporal cortex, and that the explanation for acute confusion might therefore be similar to that given for patients with right parietotemporal or frontal lesions. Devinsky and colleagues (65), however, reported that in 4 of 4 personally observed patients with acute confusion from posterior cerebral artery territory infarction, and in 14 of 15 additional patients cited in the literature, left-sided lesions predominated. Confusion in these cases cannot be explained by right hemisphere dominance for attentional mechanisms. If acute confusion in these cases resulted from bilateral ischemia or associated brainstem or diencephalic ischemia, one would not expect such a predominance of left hemisphere lesions. Among the explanations the authors offer for left lateralization in these cases is the involvement of retrieval or sequencing of language-encoded memories. The marked predominance of left-sided lesions among patients with amnesia from posterior cerebral artery territory infarctions is consistent with this view (66).

Acute confusional states accompanying focal lesions in different regions of the brain may thus have different underlying mechanisms. That clinical differences among the confusional states caused by lesions in different locations have not been better identified to date probably reflects the difficulty of examining inattentive patients. In contrast, a multitude of distinct deficits have been described affecting hemispatial attention. For example, hemineglect may be restricted to one modality, to personal or peripersonal space

(67), or to one coordinate system (vertical, radial, or lateral) (25). Furthermore, hemispheric differences in attention are not merely of degree but of kind. The left hemisphere may be better at attending to details and the right to distributing attention over a large region (68). It is therefore no longer possible to consider unilateral neglect to be a single deficit that varies only in degree. Similarly, the acute confusional state is a clinical entity that has many possible underlying mechanisms.

THE BRILLIANCE OF ATTENTIONAL ORGANIZATION

Attention is a complex multicomponential process, not a single brain function that occurs in a particular hemisphere or region. We are unable to be aware of all internal and external stimuli simultaneously, so that we must continually select among competing stimuli and response alternatives; attention is the process that allows for triage based on the importance of the stimuli. Our brief and selective review suggests anatomic correlates for the components of attention that Geschwind identified. *Selectivity* is the process whereby some stimuli (both internal and external) succeed in coming into awareness, and it probably reflects in part successful competition to attain processing in higher-order association cortex. *Coherence* is the ability to maintain related stimuli in awareness over time while avoiding distraction by irrelevant internal and external stimuli, a function normally attributed to the frontal lobes. *Distractibility* reflects the ability of some stimuli to enter into awareness, presumably by virtue of the spread of activation to entrain reticular, thalamic, and limbic activity. Distracting stimuli, distinguished by such features as loudness, brightness, or pain, may require only low-level processing, whereas other stimuli, such as name recognition, may become distracting only after cortical analysis. To be distracted by significant stimuli, we must continually monitor "as many unattended stimuli as possible, both externally and internally" (1), a process Geschwind called *universality*. The fact that we continually process stimuli of which we are not aware is dramatically demonstrated by the phenomenon of implicit memory, which has been investigated extensively in recent years (69). Similar phenomena occur in patients with neglect, whose behavior can be shown to be affected by neglected stimuli (70,71). Marshall and Halligan's (70) patient with left-sided neglect was shown line drawings of two houses, the left side of one being on fire. She deemed the drawings identical but consistently chose the one not on fire when asked to select the one she would prefer to live in. In this instance, monitoring was present but did not reach awareness when it should have. Concurrent monitoring of internal stimuli enables weight to be given to stimuli according to the needs of the organism *(sensitivity)*. Attention then becomes an emergent property of numerous brain areas engaged in multiple tasks. The network analogy (27) helps explain how brain regions specialized for particular aspects of stimulus processing can contribute to awareness via connections with the various critical components of attentional systems, and how they also provide the flexibility that such a system requires. Computational models of brain function are beginning to address issues related to selective attention, but just at the level of a single modality (72,73). The mechanisms by which multiple stimuli of different modalities compete for awareness remain to be elucidated, although almost certainly they will involve the brain regions discussed in this brief review of unilateral neglect.

CONCLUSIONS

The phenomena that we recognize as constituting attention thus result from highly complex interactions among many brain regions. The difficulties involved in defining the phenomena and their complexity understandably discouraged investigation in this area for years. Geschwind had no respect for those who argued that a behavioral phenomenon should not be investigated because it was too complex. Had he been discouraged by complexity, he would not have attempted to explain the developmental and anatomic bases of aphasia, apraxia, and agnosia in 1965, and many neurologists might have continued to consider these disorders too complex for meaningful scientific study. Although his direct contribution to the study of attention was perhaps small, Geschwind infused his students with the courage to study this difficult subject. His description more than a decade ago of the systems underlying attention reflects his own enthusiastic response to this complexity: "In most subhuman species the attentional systems represent the highest level of cognitive accomplishment, but my guess is that the human attentional systems surpass them in the brilliance of their organization."

Acknowledgment

This work was supported in part by the Department of Veterans Affairs.

REFERENCES

1. Geschwind N. Disorders of attention: a frontier in neuropsychology. *Trans R Soc London, Ser B* 1982;298:173–185.
2. Geschwind N. Disconnexion syndromes in animals and man. (2 parts). *Brain* 1965;88:237–294; 585–644.
3. Welsh K, Stuteville P. Experimental production of unilateral neglect in monkeys. *Brain* 1958;18:497–522.
4. Bianchi L. The functions of the frontal lobes. *Brain* 1895;18:497–522.
5. Kennard MA, Ectors L. Forced circling movements in monkeys following lesions of the frontal lobes. *J Neurophysiol* 1938;1:45–54.
6. Pandya DN, Kuypers HGJM. Cortico-cortical connection in the rhesus monkey. *Brain Res* 1969;13:13–36.
7. Denny-Brown D, Chambers RA. The parietal lobe and behavior. *Res Publ Assoc Res Nerv Ment Dis* 1958;36:35–117.
8. Peele TL. Acute and chronic parietal lobe ablations in monkeys. *J Neurophysiol* 1944;7:269–286.
9. Schwartz AS, Eidelberg E. "Extinction" to bilateral simultaneous stimulation in the monkey. *Neurology* 1968;18:61–68.
10. Heilman KM, Pandya DN, Geschwind N. Trimodal inattention following parietal lobe ablations. *Trans Am Neurol Assoc* 1970;95:259–261.
11. Heilman KM, Pandya DN, Karol EA, Geschwind N. Auditory inattention. *Arch Neurol* 1971;24:323–325.
12. Heilman KM, Valenstein E. Auditory neglect in man. *Arch Neurol* 1972;26:32–35.
13. Heilman KM, Valenstein E. Frontal lobe neglect in man. *Neurology* 1972;22:660–664.
14. Watson RT, Heilman KM, Cauthen JC, King FA. Neglect after cingulectomy. *Neurology* 1973;23:1003–1007.
15. Watson RT, Heilman KM, Miller BD, King FA. Neglect after mesencephalic reticular formation lesions. *Neurology* 1974;24:294–298.
16. Watson RT, Valenstein E, Heilman KM. Thalamic neglect: the possible role of the medial thalamus and nucleus reticularis thalami in behavior. *Arch Neurol* 1981;38:501–507.
17. Gainotti G, Messerli P, Tissot R. Qualitative analysis of unilateral and spatial neglect in relation to laterality of cerebral lesions. *J Neurol Neurosurg Psychiatry* 1972;35:545–550.
18. Costa LD, Vaughan HG, Horowitz M, Ritter W. Patterns of behavior deficit associated with visual spatial neglect. *Cortex* 1969;5:242–263.
19. Albert MD. A simple test of visual neglect. *Neurology* 1973;23:658–664.
20. Gasparrini W, Satz P, Heilman KM, Coolidge FL. Hemispheric asymmetries of affective processing as determined by the Minnesota Multiphasic Personality Inventory. *J Neurol Neurosurg Psychiatry* 1978;41:470–473.
21. Heilman KM, Schwartz HD, Watson RT. Hypoarousal in patients with the neglect syndrome and emotional indifference. *Neurology* 1978;28:229–232.
22. Heilman KM, Van den Abell T. Right hemisphere dominance for mediating cerebral activation. *Neuropsychologia* 1979;17:315–321.
23. Heilman KM, Van den Abell T. Right hemisphere dominance for attention: the mechanism underlying hemispheric asymmetries of inattention (neglect). *Neurology* 1980;30:327–330.
24. Watson RT, Miller BD, Heilman KM. Nonsensory neglect. *Ann Neurol* 1978;3:505–508.
25. Heilman KM, Watson, RT, Valenstein, E. Neglect and related disorders. In: Heilman KM, Valenstein E, eds. *Clinical neuropsychology.* New York: Oxford University Press, 1994;279–336.
26. Mesulam M-M, Van Hoesen GW, Pandya DN, Geschwind N. Limbic and sensory connections of the IPL (area PG) in the rhesus monkey: a study with a new method for horseradish peroxidase histochemistry. *Brain Res* 1977;136:383–414.
27. Mesulam M-M. A cortical network for directed attention and unilateral neglect. *Ann Neurol* 1981;10:309–325.

28. Mountcastle VB, Lynch JC, Georgopoulos A, Sakata H, Acuna C. Posterior parietal association cortex of the monkey: command function from operations within extrapersonal space. *J Neurophysiol* 1975;38:871–908.
29. Goldberg ME, Robinson DC. Visual responses of neurons in monkey inferior parietal lobule: the physiological substrate of attention and neglect. *Neurology* 1977;27:350.
30. Heilman KM, Watson RT, Valenstein E. Localization of lesions in neglect. In: Kertesz A, ed. *Localization in neuropsychology*. New York: Academic Press, 1983;471–492.
31. Lynch JC. The functional organization of posterior parietal association cortex. *Behav Brain Sci* 1980;3:485–534.
32. Heilman KM, Watson RT, Valenstein E, Goldberg ME. Attention: behavior and neural mechanisms. In: Mountcastle VB, Plum F, Geiger SR, eds. *Handbook of physiology*. Bethesda, MD: American Physiological Society, 1987;461–481.
33. Roland PE. The posterior parietal association cortex in man. *Behav Brain Sci* 1980;3:513–514.
34. McCulloch WS. The functional organization of the cerebral cortex. *Physiol Rev* 1944;24:390–407.
35. Jones EG, Powell TPS. An anatomical study of converging sensory pathways within the cerebral cortex of the monkey. *Brain* 1970;93:793–820.
36. Mesulam M-M. Patterns in behavioral neuroanatomy: association areas, the limbic system, and hemispheric specialization. In: Mesulam M-M, ed. *Principles of behavioral neurology*. Philadelphia: FA Davis, 1985;1–70.
37. Lamotte RH, Acuna C. Defects in accuracy of reaching after removal of posterior parietal cortex in monkeys. *Brain Res* 1978;139:309–326.
38. Faugier-Grimaud S, Frenois C, Stein DG. Effects of posterior parietal lesions on visually guided behavior in monkeys. *Neuropsychologia* 1978;16:151–168.
39. Petrides M, Iversen SD. Restricted posterior parietal lesions in the rhesus monkey and performance on visuospatial tasks. *Brain Res* 1979;161:63–77.
40. Luh KE, Butter CM, Buchtel HA. Impairments in orienting to visual stimuli in monkeys following unilateral lesions of the superior sulcal polysensory cortex. *Neuropsychologia* 1986;24:461–470.
41. Watson RT, Valenstein E, Day A, Heilman KM. Posterior neocortical systems subserving awareness and neglect: neglect associated with superior temporal sulcus but not area 7 lesions. *Arch Neurol* 1994;51:1014–1021.
42. Ungerleider LG, Mishkin M. Two cortical visual systems. In: Ingle DJ, Goodale MA, Mansfield JW, eds. *The analysis of visual behavior*. Cambridge, MA: MIT Press, 1982;549–586.
43. French JD, Hernandez-Peon R, Livingston RB. Projections from cortex to cephalic brain stem (reticular formation) in monkey. *J Neurophysiol* 1955;18:74–95.
44. Mesulam M-M, Waxman SG, Geschwind N, Sabin TD. Acute confusional states with right middle cerebral artery infarctions. *J Neurol Neurosurg Psychiatry* 1976;39:84–89.
45. Weinstein EA, Kahn RL. *Denial of illness*. Springfield, IL: CC Thomas, 1955.
46. Weinstein EA, Keller NJA. Linguistic patterns of misnaming in brain injury. *Neuropsychologia* 1963;1:79–90.
47. Alexander MP, Stuss DT, Benson DF. Capgras syndrome. *Neurology* 1979;29:334–339.
48. Geschwind N. The varieties of naming errors. *Cortex* 1967;3:97–112.
49. Chédru F, Geschwind N. Writing disturbances in acute confusional states. *Neuropsychologia* 1972;10:343–353.
50. Chédru F, Geschwind N. Disorders of higher cortical functions in acute confusional states. *Cortex* 1972;8:395–411.
51. Battersby WS, Bender MB, Pollack M. Unilateral spatial agnosia (inattention) in patients with cerebral lesions. *Brain* 1956;79:68–93.
52. Boudin G, Barbizet J, Lauras A, Lortat-Jacob O. Ramollissements temporaux droits: manifestations psychiques révélatrices. *Rev Neurol* 1963;108:470–475.
53. Juillet P, Savelli A, Rigal J, Sabourin M, Jenny B. Confusion mentale et lobe temporale droit: à propos de quatre observations. *Rev Neurol (Paris)* 1964;111:430–434.
54. Mangun GR, Hillyard SA, Luck SJ, et al. Monitoring the visual world: hemispheric asymmetries and subcortical processes in attention. *J Cogn Neurosci* 1994;6:267–275.
55. Dunne JW, Leedman PJ, Edis RH. Inobvious stroke: a cause of delirium and dementia. *Aust NZ J Med* 1986;16:771–778.
56. Kinsbourne M. A model for the mechanism of unilateral neglect of space. *Trans Am Neurol Assoc* 1970;95:143.
57. Mullally W, Huff K, Ronthal M, Geschwind N. Frequency of acute confusional states with lesions of the right hemisphere. *Ann Neurol* 1982;12:113.
58. Schmidley J, Messing R. Agitated confusional states in patients with right hemisphere infarctions. *Stroke* 1984;15:883–885.
59. Caplan LR, Kelly M, Kase CS, et al. Infarcts of the inferior division of the right middle cerebral artery: mirror image of Wernicke's aphasia. *Neurology* 1986;36:1015–1020.
60. Mori E, Yamadori A. Acute confusional state and acute agitated delirium: occurrence after infarction in the right middle cerebral artery territory. *Arch Neurol* 1987;44:1139–1143.
61. Fassbender K, Schmidt R, Mossner R, Daffertshofer M, Hennerici M. Pattern of activation of the hypothalamic-pituitary-adrenal axis in acute stroke: relation to acute confusional state, extent of brain damage, and clinical outcome. *Stroke* 1994;25:1105–1108.
62. Olsson T, Marklund N, Gustafson Y, Näsman B. Abnormalities at different levels of the hypothalamic-pituitary-adrenocortical axis early after stroke. *Stroke* 1993;23:1573–1576.
63. Horenstein S, Chamberlain W, Conomy J. Infarctions of the fusiform and calcarine regions: agitated delirium and hemianopia. *Trans Am Neurol Assoc* 1967;92:85–89.

64. Medina JL, Chokroverty S, Rubino FA. Syndrome of agitated delirium and visual impairment: a manifestation of medial temporo-occipital infarction. *J Neurol Neurosurg Psychiatry* 1977;40:861–864.
65. Devinsky O, Bear D, Volpe BT. Confusional states following posterior cerebral artery infarction. *Arch Neurol* 1988;45:160–163.
66. von Cramon DY, Hebel N, Schuri U. Verbal memory and learning in unilateral posterior cerebral infarction: a report of 30 cases. *Brain* 1988;111:1061–1077.
67. Halligen PW, Marshall JC. Neglect for near but not far space in man. *Nature* 1991;350:498–500.
68. Robertson LC, Lamb MR, Knight RT. Effects of lesions of temporal-parietal junction on perceptual and attentional processing in humans. *J Neurosci* 1988;8:3757–3769.
69. Schacter DL. Implicit memory: history and current status. *J Exp Psychol [Learn Memory]* 1987;13:501–518.
70. Marshall JC, Halligan PW. Blindsight and insight in visuospatial neglect. *Nature* 1988;336:766–767.
71. Berti A, Rizzolatti G. Visual processing without awareness: evidence from unilateral neglect. *J Cogn Neurosci* 1992;4:345–351.
72. Cohen JD, Romero RD, Farah MJ, Servan-Schreiber D. Mechanisms of spatial attention: the relation of macrostructure to microstructure in parietal neglect. *J Cogn Neurosci* 1994;6:377–387.
73. Felleman DJ, Van Essen DC. Distributed hierarchical processing in the primate cerebral cortex. *Cereb Cortex* 1991;1:1–47.

19
Autism and Related Disorders of Development

Martha Bridge Denckla

Kennedy Krieger Institute, Baltimore, Maryland 21205.

Because Dr. Geschwind focused his attention during the last 4 years of his life (1980 to 1984) on disorders of development, especially developmental dyslexia, the content of this chapter overlaps unavoidably with Chapter 15. Suffice it to say that from the very start, Dr. Geschwind extended his hypotheses concerning dyslexia to other, neighboring clinical disorders of spoken language, which were also suspected of having their origins in the left hemisphere. It is in the differential diagnosis of delayed speech and language that the perplexing, intriguing disorder of autism must be considered.

Autism encompasses delayed speech/language, as well as a constellation of attentional, sensorimotor, social, and complex cognitive manifestations. Autism remains a diagnosis concealing many mysteries of brain development gone awry. Long before his efforts in the 1980s, Dr. Geschwind encountered and pondered the mystery of autism. When I was a resident training with him in the 1960s, he took me along on his consultations to a children's unit at the state mental hospital. I can recall a 3-year-old boy whose clinical picture suggested classic early infantile autism but who had a history of viral limbic encephalitis. Dr. Geschwind's response to this case (which he elaborated on during the car trip back) was to speculate that Korsakoff's amnestic syndrome (secondary to limbic encephalitis) in a 3-year-old might devastate all of the learning that had occurred since birth, because there would be no "remote" period of life for one so young. Therefore, social and interpersonal skills, as well as all learned language skills, would be lost, resulting in autism.

I was duly impressed by that case discussion, but, because I was more immediately concerned with my residency and, later, my early career, which focused on "easier" developmental disorders like dyslexia and hyperactivity, I put aside all but sporadic thoughts about autism. This changed when I took a position at the National Institute of Neurological and Communicative Disorders and Stroke, as it was called then, that required me to identify what research was needed on autism and to facilitate its accomplishment. I took the new job in 1981, when Dr. Geschwind was in his "developmental" period. That was a happy coincidence, indeed, because meetings often brought him to Bethesda and our discussions of topics of mutual interest could be easily grafted onto dinners or breakfasts. (Those occasions, so delightful for me, were greeted with less enthusiasm by my youngest son, who noted that when Norman came to our house, it was difficult for anyone else to capture my attention or, indeed, for anyone else to get a word in edgewise!) During that period (1981 to 1984), Norman and I had frequent discussions about developmental disorders other than dyslexia, including autism, which was my focus at that time.

BRIEF HISTORY OF AUTISM UP TO THE 1980S

Autism was first described barely over 50 years ago; in 1943, Kanner (1) reported on 11 children whom he characterized as unable to relate to other human beings, delayed in their acquisition of speech, uncommunicative with the little speech that had developed, repetitious and stereotyped in their play, and obsessed with sameness. For Kanner, autism (*infantile autism* was his term) was different from childhood schizophrenia and from virtually every other form of childhood-onset psychopathology. A similar but less severe syndrome was described 1 year later by an Austrian psychiatrist, Asperger (2), who called it *autistic psychopathy*. Because his description was in German, it received little attention from English-speaking physicians until 1981, when Wing (3) used an account of six British cases of what she called *Asperger syndrome* to spread awareness of this variant of social impairment accompanied by deviant, but not initially delayed, language, and restricted, repetitive activities. Common to both infantile autism and Asperger syndrome, and thus constituting the core features of what is now termed the *autistic spectrum*, are interpersonal, nonverbal communicative, imaginative, and exploratory deficits. The pathophysiological bases of the two disorders have not yet been established, even at the level of "primary" psychological deficits (much less their biological etiologies).

Between 1943 and the late 1970s, perhaps as a reflection of the Freudian *Zeitgeist* that prevailed in British and American psychiatry, Kanner's several vacillating early etiologic interpretations (back and forth from biological to psychodynamic) of infantile autism came to rest on the psychodynamic cause. Aided and abetted by the eloquent writing of Bettelheim (4), the dominant interpretation of autism for over 30 years was that it was an emotional disturbance of psychotic proportions caused by neglect of the child's emotional needs by cold ("refrigerator") parents. Psychoanalysis or psychoanalytically driven therapies for autistic children were still used in Boston in 1976 when I returned there to direct the Learning Disabilities Clinic at Children's Hospital, and they continued into the late 1980s in France (Martine Flament, personal communication).

One of the most influential British child psychiatrists, Rutter (5), helped to refocus the emphasis on the behavioral pathophysiology of autism by stressing the language disorder associated with autism, with its echolalia and pronominal reversals, and its implications in terms of brain maldevelopment. Further, Rutter took the lead in noting that the association between autism and organic brain disease appeared more significant than for any other developmental disorder. After Rutter and his colleagues demonstrated that intelligence in autistic youngsters could be reliably measured, most autistic children were found to be mentally retarded. Other work showed that seizures developed by adolescence in about 25% of autistic children, even those with "normal" neurological examinations (6). In a review that brought together all of the research of the preceding 15 years, De Myer and colleagues (7) pointed out that infantile autism was diagnosed clinically as "secondary to" infantile spasms/hypsarhythmia, often with tuberous sclerosis underlying both conditions, or it was diagnosed after congenital rubella or viral-limbic encephalitis.

Some neuroanatomic and biochemical themes were emerging in the 1970s and early 1980s. First, in 1975 Hauser et al. (8) reported pneumoencephalographic evidence of bilateral temporal horn enlargement, greater on the left side, in patients with infantile autism. Second, in 1982 Young and colleagues (9) reported serotonergic abnormalities in autistic patients. As genetic approaches became central to medicine, Folstein and Rutter (10) documented a genetic risk for autism in a study of 21 pairs of DZ (dizygotic) and MZ (monozygotic) twins (each pair containing at least one autistic twin); no concordance was found among DZ pairs, whereas both twins were autistic in 36% of MZ pairs.

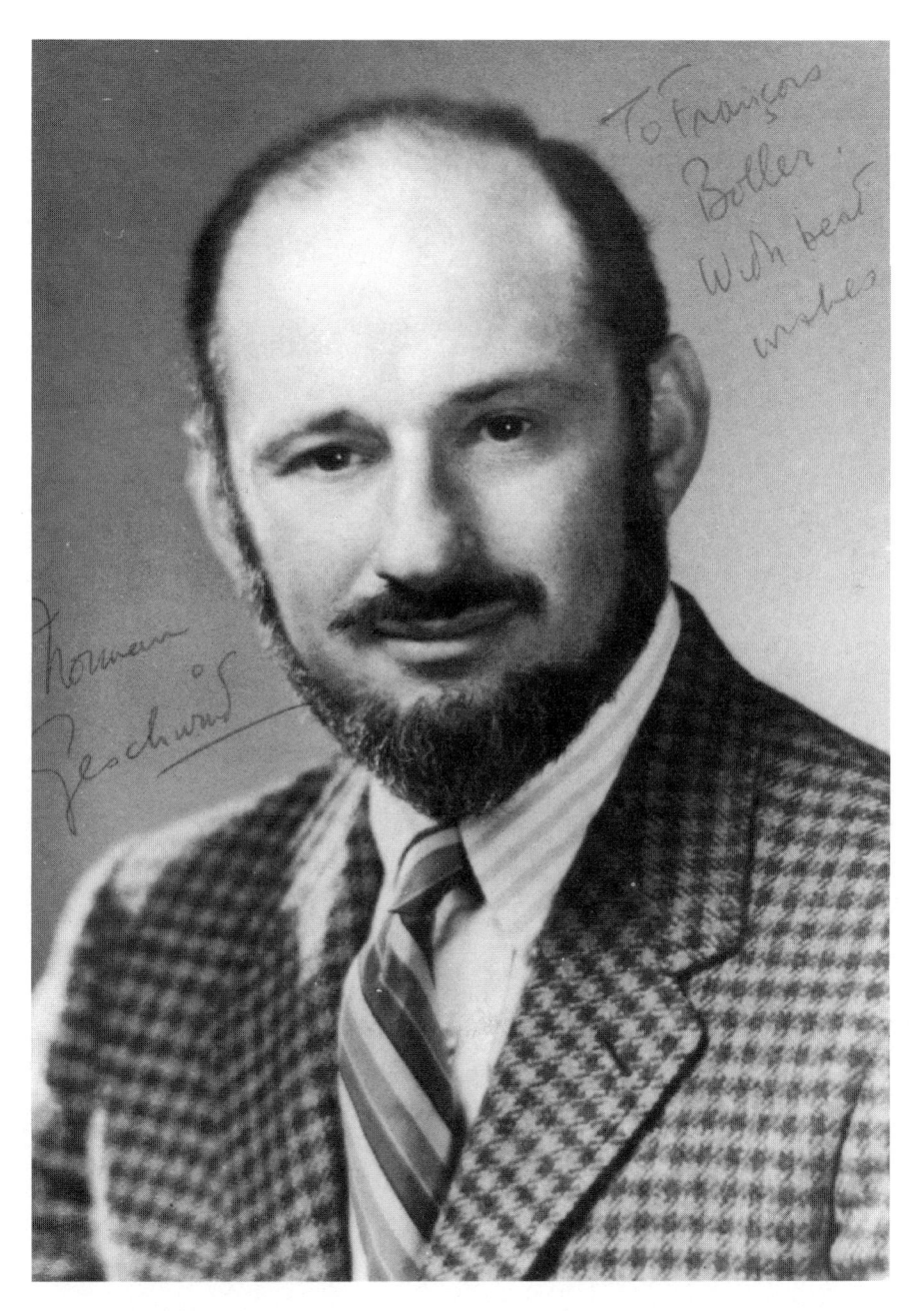

Norman Geschwind, 1964 (Courtesy of François Boller, M.D. Ph.D.)

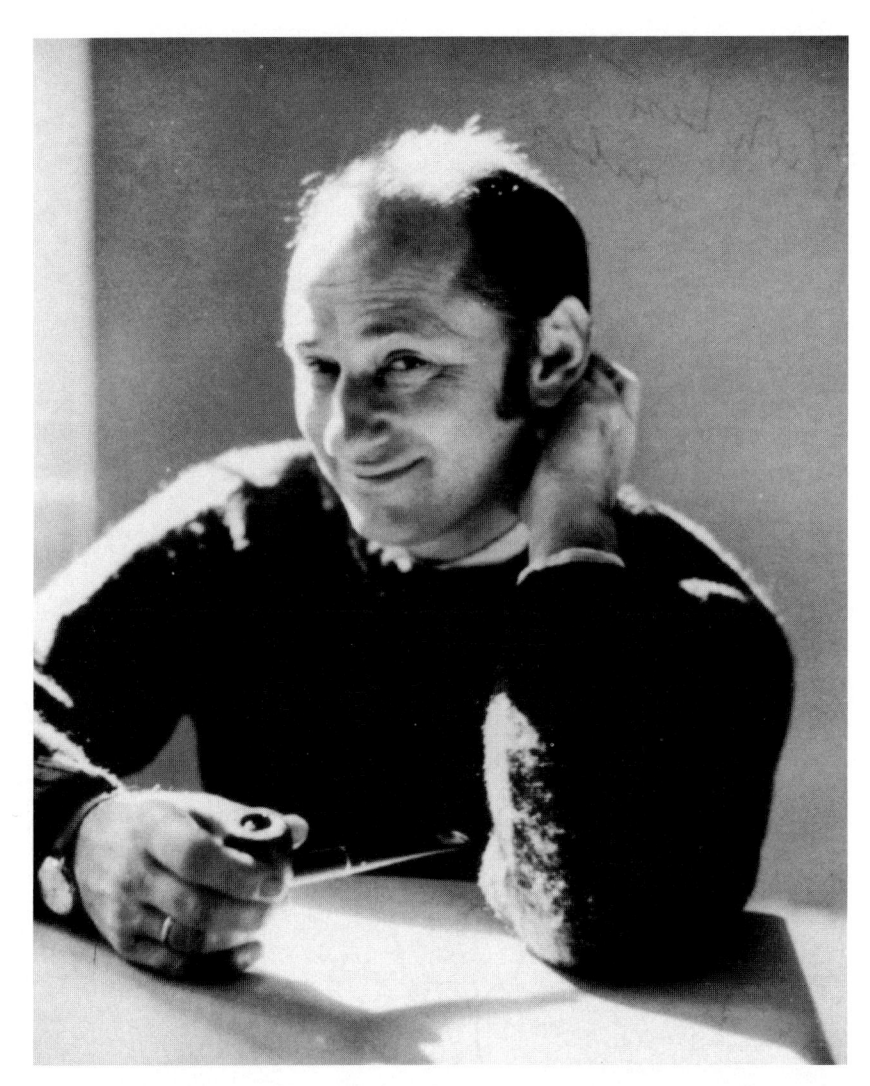

Norman Geschwind, 1968 (Courtesy of Kenneth Heilman, M.D.)

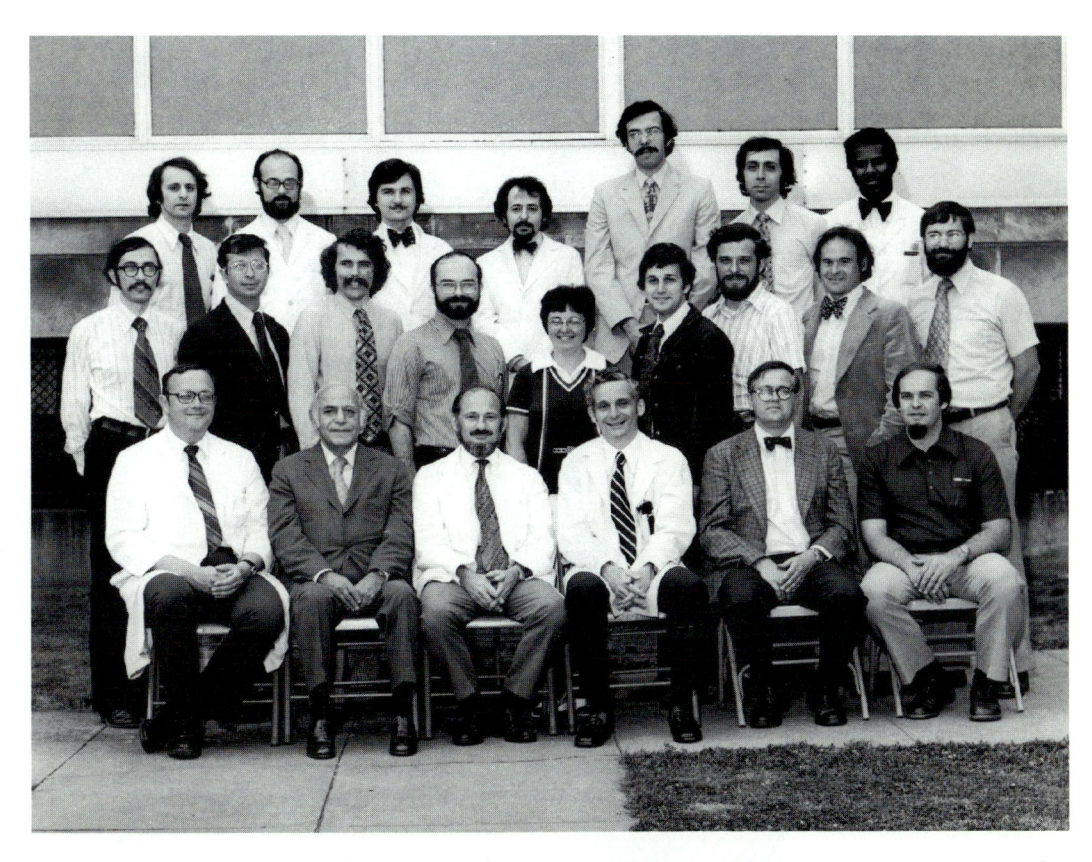

Boston City Hospital Neurologic Unit, 1973. *Back row*: (left to right) Steve Waxman, Elliot Ross, Albert Galaburda, Marcel Mesulam, Mike Biber, Robert Morin, Patrick Griffith. *Middle row*: Edgar Oppenheimer, Arthur Safran, James Nealis, Tom Stanley, Eileen Ouellette, Andrew Herzog, Brent Vogt, Brooke Seckel, Joseph Donnelly. *Front row*: Thomas Sabin, Sam Epstein, Norman Geschwind, Paul Rossman, Tom Kemper, Gary Van Hoesen. (Courtesy of Arthur Safran, M.D.)

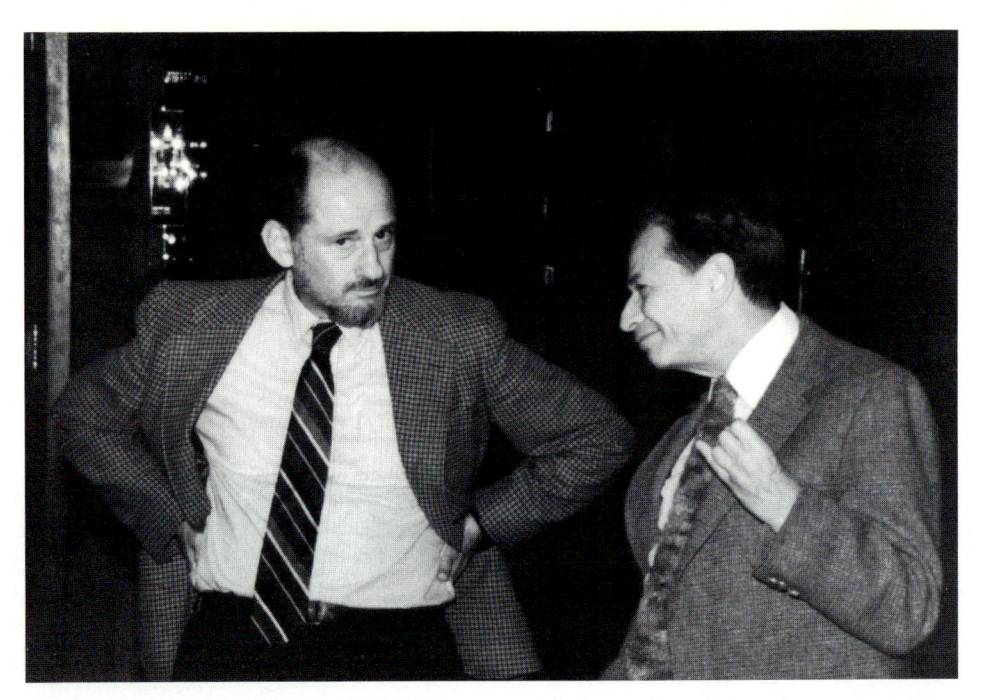

Norman Geschwind with Harold Goodglass, 1982 (Courtesy of Harry Whitaker, Ph.D.)

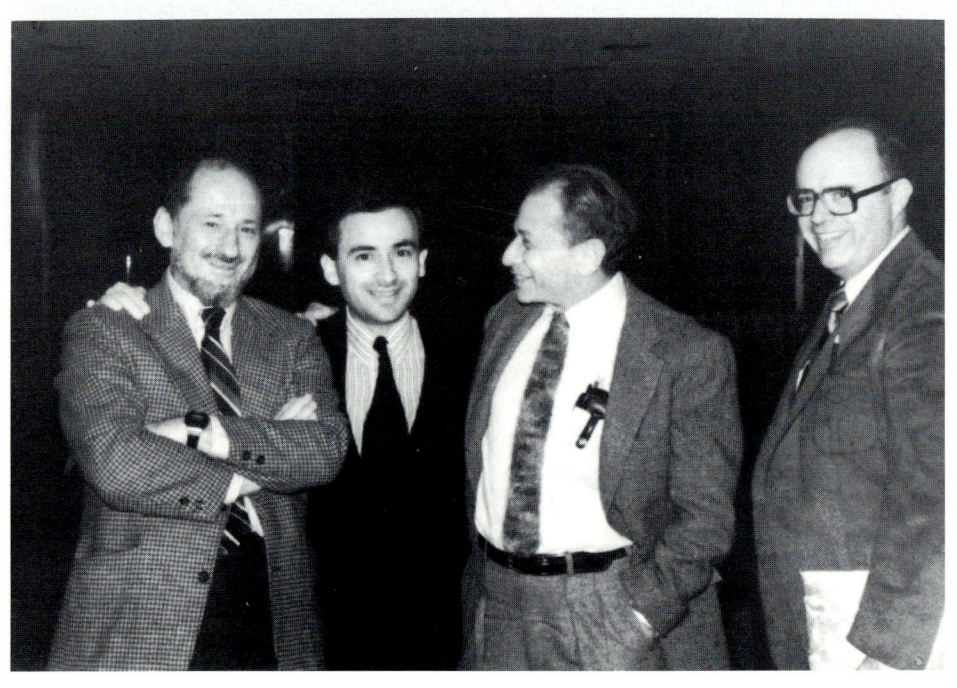

Norman Geschwind, Antonio Damasio, Harold Goodglass and M. Phil Bryden, 1982 (Courtesy of Harry Whitaker, Ph.D.)

As the 1970s drew to a close, one of Dr. Geschwind's most distinguished disciples, Antonio Damasio, proposed a neurologic model for autism (11). This model was influenced by observations (first brought to his attention by Hanna Damasio, according to my informants) of parkinsonian-like gait disturbances in autistic children (12). Antonio Damasio collaborated with child psychiatrist Maurer to generate a "neostriatal-mesolimbic" theory of autism (11,12). Disturbed quality of movement and disturbed attention were key features of autism that had not previously been emphasized by those who believed in an organic basis to autism. Because Rutter, Wing, and other psychiatrically trained physicians had emphasized the primacy of disordered communication (verbal and nonverbal) in autism, a "lateralization" theme had begun to divide the ranks of researchers who had but recently been allied against those who interpreted autism psychodynamically, even denying the primacy of a "social deficit" because its neurological basis was insecure (13). Anomalous right–left asymmetries in autism, as in dyslexia, were being reported (14). On the other hand, Boucher and Warrington (15), in following up on the earlier pneumoencephalographic evidence that implicated mesial temporal structures, noted similarities to the amnestic syndrome (reminiscent of Geschwind's comments in the mid 1960s). Damasio agreed that social deficiency was secondary, awarding neurological primacy to a group of functions that arise from a bilateral ring of mesocortex and neostriatum and that are neurochemically related as the terminal zones of the dopaminergic pathway (11). Damasio's formulation of autism depended on allocating those autistic features that he as a neurologist had brought to the fore (motor and attentional) to neostriatum; although neostriatum and mesocortex are affiliates, he saw the need to assign the core of autistic disturbances to a disrupted relay between limbic and neocortical regions and hence, disrupted associations of affect with sensory stimuli. Damasio speculated that a variety of perinatal cardiorespiratory catastrophes, genetically determined aberrations of either vascular or neuronal architecture, or any of a host of infectious or metabolic diseases might cause autism (11).

Damasio emphasized the dopaminergic system within the bilateral mesolimbic-cortex/neostriatum and was not concerned with cerebral asymmetry. Furthermore, he extrapolated from lesions of mesolimbic/neostriatal regions acquired in adulthood, which are characterized by "frontal" deficits. This formulation did not fit well with the clinical picture of most autistic children and failed to address possible amnestic aspects.

Not surprisingly, lack of agreement over the essential features of autism hampered research. Different brain regions received the research spotlight in direct proportion to the ease with which deficits in language, social, attentional, or motor functions could be documented. From a developmental perspective, the earliest deviant feature or features in autistic infants should inform the neurobiological research. On the other hand, a clinical picture of such complexity might make sense only in terms of an array of consequences of a particular neuropathogenetic mechanism. As of 1980, the year when Geschwind focused his formidable powers of synthesis and analysis on disorders of brain development, there was no consensus on the neuroanatomic or neuropsychological deficits in autism; the only other approach of child psychiatrists was to "round up the usual suspects"—neurotransmitters. In approaching this problem, Geschwind had available the then-prevailing emphasis on cognitive and, particularly, linguistic deficits and neuroimaging data that highlighted anomalies of hemispheric asymmetry. Demonstrating his ability "to see similarities where others see only differences" (one-half of Aristotle's definition of intelligence), Geschwind brought together the feature of anomalous hemispheric asymmetry [computed tomography (CT) data] and two other clinical characteristics of people with autism—the preponderance of males and non-right-handers (16).

Given all the exotic and puzzling features of autism that were researched and debated, it is little wonder that these two characteristics did not capture the attention of investigators. Besides, mental retardation (present in the majority of autistic children) is associated with non-right-handedness, and developmental language disorders have long been known to occur with greater frequency in males.

GESCHWIND'S CONTRIBUTIONS TO AUTISM RESEARCH AND CLINICAL ISSUES

By 1980, the neurologic basis of autism was no longer disputed. Thus, which structures in the brain were dysfunctional in autism and what might cause this dysfunction could be addressed within the larger context of the developmental disorders, of which dyslexia was the best example (see Chapter 15). Dr. Geschwind's contributions to our understanding of all the developmental disabilities, as exemplified by the prototypical dyslexia, lay in his brilliant contextualization of these phenomena.

It is all there, in the great three-part, posthumously published opus by Geschwind and Galaburda (16; autism receives particular mention on pages 428, 431, 433, 451–453, 455, 522, 536, and 546). In a sense, Dr. Geschwind "normalized" dyslexia and autism, at least for the human species (if not for the individual) in his hypothesis that these disorders represent the price we (humans) pay for specialized genius. He referred to the concept as "the pathology of superiority." Sometimes within a person, but more often within a family, great specialized talents coexist with diminished aptitudes. Anomalies also bring diversity. The sweep of this philosophic aspect of his contribution is matched by the breadth of biological data that he synthesized into the theory of anomalous dominance. Many would review the literature of the last decade and say that Dr. Geschwind was just plain wrong. Yet of those many, few accurately summarized his theory. Usually, detractors failed to note the subtle timing-related features of the theory, or they expected all aspects of the clinical triad (anomalous dominance, autoimmune disorder, and learning disability) to be obvious in a single person rather than in a single family. My own family (too late for me to tell Dr. Geschwind about it) illustrates the assortment of elements: When I was age 45, I was given the diagnosis of "by far the most common of all forms of autoimmunity"—Hashimoto's thyroiditis (which had probably been present for decades). I have one frankly left-handed son and two ostensibly right-handed (but partially left-preferring) sons. In addition, one of my sons has well compensated dyslexia with many "classic" features of phonologic deficit [including anomalous auditory evoked potentials on brain electrical activity mapping (BEAM)]. Dr. Geschwind believed that "the same influences which *in utero* cause disturbance of development of particular portions of the brain have a parallel effect on the development of the immune system. The mother with autoimmune thyroid disorder . . . is very likely to have many other alterations . . . since in her own development sex hormone changes may have altered the development of her immune system. . . . Their male children would be particularly at risk because the male fetus produces very high amounts of testosterone *in utero* and the additional maternal contribution will be more likely to push them over some threshold. . . . The hypothyroid mother is different from others in ways that may affect offspring, and . . . the hypothyroidism may not be directly causative. . . . The same influences that disturb brain development also disturb pregnancy—again these are parallel effects." (All quotations in this paragraph are from a letter dated February 4, 1983, from Dr. Geschwind to a patient's mother. See Case 3 abstract, later.)

Of course, it is extraordinarily difficult to sort out these "parallel effects," especially when anomalous dominance occurs in right-handers (who probably constitute more than half of the population with anomalous dominance) and when the borders of autoimmune phenomenology are fuzzy as well. (What are we to make of migraine?) It is also possible that only a fraction of cases in any developmental disability category (e.g., only some cases of autism) fit the Geschwind theory and that we cannot detect them within the "noise" of heterogeneity. Another possibility is that still more (insult added to injury) has to be added to the Geschwindian hormonal–autoimmune interaction before normal variation shades over into "disorder." As a clinician who is privileged to assess many very high-functioning patients with specific cognitive deficits relative to their overall cognitive strengths (and who therefore do not meet society's criteria for "disability"), I am more impressed with the validity of Geschwind's theory as applied to human diversity. So here we are again, back to where biology confronts philosophy!

Dr. Geschwind's clinical approach overwhelmingly emphasized the patient's history. His bedside examination, as I recall, went in pursuit of what the history suggested. As more of a "button-sorter," I myself do more "blind" examination of patients and get to the history later). I am like an "archaeologist of development," unwilling to surrender any bit of "broken crockery" that might make sense when presented to someone with Geschwindian-type brilliance. In Dr. Geschwind's case notes, I have found one instance in which Dr. Geschwind saw fit to document mirror movements [asymmetrical, in that "when she moved the left hand . . . involuntary movements were seen on the right side" (October 23, 1981, summary of case MP)]. In this case summary, Dr. Geschwind explains how he has "drawn the conclusion that disorder of the nervous system is the primary cause" of the 23-year-old patient's "persistent disorders in behavior and thought." He has very little to go on in this case, although the patient's history offers him a dyslexic father, other family members with strabismus, and in the young patient herself several abnormal electroencephalograms (EEGs) and metabolic deviations. He is very explicit in this case about the added impact that the left-sided signs, including the subtle developmental sign just described, had on his thinking. In this case summary, Dr. Geschwind illustrates an axiom that is exemplified in my metaphor of the clinician as archaeologist and that I heard him repeat many times, "Where we are so ignorant, we cannot afford to throw away information." Of course, he put this axiom into practice by carefully listening to what patients offered as relevant information, even when their comments did not conform to usual and customary medical thinking. Dr. Geschwind never scoffed at the apparently irrational or irrelevant; he would ruminate on even the most bizarre associations and try to place them in some broader biological context. I was reminded of that legacy in May 1995, at the annual dinner meeting of the Behavioral Neurology Society, when Dr. Kenneth Heilman, another brilliant disciple of Geschwind, admonished us to listen thoughtfully to the after-dinner speaker's account of "sensory integration" therapy for developmental disabilities. With a perfect Geschwindian attitude, Heilman remarked that the apparent "irrelevance" of vestibular stimulation might conceal an ameliorative effect on attention that, although not the whole therapeutic story, might be as "rational" as stimulant medication.

Dr. Geschwind's most enduring contributions to the clinical and clinical-research aspects of the field of developmental disabilities (or developmental cognitive neurology) lie in the attitudes and habits of thought he modeled for those of us who trained with him.

ILLUSTRATIVE CLINICAL CASES

Case 1 abstract (A.S.). Dr. Geschwind's consultation letter starts out by stating that because the patient's history is already well known to report recipients, he will not review it except to comment. He then proceeds to express skepticism about the significance of the mother's difficult labor and delivery, and he points out that high birth weight and developmental delays in both speech and motor functions were shared by the patient and his brother. Dr. Geschwind places diagnostic emphasis on the following facts: (a) the patient has an autistic brother, (b) the patient has a deaf autistic cousin, (c) the patient's mother is left-handed and hypothyroid, and (d) the maternal family includes several "seriously depressed" persons, one of whom is the patient's mother. Dr. Geschwind then points out that there is more non-right-handedness and neurological disorder on the paternal side. The patient himself had precocious singing ability, which was manifest in toddlerhood, when he had only echolalic speech and exhibited much rocking behavior. On examination, A.S. was found to be a "large and pleasant" but immature-for-age boy who was interested in word games like crossword puzzles, spoke quite well and read beautifully, but was poorly coordinated and could not "manipulate old knowledge" to calculate or interpret proverbs. (He had been a precocious "reader," hyperlexic in the sense that at an early age he could read words out loud even though he did not understand them).

Dr. Geschwind recommended tests to evaluate the patient for autoimmune disease (e.g., assay of antinuclear antibody) and suggested a BEAM test be obtained and interpreted by Dr. Frank Duffy at Children's Hospital. In terms of treatment, he recommended stabilization of the young autistic boy's environment (cautioning against his accompanying the father on the latter's sabbatical) and discontinuation of thioridazine, implicated in A.S.'s excessive hunger and thirst while not clearly beneficial to the patient. A trial of stimulant medication was suggested on the grounds that some of the patient's characteristics were similar to those of "hyperactive children" (report on A.S., April 23, 1981).

Case 1 discussion (A.S.). Dr. Geschwind makes or confirms (the letter does not state prior diagnosis) the diagnosis of autism. The patient's personal and familial history is clearly uppermost in his mind when he formulates the case. The laboratory tests he orders are directed towards possible etiology, both the biological "what" and localization-oriented, neurological "where." His treatment recommendations emanate from what he sees before him as the clear-and-present clinical picture and specific problems of the patient and his family. As a treating physician, he concerns himself with the social arrangement that is best for this immature and isolated boy, who needs "close supervision," and with the possibility for improving the psychopharmacologic benefit-to-risk ratio. Dr. Geschwind is straightforward about the empiricism involved in drug therapy and the non-isomorphism of "diagnosis" (syndromic or etiologic) and symptom relief. He explains in clear, layperson-friendly language the rationale behind his psychopharmacologic thinking. Similarly, he elucidates in teaching style the clinical features that led to the diagnosis and recommendation of certain laboratory tests (letter to mother of A.S., April 29, 1981).

Dr. Geschwind did make one error in this consultation, although it was an error commonly made then, when he echoed the misconception that autistic patients lack interest in sex. In fact, after they have reached puberty, their interest in sex may be likened to a "double-edged sword," driving some patients to work hard to improve socially but provoking others to engage in deviant and socially unacceptable sexual behaviors. For example, some autistic adolescents masturbate in public, sometimes exhibiting peculiar fetishes. Such behaviors pose a significant management problem for their caregivers.

Some autistic adolescents are hyposexual, but nobody has investigated whether they are among those with adolescent-onset epilepsy, specifically complex partial seizures.

Case 2 abstract (S.G.M.). This patient was an 18-year-old boy about whose history "only some major points" were summarized. After a postvaccination fever at 18 months of age, the patient had exhibited withdrawal and deterioration of speech. The child had lost all speech by age 4, when he began rocking and twirling behaviors, yet he learned to ride a bicycle quite well. Since age 4, S.G.M. had developed reasonably good self-care skills and the ability to carry out commands (if repeated), but he had spoken only occasionally and briefly. Six episodes of loss of consciousness had been reported, but whether these were seizures or fainting spells remained unclear as of 1979, when Dr. Geschwind noted that the boy had shown some minor improvement in attention after a few weeks of methylphenidate treatment, just before the visit to Beth Israel Hospital to see Dr. Geschwind. Nothing in the patient's family history contributed to the diagnostic process. The boy was mostly but not exclusively right-handed, and he had allergies. S.G.M. was not cooperative enough to be thoroughly examined, but no "elementary neurologic signs" were found. The patient was observed to remove his shoes after his father repeatedly asked him to do so, but the boy neither spoke nor appeared to comprehend when Dr. Geschwind spoke to him, and the patient never made eye contact with Dr. Geschwind. The boy rocked "somewhat" and displayed "an occasional, curious smile."

Dr. Geschwind concluded (apparently after some discussion with Dr. Charles Barlow and with me) that the patient did not have aphasia but a disorder that "most closely approximates to childhood autism." He concurred that a CT scan and EEG were warranted and that if methylphenidate or dextroamphetamine failed, empiric trials of other catecholaminergic drugs were advisable. Language evaluation was recommended, with an eye to decisions about language therapy. Dr. Geschwind's notes ended with a reference to a conversation with me in which I apparently emphasized both the importance and the difficulty of finding a prosocial environment (such as a residential school) for this presumably autistic boy (letter to Dr. Leo Alexander, March 15, 1979).

Case 2 discussion (S.G.M.). Dr. Geschwind mentions that this young man masturbates, but he does not return to this point in relation to sexuality in autistic persons (compare Case 1, A.S.). He expresses surprise that the child "regressed" postvaccination at age 18 months; although he does not spell it out, he seems to be under the impression that autism is uniformly manifested by delay in social/language development and to be unaware of the "regressive" subgroup. The patient's history appears to have let him down in this case, so he turns to management issues and appeals to colleagues for guidance. This case demonstrates the side of Geschwind that is less well known than his pyrotechnic brilliance as a teacher—the side that "knows what he does not know" and is unpretentious and capable of a disarming humility (letter to parents of S.G.M., March 15, 1979).

Case 3 abstract (D.M.). The mother of D.M. wrote to Dr. Geschwind on my advice (she incorrectly spelled my name as "Denkla," which occasioned her first bit of teaching from Dr. Geschwind) in a letter dated February 4, 1983. In her letter, she described her firstborn son, whom she explained was born "scrawny, jaundiced, with no suck reflex and an 'overblown' startle." Although right-handed and an early, excellent talker and reader, he learned to write late and never performed normally in mathematics. He rode a bicycle, swam, assembled models, and painted "in miniature," but he could not play ball or handwrite. His social skills were seriously impaired, as were "executive functions." He was unusually extreme in his reactions (underreactive or overreactive) to various sensory stimuli. His maternal grandmother and mother both suffered from hypothyroidism and had difficult first pregnancies (first-trimester exhaustion, fainting, shortness of breath, cardiac arrhythmia). D.M. ran high fevers of unknown cause, was suspected of having viral meningitis at age 6 and again at age 7, suffered from atopic allergies and severe migraines until adulthood, and possibly had one seizure at 7 years of age. He had bowel dysfunction (constipation and abnormal clay-colored bowels).

Dr. Geschwind responded in a long didactic letter to the mother of D.M., herself an active official of an organization devoted to research on learning disabilities, on July 13, 1983. The letter is extraordinary. He presents the subtle and sophisticated issues of gestational timing and testosterone effects with lucid simplicity to a deeply interested but untrained consumer of medical-neurological reasoning. He suggests that D.M. (then age 32) would indeed be an appropriate person to refer to the Behavioral Neurology Unit. A November 7, 1983, report from Dr. Marsel Mesulam details impairments found in "analogical reasoning, abstraction, mental flexibility, response set maintenance, resistance to interference," and inhibition; aside from bilaterally deficient fine motor control and speech, findings from neurological examination of the patient were normal. The pattern revealed by the clinical assessment, in concert with the history, suggested that the right hemisphere was the source of D.M.'s difficulties. A BEAM study done by Dr. Frank Duffy was "not entirely normal . . . not interpretable in reference to any known standard condition," although evoked potentials suggested right-sided abnormality of brain responses. D.M.'s disorder was thought to "fit" in the category of "right hemisphere learning disabilities," the subject of a paper by Weintraub and Mesulam (17).

Later, in 1989, D.M. and 18 other members of his family were studied by another EEG technique (K. Bonnet, New York University School of Medicine). All symptomatic family members displayed left dorsolateral-frontal and left parietotemporal abnormalities. None of the asymptomatic relatives exhibited any abnormalities whatsoever. Review of the 1983 BEAM study done on D.M. revealed background left-sided mild slowing. Again, EEG findings did not converge on the clinical picture.

D.M., now nearly 45, has learned many languages but has held no jobs and formed no relationships. He has had major depressive episodes. In the eyes of clinicians who see many patients with disorders that fall within the autistic spectrum, D.M. appears to fit the criteria for Asperger syndrome, which is in turn very hard to distinguish from "nonverbal learning disability," a concept close to "right-hemisphere-based learning disability" (18).

Case 3 discussion (D.M.). Although D.M. had Asperger syndrome rather than classic autism, I include this case out of interest because I was so much involved with the referral and subsequent discussions and because the correspondence with the patient's mother was very elaborate.

Dr. Geschwind and I had a major disagreement over the diagnosis in this case; he opposed the "stress on Asperger's" as a differential diagnosis, separate from classic early infantile autism (within what we now call the autistic spectrum) and across a border from the learning disability called "nonverbal" (18) or simply "of the right hemisphere." Dr. Geschwind was worried about "endless bureaucratic arguments about criteria" and (correctly) commented that "even so apparently clear a category as dyslexia leads to endless problems" (letter to mother of D.M., July 13, 1983). My rebuttal to Dr. Geschwind was that, by his own standards, among which is the primacy of history of the disorder, Asperger syndrome had won the right to be differentiated from autism because speech/language delay is not a feature of Asperger's. Even though two hypothetical adolescents, one with Asperger's and one with classically unfolding but very high-functioning autism, may have clinically indistinguishable disorders when seen in adolescence, they were enormously different at age 3 years. In addition, Geschwind himself discussed D.M. with emphasis on his higher verbal IQ than performance IQ, a pattern seen in the majority of adults with Asperger's, whereas the reverse is characteristic of high-functioning autistic adults (like the famous Temple Grandin, Oliver Sacks' "Anthropologist on Mars"). Geschwind went on, in the very same letter to D.M.'s mother, to state that Asperger patients "may share what I have postulated to be the early developmental structural changes that I think will be the hallmark of autism but not the later effects in some cases on language areas." It is in this letter that he stated clearly that autism's "prime feature in my view is difficulties in response to others." Dr. Geschwind apparently thought that these "difficulties in response to others" could be explained by interference of the right hemisphere early in pregnancy, whereas late-pregnancy events were thought to underlie the left hemisphere disturbances exemplified by "dyslexia." My point about this formulation was that it did not adhere sufficiently strictly to Dr. Geschwind's own principle (stated in an earlier letter dated February 4, 1983, to D.M.'s mother) that "my own strategy has been to attempt to pin down exactly which parts of the brain could be involved in the abnormal behaviors." By this standard, the elision (as it were) between Asperger's and right-hemisphere-based learning disability (or nonverbal learning disability) seems to me to ignore the autistic spectrum features of the former; that is, the disturbances in repertoire of activities and interest, and the peculiar behavioral rigidity that suggest a disturbance far removed from the right hemisphere's contributions. Shared prosodic, pragmatic, and affect recognition deficits may implicate the right hemisphere in both autism and nonverbal learning disability, but something more fundamental is amiss in Asperger syndrome. To be fair to Dr. Geschwind, the neuroanatomic data implicating the cerebellum were not available to him to influence his thinking, although he made note of the "late-developing" gestational status of the cerebellum. We must keep in mind that Asperger syndrome was not very thoroughly explored or well delineated clinically before 1985. It is also important to note that the controversy about Asperger syndrome, a controversy in which Dr. Geschwind and I engaged so amicably, is not settled today; neither are the identity and source of nonverbal learning disabilities (the latter is a major subject of my own ongoing research efforts). In addition, the tone and manner that Dr. Geschwind used in arguing his point of view are exemplified by our exchanges of opinion about D.M. At one point, after D.M. had been evaluated by the Beth Israel Neurological Unit, Dr. Geschwind telephoned to tell me that, with respect to certain features of the patient that he had doubted could be so, my predictions were correct. Dr. Geschwind, true to his name (which means "quick" in German), was always quick even to say "I was wrong; you were right!"

Dr. Geschwind's great strengths and minor weaknesses as a clinician are exemplified in his correspondence about D.M. His minor weaknesses revolve around his relative disregard for what he considered "hair-splitting" clinical details; his great strengths lie in how carefully he listened to patients' histories, how he pulled together seemingly unrelated facts, and how clearly he reported back to patients.

GESCHWIND'S INFLUENCE ON MAJOR RECENT ADVANCES IN THE FIELD

During the past decade, views on the fundamental core deficit in autism still assume a neurological basis, but they have otherwise come nearly full circle to Kanner's suggestion of "an innate inability to form the usual biologically provided affective contact with people." Other developments in the fields of behavioral neurology, neuropsychology, and neuropsychiatry (many of which were the work of researchers trained by

Geschwind) have facilitated a reexamination of social cognition in autism. Within the community of autism-centered researchers, there has been increasing awareness that comparison groups of language-impaired children, mentally retarded children, or both are rarely as socially impaired, as stereotypically restricted, as unimaginative in play, or as resistant to novelty as are autistic children (13). Finer-grained studies of early social cognitive competence have furthered refined, often in surprising ways, our understanding of the domains in which autistic children are impaired. Attachment, self-recognition, person-versus-inanimate-object discrimination, and a hierarchy of social responsiveness based on the usual degrees of familiarity with people are all normal in autistic children. Deficient in these children are gestural imitation, joint attention, affect recognition, pragmatic language, symbolic play, and theory of mind (20). As with any other developmental disorder, not all these deficits are demonstrable at every age; that is, the disorder seems a little different at each stage of maturation, and improvements in earlier-apparent deficits often occur.

Theory of mind, which refers to the autistic person's failure to predict how another person will be misled or mistaken by superficial perceptions, has become the most widely popular description of what autistic persons lack, although it is one of those explanations that I can imagine Dr. Geschwind greeting with derision (as he did when offered terms like *communication* and *abstraction*). This verbally mediated theory of mind itself necessitates an analysis in terms of a social-empathic versus cognitive deficit. Is it a deficit in feeling how another person feels or "mentally rotating" into another person's cognitive perspective? Besides being untestable in nonverbal autistic persons, theory of mind represents a complex appreciation that "things are seldom what they seem," more closely allied to the symbolic "let's pretend" play deficit than to the earlier infantile preverbal imitative and joint-attention aspects of autism.

The reader will note the reemergence of themes mentioned by Damasio (11)—motor (imitative) and attentional (joint attention) issues—in the early manifestations of autism. It is possible that symbolic play and theory of mind, both of which involve the ability to "imagine" what else a perception could represent, may belong to the other module of cognition implicated in research over the last decade, that labeled *executive function*. Unfortunately, executive function is a neuropsychological domain that has been implicated too often, and thus is suspiciously nonspecific, in several developmental disorders. In this respect, the executive function domain is consistent with its presumed neuroanatomic substrate, the prefrontal cortex, which neuroimaging (e.g., positron emission tomography) "landscapes" repeatedly indict in a wide variety of neuropsychiatric disorders (20). In any event, when high-functioning autistic adolescents (who are everyone's favorites to assess for practical reasons, although they are in the minority) are presented with the Wisconsin Card Sorting Task and the Tower of Hanoi planning task, they perform more poorly on these executive challenges than they do on tests of affect perception and theory of mind problems. Yet (as was the problem with Damasio's model) early-acquired bifrontal lesions do not produce autistic behavior (21,22), and "frontal executive" deficits may be secondary, later-developing remote effects of more fundamental autistic impairments.

Progress has been made over the past decade, but disagreement persists between those who cling to the notion that a "higher cortical association area" (parietal, prefrontal, or both) underlies autism (though they no longer insist that a language disorder is primary in autism) and the majority, who emphasize a "bottom-up" neurological model. Among that majority, the mesolimbic temporal cortex is the "highest" structure most emphasized, although the cerebellum has its advocates as an organ of cognition relevant to autism (23). In these majority views, most investigators are reinforced by the past decade's advances in neuroanatomy, both painstaking, classic postmortem studies and *in vivo*, structural neuroimaging investigations made possible by magnetic resonance imaging (MRI). Dr. Geschwind was indirectly responsible for the only source of funding that supported Bauman and Kemper's landmark postmortem examinations of autistic brains (24), because he referred me to a private benefactor who was interested in supporting worthwhile research on autism, and I directed this benefactor to Bauman. The information derived from the autopsy studies of Bauman, Kemper, and others is widely regarded as the most solid evidence amassed over the past decade of the structural features of the brains of autistic persons. Autistic brains are large and heavy. The limbic system (amygdala, hippocampus, or both) has too many closely packed small cells. In the cerebellum, Purkinje cells are abnormal, and the relationship of the cerebellum to its olivary nucleus reflects abnormalities consistent with anomalous development that takes place before 30 weeks (gestational age) in the human fetus. Amygdala, hippocampus, septum, mammillary bodies, and cerebellum are neuropathologically abnormal. Despite functional and neuropsychological studies that implicate late information processing, executive dysfunction ("frontal"), and other "higher" deficits, the neuropathological findings fail to show neocortical abnormalities. The "neocortical" deficits may possibly emerge later, secondary to abnormalities of the infantile limbic system (as has been established in primate models, in which early limbic abnormalities lead to later, apparently neocortical ones).

Magnetic resonance imaging volumetric data document large cerebral hemispheric volume that is, in turn, based on larger amounts of parieto-temporo-occipital white matter. Diencephalic and lenticular volumes are large. There is no lateralization to the findings (23).

Brain–behavior relationships emanating from the neuroanatomic data (postmortem and *in vivo*) fail to explain the apparent left hemisphere deficit profiles still reported in clinical studies of autistic populations (25,26). Affective deviations do map nicely onto the amygdala, "frontal" deficits may be traced secondarily developmentally to the hippocampus (as mentioned earlier), and sluggish, restrictive "overfocus" of attention may be associated with cerebellar deficiencies (23). Still unresolved is whether the verbal deficits and non-right-handedness, like the mental retardation that coexists in most patients with autism, are nonessential comorbidities that implicate a neurobiological mechanism of pathogenesis "parallel" to, rather than central to, the issues. Even with the overwhelming emphasis on the role of genetics in the pathogenesis of autism, the striking male-to-female sex ratio and the nonconcordant-for-autism sets of monozygotic (MZ) twins continue to raise Geschwindian questions about epigenetic "triggers" and gene-environment interactions. The possible role of immune factors continues to be mentioned; there are even indications that immune system responsiveness and elevated serotonin levels (that most haunting of autism-related neurotransmitter abnormalities) are correlated with autism (23). As is the case with dyslexia, however, the heterogeneity of autistic persons continues to confound efforts to find direct or indirect genetic and/or epigenetic (e.g., immune) causes. Clinical studies have tried to approach the issue of epigenetics by comparing the neuropsychological profiles of siblings of autistic persons with the profiles of siblings of other IQ-matched, developmentally disabled persons. Male relatives of autistic females (who are consensually regarded as the most severely cognitively and socially impaired autistic persons) were not found to be mentally retarded but were verbally impaired relative to their own parents and to siblings of persons with Down syndrome, suggesting again the testosterone effect on cerebral lateralization (26), which is not necessarily to be found at the neocortical level. Limbic and cerebellar asymmetries have not yet been investigated, as I am sure Dr. Geschwind would have advised.

As of the 1995 "state-of-the-art" National Institutes of Health conference on autism (23), the decade's advances were equaled by its controversies. The oldest techniques (postmortem whole-brain sections) and the newest (MRI) have made the most solid moves forward. Geschwind, indirectly instrumental in the funding of Dr. Bauman's research, was the direct promoter of the type of painstaking neuroanatomic description in which Dr. Bauman collaborated with the very same Dr. Kemper who examined dyslexic brains with Dr. Galaburda (27). This "classic" emphasis on the fine-grained structural neuroanatomy is a Geschwind legacy. An equally important Geschwind legacy is his lively and controversial hypothesis that the cause of autism is a pathophysiological process involving anomalous dominance, male hormones, and immunoreactivity. What we still do not know, as of this writing, is how broad a set of phenotypes to include as "familial" manifestations.

We are not sure how wide a net to cast, not only within but also outside the autistic spectrum. Perhaps we should include apparent opposites—verbally erudite persons who have subtle socially odd behaviors and persons who have relatively deficient language skills (including reading disabilities). We are left with research strategies that attempt to demonstrate hormonal and/or autoimmune relevance of specific selective impairments of brain function. We can continue to use clinical manifestations as clues to localization, which in turn suggests the type and timing of gestational interference, and we can take advantage of prototypes afforded by advances in molecular genetics and work from "inside out," tracing the neurodevelopmental pathway from gene to brain to dysfunction, as modified by hormonal and autoimmune factors. I believe that Dr. Geschwind would have encouraged us to attack the mysteries of autism on all fronts.

Acknowledgments

This work was supported by grant #P50 HD25806 from the National Institutes of Health. The author wishes to acknowledge Miss P. D. Yerby for her help in the preparation of this manuscript.

REFERENCES

1. Kanner L. Autistic disturbances of affective contact. *Nerv Child* 1943;2:217–250.
2. Asperger H. Die "autistichen psychopathen" im Kindesalter. *Archiv Psychiatrie Nervenkrankheiten* 1944;127: 76–1356. Translated and annotated by Frith U, ed. *Autism and Asperger syndrome*. Cambridge, England: Cambridge University Press;37–92.
3. Wing L. Asperger's syndrome: a clinical account. *Psychol Med* 1981;2:115–129.
4. Bettelheim B. *The empty fortress: infantile autism and the birth of the self*. New York: Free Press, 1967.
5. Rutter M. The development of infantile autism. *Psychol Med* 1974;4:147–163.
6. Rutter M. Language, cognition and autism. In: Katzman R, ed. *Development and acquired disorders of cognition*. New York: Raven Press, 1979;247–264.
7. De Myer MK, Hingtgen JN, Jackson RK. Infantile autism reviewed: a decade of research. *Schizophr Bull* 1981;7(3):388–451.
8. Hauser S, Delong R, Rosman P. Pneumographic findings in the infantile autism syndrome. *Brain* 1975;98:667–688.
9. Young JG, Kavanagh ME, Anderson GM, Shaywitz BA, Cohen DJ. Clinical neurochemistry of autism and associated disorders. *J Autism Dev Disord* 1982;12:147–165.
10. Folstein S, Rutter M. Infantile autism: a genetic study of twenty-one twin pairs. *J Child Psychol Psychiatry* 1977;18:297–321.
11. Damasio AR, Maurer RG. A neurological model for childhood autism. *Arch Neurol* 1978;35:777–786.
12. Vilensky JA, Damasio AR, Maurer RG. Gait disturbances in patients with autistic behavior: a preliminary study. *Arch Neurol* 1981;38:646–649.
13. Fein D, Pennington B, Markowitz P, Braverman M, Waterhouse L. Towards a neuropsychological model of autism. *J Am Acad Child Psychiatry* 1986;25:198–212.

14. Hier DB, LeMay M, Rosenberger PB. Autism and unfavorable left-right asymmetries of the brain. *J Autism Dev Disord* 1979;9:153–159.
15. Boucher J, Warrington EK. Memory deficits in early infantile autism: some similarities to the amnesic syndrome. *Br J Psychol* 1976;67:73–87.
16. Geschwind N, Galaburda AM. Cerebral lateralization, biological mechanisms, associations, and pathology: a hypothesis and a program for research. *Arch Neurol* 1985;42(pts I–III):428–459, 521–552, 634–654.
17. Weintraub S, Mesulam MM. Learning disabilities of the right hemisphere: emotional, interpersonal and cognitive components. *Arch Neurol* 1983;40:463–468.
18. Rourke BP. *Nonverbal learning disabilities: the syndrome and the model.* New York: Guilford Press, 1989.
19. Rogers SJ, Pennington BF. A theoretical approach to the deficits in infantile autism. *Dev Psychopathol* 1991;3:137–162.
20. Denckla MB. Prefrontal-subcortical circuits in developmental disorders. In: Krasnegor N, Lyon R, Goldman-Rakic P, eds. *Development of prefrontal cortex: evolution neurobiology and behavior.* Baltimore: PH Brookes, 1995.
21. Price BH, Daffner KR, Stowe RM, Mesulam MM. The comportmental learning disabilities of early frontal lobe damaged. *Brain* 1990;113:1383–1393.
22. Eslinger PJ, Grattan LM. Perspectives on the developmental consequences of early frontal lobe damage: introduction. *Dev Neuropsychol* 1991;7(3):257–260.
23. Denckla MB. Brain mechanisms. In: Bristol M, ed. State of the science in autism: *Report to the National Institutes of Health* 1996;26(2):134-140.
24. Bauman ML, Kemper TL. Histoanatomic observations of the brain in early infantile autism. *Neurology* 1985;35:866–874.
25. Klin A. Asperger syndrome. *Child Adol Psychiatry Clin North Am* 1994;3:131–148.
26. Klin A, Volkmar FR. *Assessment, diagnosis and intervention of Asperger syndrome: guidelines for parents.* Pittsburgh, PA: Learning Disabilities Association of America, 1995;5–7.

20

Frontal Lobe Syndrome

François Boller

INSERM U324, Centre Paul Broca, 75014 Paris, France.

The stricter the rules, the easier it is. In 19th century academic Prussia, you could diagnose a major frontal lobe lesion at a glance. (Paraphrase of statement by Norman Geschwind, about 1969.)

The word *frontal* does not appear even once in Norman Geschwind's curriculum vitae. Yet Geschwind was quite aware of the importance of the frontal lobes, structures that, as he was fond of saying, "occupy half the brain." In my opinion, Norman Geschwind would have loved that paradox.

This chapter will present some of the historical background that led to the state of knowledge about the frontal lobes at the time of Norman Geschwind's teaching. It will present his views on the topic, as can be inferred from his office notes and correspondence, and from personal recollections.

HISTORY OF THE FRONTAL LOBE SYNDROME

A great deal has been written about the frontal lobe syndrome by authorities such as Denny-Brown (one of Norman Geschwind's teachers) (1) and by many others (2–4). I have chosen to comment on three unconventional landmark episodes that, just like frontal lobe patients, did not "follow the rules," but which made major contributions to our understanding of the functions of the frontal lobes.

It may well be said that the story started in New England in 1848, not on the polished mahogany desks of Harvard or the wards of Massachusetts General Hospital but in Cavendish, Vermont, in the sweat-and-blood context of the Rutland & Burlington Rail Works. This is where Phineas Gage miraculously survived a major head injury to become the first well-documented case of frontal lobe syndrome in history, thanks to Harlow's vivid description and thanks also to the stupendous reconstructive work of Hanna Damasio and her colleagues (5).

The next episode took place in Germany in 1864, once again far from formal academic surroundings. As the legend goes, Fritsch, while dressing a wounded man in the battlefields of the Prussian-Danish War, "discovered" that irritation of the brain causes twitching of the opposite side of the body. Fritsch continued his work with Hitzig (6) in an unconventional fashion (the two performed their first studies on dogs in Hitzig's home, operating on Frau Hitzig's dressing table) (7). Incidentally, Fritsch, a wealthy man, spent many of the subsequent years traveling around the world and is therefore remembered only because of this particular piece of work.

Another event *did* take place in academic settings—but in Palermo and Naples, cities not readily associated with the field of neuroscience. I am alluding to the work of

Leonardo Bianchi. Together with Mingazzini, whose work on the corpus callosum Geschwind knew well, and Luciani, who was best known for his work on the cerebellum, Bianchi was undoubtedly one of the first Italian precursors of modern neuroscience to become internationally famous, mainly because of his work on the frontal lobes. Bianchi based his work on that of the founders of neuroscience who had preceded him, particularly Theodor Meynert, Eduard Hitzig, and David Ferrier. Starting in 1888, first in Palermo and then in Naples, Bianchi performed a series of experiments consisting of electrical stimulation or surgical removal of the frontal lobes of monkeys and dogs. His papers, which included a good description of what is known today as the frontal lobe syndrome, soon made him famous all over Europe and even in the United States, in part because of an article that appeared in *Brain* (8) and later because of a book *("La meccanica del cervello e la funzione dei lobi frontali")*, which was translated into French and English (9). Bianchi confirmed Ferrier's observation that animals whose frontal lobes were removed either kept their elementary motor and sensory functions intact or recovered them soon after the operation. Bianchi, however, was impressed by the severe psychological deficits that had not been clearly described by previous investigators but were sufficiently severe to interfere with the mental capacities of the animals: "Removal of the frontal lobes does not so much interfere with the perceptions taken singly, as it does disaggregate the personality." This statement clearly suggests the complex relationships between frontal lobe lesions and major behavioral changes.

These early scientists were some of the many whose work laid the foundation for our current understanding of the frontal lobes. What were Norman Geschwind's thoughts on this matter?

NORMAN GESCHWIND'S WRITINGS ON THE FRONTAL LOBES

As stated previously, the word *frontal* does not appear in Geschwind's curriculum vitae. Naturally, his many papers on aphasia, particularly on the disconnection syndrome and on motor and transcortical motor aphasia, often discussed Broca's area, the anterior portion of the corpus callosum and its projections and other structures anterior to the Rolandic fissure. He did not publish, however, any papers specifically on the prefrontal cortex, and the personal recollections of various persons who worked closely with him for many years (i.e., Frank Benson, Joaquin Fuster, and Marjorie LeMay) would suggest that he did not talk much about it.

Yet I am sure that all those who trained with Norman Geschwind heard a great deal about the frontal lobes and the frontal lobe syndromes. That this is so is reflected in some of the office notes kindly provided by the editors of this book. For example, in a set of notes dated February 12, 1982, Geschwind refers to a patient he first saw in June of 1981 and again in February 1982. The notes do not specify the cause of the patient's disorder; they merely mention "late changes following a local damage." On the first visit the patient was depressed, but on the second visit he seemed quite unconcerned about his health and financial problems. In addition, the patient displayed inappropriate behavior, lack of emotional response, "irritable euphoric apathy" (a phrase I frequently heard Geschwind use), and illogical thinking, all of which are "so characteristic of classical patients with frontal lobe syndrome." The patient's wife was advised that her husband might be dangerous (e.g., cause fires, have automobile accidents) and was urged to have herself appointed as his legal guardian. In correspondence with a colleague, Norman

Geschwind quoted numerous examples of sexual misconduct he had witnessed (or heard about) in patients with frontal lobe damage.

In addition to reflecting a detailed understanding of the frontal lobe syndromes, these notes clearly demonstrate one of the most characteristic features of Norman Geschwind as a teacher: his frequent illustration of his scientific arguments with "live" anecdotes. This brilliant stratagem successfully aimed at enlivening topics that might otherwise seem dreary and oppressive.

On April 18, 1979, Norman Geschwind wrote to a colleague about a general from the Soviet Army (age not specified) whom they had both seen. In that letter, Norman Geschwind strongly objected to the simplified view that the frontal lobes are "those areas of the brain related to intellectual functioning" and suggested omitting the whole sentence altogether "since you probably don't really want to get into a long discussion of frontal lobe function." In an unrelated but interesting part of that letter, in which Geschwind discussed the differential diagnosis of dementia, he mentioned atherosclerotic dementia (indicating that the term is no longer used), multi-infarct dementia, and senile dementia but made no mention of Alzheimer's disease. At that time, the arguments questioning the distinction between presenile and senile dementia were just starting (10) and the matter was far from resolved (is it resolved now?).

Norman Geschwind's thoughts are particularly well documented about one aspect of the frontal lobe syndrome which Lhermitte called *utilization behavior* (11). Geschwind wrote to Lhermitte to let him know that although Geschwind had known about this kind of behavior for years, he found Lhermitte's description and interpretation "profoundly original." Geschwind provides an interesting explanation for this behavior by comparing the patients' reactions to the field-dependence observed by psychologists in some persons. Incidentally, a strong relationship between certain environmental and mood factors and utilization behavior has been confirmed by recent research (12). After several comments that also cover grasping, sucking behavior, and the magnet reaction, Geschwind quoted Goethe's statement that "the most difficult things to see are not those which are hidden, but those which lie directly in front of our eyes." That statement describes exceedingly well Norman Geschwind's unique ability to make complicated facts and behaviors seem obvious once he explained them.

NORMAN GESCHWIND'S FORMAL TEACHING ON THE FRONTAL LOBES

I distinctly recall Norman Geschwind's Harvard Medical School lecture on the frontal lobes. He characterized the "frontal lobe syndrome" as a failure to learn and follow the rules imposed by society on everyday life. This failure to learn the rules refers to an inability to put them into practice, rather than to a failure of encoding or storage. "What did I tell you?" the doctor asks the patient caught drinking at the water fountain despite having been told in detail why he should refrain from drinking for a while. "You told me not to drink," says the patient while he resumes his drinking, not in the least concerned or defiant. The quotation at the beginning of the chapter is extrapolated from another illustration of the syndrome and Norman Geschwind's conclusion that in 19th-century Prussia, if a professor ever arrived at work without having first polished his shoes perfectly, one could be certain that he had a frontal lobe syndrome (which would likely be due to either a tumor or neurosyphilis).

CURRENT TRENDS IN FRONTAL LOBE RESEARCH: WHAT WOULD NORMAN GESCHWIND THINK?

A considerable amount of research in the past 20 years has involved the frontal lobes, one of the most active aspects of research and speculation in neuropsychology. Many among the current leading investigators (such as Frank Benson, Jeffrey Cummings, Antonio Damasio, Deepak Pandya, and Donald Stuss) either trained with Norman Geschwind or were otherwise closely associated with him. Much has been written about disturbances of executive functioning and the "dysexecutive syndrome" that is often found in patients with frontal lobe lesions (13), but I do not know if Geschwind ever used that term, which, owing to its inclusion in the *Diagnostic and Statistical Manual of Mental Disorders,* Fourth Edition (DSM IV), is now standard nomenclature (14). Unfortunately, I never had a chance to hear Geschwind comment on such models proposed by cognitive psychologists as the working memory model (15), and nobody knows how he would have reacted to subsequent models (16). It can be safely assumed that he would have objected to the automatic assimilation between dysexecutive syndrome and frontal lobe disease made by some (mostly nonneurologists). Like most of us, he likely would have pointed out that patients with demonstrated frontal lobe lesions do not always have dysexecutive syndrome, and vice versa. He probably would have been fascinated by recent advances in functional imaging that permit the demonstration of, for instance, the complex pattern of activation that occurs during the performance of "simple" tests such as the Stroop test (17,18).

As this chapter shows, Norman Geschwind was acutely aware of, and intellectually attracted by, what Teuber called "the riddle of the frontal lobe function" (19).

REFERENCES

1. Denny-Brown D. The frontal lobes and their function. In: Williams D, ed. *Modern trends in neurology.* London, England: Butterworths, 1951.
2. Meyer A. The frontal lobe syndrome, the aphasias and related conditions: a contribution to the history of cortical localization. *Brain* 1974;97:565–600.
3. Fuster J. *The prefrontal cortex,* 2nd ed. New York: Raven Press, 1989.
4. Benton A. The frontal lobes: a historical sketch. In: Boller F, Spinnler H, Hendler J, eds. *The frontal lobes,* vol 9 in Boller F, Grafman J, eds. *Handbook of neuropsychology.* Amsterdam, The Netherlands: Elsevier, 1994;3–15.
5. Damasio H, Grabowski T, Frank R, Galaburda A, Damasio A. The return of Phineas Gage: the skull of a famous patient yields clues about the brain. *Science* 1994;264:1102–1105.
6. Fritsch T, Hitzig E. Uber die elektrishe Erregbarkeit des Grosshirns. *Arch Anat Physiol* 1870;4:300–332.
7. Kuntz A, Eduard Hitzig. In: Haymaker W, Schiller F, eds. *The founders of neurology.* Springfield, IL: Charles C Thomas, 1970;229–233.
8. Bianchi L. The functions of the frontal lobes. *Brain* 1885;18:497–522. (Reprinted by the Centro Ricerche Sen. Leonardo Bianchi, Edizioni del Centauro, Udine, Italy, 1995.)
9. Bianchi L. *The mechanism of the brain and the function of the frontal lobes.* New York: William Wood, 1922. (Reprinted by the Centro Ricerche Sen. Leonardo Bianchi, Edizioni del Centauro, Udine, Italy, 1995.)
10. Katzman R, Terry R, Bick K, eds. Alzheimer's disease: senile dementia and related disorders. In: *Aging,* vol 7. New York: Raven Press, 1978;595.
11. Lhermitte F. "Utilization behavior" and its relation to lesions of the frontal lobes. *Brain* 1983;106:237–255.
12. Spinnler H. Lack of frontal inhibitory mechanism: utilization and behavior. *Unpublished manuscript.*
13. Tranel D, Anderson SW, Benton A. Development of the concept of "executive function" and its relationship to the frontal lobes. In: Boller F, Spinnler H, Hendler J, eds. *The frontal lobes,* vol 9 in Boller F, Grafman J, eds. *Handbook of neuropsychology.* Amsterdam, The Netherlands: Elsevier, 1994;125–149.
14. American Psychiatric Association. *Diagnostic and Statistical Manual of Mental Disorders,* 4th ed. Washington, DC: American Psychiatric Association, 1994.
15. Baddeley AD, Hitch G. Working memory. In: Gower G, ed. *The psychology of learning and motivation: advances in research and theory,* vol 8. New York: Academic Press, 1974.
16. Grafman J. Alternative frameworks for the conceptualisation of prefrontal lobe functions. In: Boller F, Spinnler

H, Hendler J, eds. *The frontal lobes,* vol 9 in Boller F, Grafman J, eds. *Handbook of neuropsychology.* Amsterdam, The Netherlands: Elsevier, 1994;187–203.
17. Bench CJ, Frith CD, Grasby PM, et al. Investigations of the functional anatomy of attention using the Stroop test. *Neuropsychologia* 1993;31:907–922.
18. Boller F, Traykov L, Dao-Castellana M, et al. Cognitive functioning in "diffuse" pathology: role of prefrontal and limbic structures. In: Grafman J, Boller F, Holyoak K, eds. *Structure and functions of the human prefrontal cortex.* New York: New York Academy of Sciences. 1995;23–39.
19. Teuber H. The riddle of frontal lobe function in man. In: Warren J, Akert K, eds. *The frontal granular cortex and behavior.* New York: McGraw-Hill, 1964;416–441.

Behavioral Neurology and
the Legacy of Norman Geschwind,
edited by S. C. Schachter and O. Devinsky,
Lippincott-Raven Publishers, Philadelphia © 1997.

21
Norman Geschwind and Dementing Disorders

Robert C. Green

Emory Neurobehavioral Program, Wesley Woods Center, Atlanta, Georgia 30329.

Norman Geschwind was a remarkable clinician and teacher whose professional contributions advanced the study of the neurological substrates of behavior in many arenas. Although he focused a relatively small proportion of his energies on dementia, the breadth of his competency as a behavioral neurologist embraced the disorders of attention and memory associated with aging, and his clinical notes and bedside teachings revealed a prescient approach to dementing disorders. Dr. Geschwind's commitment to the education of several generations of behavioral neurologists also has advanced our understanding of dementia, because many of his trainees have made major contributions to this field.

GESCHWIND'S PUBLICATIONS ON DEMENTIA

When Norman Geschwind began his career, Alzheimer's disease had been recognized for decades (1,2), but there was considerable confusion about the distinctions between various forms of vascular dementia and Alzheimer's disease and about the best way of communicating those distinctions (3,4). Without the aid of computed tomography and magnetic resonance scanning, nonmotor strokes could not be accurately diagnosed during life. Further, "hardening of the arteries" and "atherosclerotic dementia" were commonly thought by clinicians to be principal causes of progressive dementia (5), despite evidence that atherosclerosis in the brain was not regularly accompanied by dementia (6). Dr. Mick Alexander, one of Dr. Geschwind's earliest students, recalls that Dr. Geschwind "didn't believe in multi-infarct dementia" but rather felt that specific "uni-infarct" stroke syndromes, such as left thalamic stroke, were frequently responsible for cognitive impairments in the elderly. Even in the 1970s and early 1980s, residents and fellows were often not taught to distinguish dementia syndromes in patients on the basis of the cognitive domains that were affected early in the clinical course of the illness. The cognitive deficits in dementia were often described as *global,* a term that Dr. Geschwind frequently and loudly rejected as vague and nonspecific. He favored searching for the specific patterns of cognitive strengths and weaknesses in each patient.

The first publication by Dr. Geschwind on dementia was a short piece summarizing the clinical approach to memory disturbances (7). In this article, which reflected his characteristic disdain for citing many references, Dr. Geschwind made several points. He noted that "early signs of disturbances of memory are often unnoticed in slowly progressive syndromes." [The insidiousness of preclinical symptoms was not obvious to most clinicians of his day and has recently become the focus of a number of important research initiatives (8)]. Dr. Geschwind emphasized that the particular clinical presentation of dementia in a patient depends upon the regions of cortex that are affected, and he succinctly summarized the differential diagnosis of disorders that can disrupt cognition, particularly in the elderly. He strongly recommended neuropsychological testing as part of the evaluation, implying that it may be useful in almost all memory-impaired patients. At first blush, this recommendation seems curious because his office notes indicate that he rarely ordered such testing when examining his own patients. Perhaps Dr. Geschwind assumed that general clinicians would need neuropsychological assistance more than behavioral neurologists.

A few years later, in a piece he wrote for a psychiatric journal to accompany an article on brain syndromes in aging and alcoholism, Dr. Geschwind elaborated on his objection to the notion of dementia as a global disorder (9). Again, he emphasized how specific clinical features could correspond to the involvement or sparing of discrete brain regions in Alzheimer's disease. These clinical observations, which were not widely disseminated at that time, have now entered the mainstream of clinical thinking about dementia, particularly Alzheimer's disease (10–17). In this article, he also objected to use of the term *chronic brain syndrome* as he frequently did in mock tantrums of withering sarcasm while making ward rounds. He also discouraged use of the term *organic brain syndrome*. He considered it somewhat ridiculous to use redundantly descriptive and imprecise syndromic nomenclature as a substitute for diagnostic categories.

In an article from that same time period, Drs. Marcel Mesulam and Geschwind noted that mildly or subclinically demented patients experienced worsening or emergent confusion after surgery (18). This important clinical observation has also become widely accepted (19).

GESCHWIND'S CASE NOTES ON DEMENTED PATIENTS

For those of us who trained with Dr. Geschwind, reviewing the transcripts of his dictated case notes elicits many memories of his fluent clinical convocations at the bedside. There is a remarkable consistency of tone throughout these notes, characterized by sympathy for the patient and patient's family, and respect for the referring physician. No matter how much Dr. Geschwind disagreed with the prior diagnosis, his letters were polite and instructive, filled with reason, and buttressed by his inexhaustible memory of past cases. He approached the evaluation of patients with dementia with conceptual clarity, diagnostic imagination, and therapeutic optimism.

In an era when theories about causal mechanisms for dementias were particularly undeveloped, Dr. Geschwind took a phenomenologic approach to dementing disorders. Eschewing the tautologic traps inherent in the use of the term *dementia,* he wrote to Dr. Nelson Butters in 1974: "It seems to me that a dementia is any disorder in which there is a decline in intellectual performance." In this and in other letters, Dr. Geschwind went on to differentiate between dementia and memory disorder, pointing out that although memory difficulties are frequently the presenting symptoms of some dementias, such as Alzheimer's disease, deficits in other cognitive domains are often the presenting symptoms of other dementing disorders. In some of his case notes, he was even more explicit. For example, in 1981 he evaluated a 72-year-old man who became agitated and aggressive 6 years after speech difficulty and word finding problems had developed. In his report on this patient, Dr. Geschwind clearly differentiated this type of dementing illness from the more characteristic presentations of Alzheimer's disease, noting that a number of patients with "focal progressive disorders" had been brought to his attention. Dr. Geschwind was not alone in his understanding of this phenomenon, but his awareness of focal dementias predated later publications by a number of investigators, including some of those who worked with him (20,21).

Dr. Geschwind used his imagination in formulating a diagnosis. He frequently speculated about how seemingly unrelated clinical syndromes were actually connected. In his view, there were "no coincidences." His remarkable ability to recall details about patients he had evaluated allowed him to perform ad hoc regression analyses on the clinical features of his patients' cases long before computers and formal clinical databases were used for such purposes. In his evaluation of patients with dementia, Dr. Geschwind was continually seeking to uncover new clinical relationships. For example, in a letter to a colleague who seemed to be relating memory disorders exclusively to dysfunction of hippocampal structures, Dr. Geschwind pointed out that other structures may mediate memory, such as the medial-dorsal nucleus of the thalamus and the mammillary bodies. That comment presaged the later emphasis on the primacy of memory networks over specific memory structures (22,23). In another letter, to neuroimmunologist Dr. Howard Weiner, he speculated about whether viruses might be associated with paraneoplastic neurological phenomena, such as the dementia associated with cancer.

Today there are a few promising strategies for treating dementing illnesses, particularly Alzheimer's disease (24,25), but during Dr. Geschwind's career, the prospects for treating these diseases were grim. Yet Dr. Geschwind managed to infuse his notes and writings with extraordinary optimism about treatment. Rejecting the therapeutic nihilism that so often surrounded the management of dementia, Dr. Geschwind always sought the marginal interventions that might improve the patient's symptoms and quality of life. For example, he was willing to try electroconvulsive therapy (ECT) in demented patients with behavioral symptoms—an idea predicated in part on his awareness of the common co-occurrence of dementia and depression symptomatology, and in part on his empiric understanding that (as he stated in a letter to a referring physician) "organic confusion . . . often responds favorably to ECT." Similarly, Dr. Geschwind favored the use of antidepressant treatment as a diagnostic probe. For example, in describing a patient with atypical dementia and parkinsonian features, he recommended separate trials of both carbidopa-levodopa and antidepressant medication, to see which symptoms might improve.

In reviewing Dr. Geschwind's case records and correspondence about patients with dementia whom he had seen, I was surprised to learn how often he recommended brain biopsies. In one such case he stated:

> I would myself recommend that a brain biopsy be carried out, since it has increasingly become our experience that, although many dementias can be diagnosed clinically, there are many others which simply have pathological bases which are surely unknown to us now, and among these there must be some which must be potentially treatable. . . . Very rarely, one finds an unusual condition such as a progressive vasculitis or sarcoidosis—conditions which might respond to . . . steroid or immunosuppressant therapy. . . . As you know, most neurologists and neurosurgeons are reluctant to take this step, and I therefore mention it hesitantly. It would, of course, certainly settle the diagnosis.

This quote reveals a clinician who was ever hopeful of finding the unusual disorder that would respond to treatment. And despite the risks associated with brain biopsies, Dr. Geschwind seems to have appreciated the fact that making a secure diagnosis, even one that is untreatable, has considerable value in itself. Although brain biopsy has not often proved to reveal otherwise unsuspected but treatable disorders (26–28), in cases of atypical dementia, the knowledge gained from biopsy has been shown to be very comforting to families caring for patients with dementia (27).

RECENT ADVANCES IN DEMENTIA

Dr. Geschwind's influence on recent work in the field of dementia is significant. The concept of disconnection has provided an intellectual framework for clinical descriptions of patients with dementia and for explaining the pathogenesis of the clinical manifestations of Alzheimer's disease. For example, the concentration of pathological markers in layer 2 of the human entorhinal cortex has been interpreted as disconnecting the hippocampus from its neocortical afferents, impairing the consolidation of new learning, and leading to the classic amnestic syndrome characteristic of Alzheimer's disease (29,30). Dr. Geschwind's writings on apraxia (31,32) have also been helpful in explaining the abnormalities of praxis associated with dementia and the clinical presentations of atypical dementias (20,33–35).

Dr. Geschwind's influence on his students has had an even further-reaching effect, as recounted in recent descriptions of the history, intellectual content, and training curricula of behavioral neurology programs (36–39). In 1966 Dr. Geschwind established, at the Boston Veterans Administration Hospital, the first American fellowship program in behavioral neurology; for many years it remained the sole fellowship of its type (Fig. 1). Then, as Dr. Geschwind's trainees and others established training programs of their own, the number of fellowships grew. A survey conducted in 1995 revealed that out of 157 residency training programs in neurology, 34 (21%) also had active behavioral neurology fellowships, and 28 more (18%) reported plans to develop fellowships (38). Of the existing 34 programs, 27 (79%) evaluated patients with dementing disorders and 9 (26%) were predominantly or exclusively concerned with dementia and age-related disorders, whereas only 6 (17%) were primarily concerned with the evaluation of strokes.

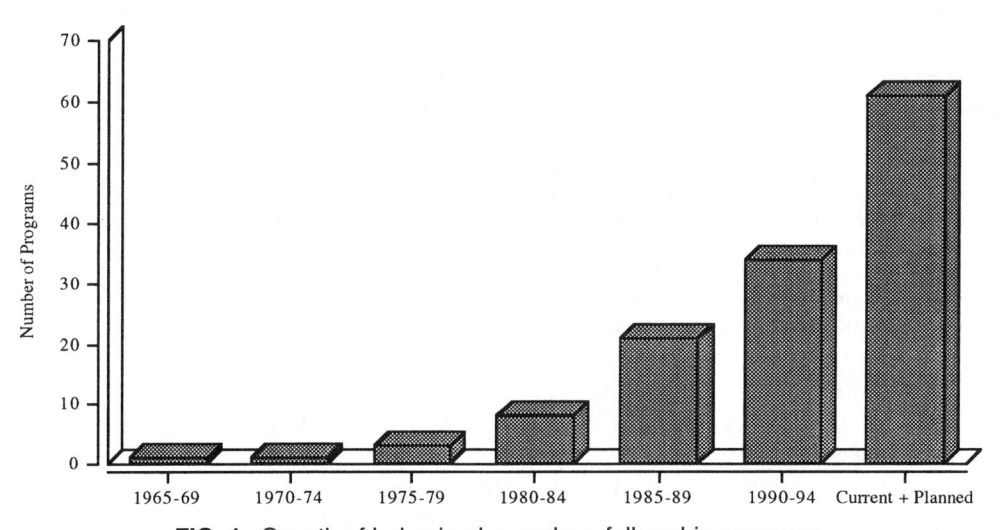

FIG. 1. Growth of behavioral neurology fellowship programs.

DEMENTIA, OLFACTION, AND VISUAL HALLUCINATIONS

In recent years, a connection has been established between deficits in olfaction and some dementing disorders, especially Alzheimer's disease. Peripheral and central olfactory pathways are dramatically affected in Alzheimer's disease (40–42). Diminished olfactory discrimination appears early in the clinical course, and diminished olfactory sensitivity occurs later (43,44). But as a resident in neurology under Dr. Geschwind in 1984, well before the publication of those findings, I learned that he had a particular and personal interest in olfaction, sparked by the fact that he himself had anosmia! Dr. Geschwind attributed his complete loss of the sense of smell to a viral syndrome some years earlier. At the time I learned this fact, I was preparing a grand rounds presentation on the neurology of taste and smell. Dr. Geschwind volunteered to be the surprise "patient" whom I would present at grand rounds. The interview in which he described the onset and course of his anosmia (Fig. 2), and a subsequent demonstration of ways to test taste and smell at the bedside were videotaped. I had never before, nor have I since, seen a medical school faculty member volunteer himself or herself as the patient for a grand rounds. Yet Dr. Geschwind fulfilled that role so generously and graciously that students, my fellow residents, and I were enthralled.

Dr. Geschwind took considerable pride in his clinical skills and in his ability to contribute to the body of scientific knowledge through shrewd clinical observations and clinicopathological correlations. He once attended a lecture by the noted neuro-ophthalmologist Dr. Simmons Lessell on visual hallucinations; during the lecture, Dr. Lessell described the hallucinating patient as "seeing something that other observers cannot see." Dr. Lessell recalls that Dr. Geschwind had called him at 11:30 that evening to discuss the lecture and, in the course of that conversation, repeated this quote back, saying "...that's not a hallucination, that's the definition of a good clinician!" It was this ability to see what others missed that delighted Dr. Geschwind, and that delight was palpable to his many colleagues, students, and friends. Dr. Geschwind respected research in the basic sciences but never wavered in his conviction that clinical research, particularly the in-

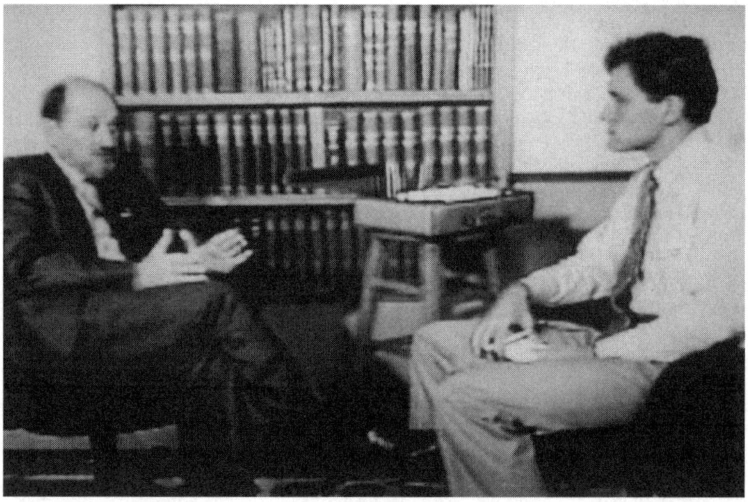

FIG. 2. Dr. Geschwind and Dr. Green; photo from the videotape of grand rounds.

depth case study, was the foundation of what has become behavioral neurology, neuropsychiatry, neuropsychology, and the many other branches of cognitive neuroscience.

Like any athlete, politician, or artist whose death comes during his or her most productive years, Dr. Geschwind is remembered as he was at the height of his talents, with his energies and humor intact and his prodigious memory undiminished. The legacy of his accomplishments is tinged only by the bittersweet awareness of what he might have accomplished had he lived longer. He was for all a shining example of a resplendent clinical scientist, teacher, mentor, and friend, one whose faith and presence we still miss.

REFERENCES

1. Alzheimer A. Uber eine eigenartige Erkrankung der Hirnrinde. *Allg Z Psychiatr* 1907;64:146.
2. Alzheimer A. Über eigenartige Krankheitsfälle des späteren Alters. *Z Gesamte Neurol Psychiatr* 1911;4: 356–385.
3. Haase G. Diseases presenting as dementia. In: Wells C, ed. *Dementia*. Philadelphia: FA Davis, 1971:163–207.
4. Pearce J, Miller E. *Clinical aspects of dementia*. London, Baillere-Tindall 1973.
5. Arab A. Plaques seniles et arteriosclerose cerebrale. *Rev Neurol* 1954;91:22.
6. Fisher CM. Dementia in cerebral vascular disease. *In: Cerebral vascular disease, sixth conference.* New York: Grune & Stratton, 1968.
7. Geschwind N. Disturbances of language, perception, and memory. In: Keefer C, Wilkins R, eds. *Medicine: essentials of clinical practice.* Boston: Little, Brown, 1970:973–980.
8. Petersen RC. Normal aging, mild cognitive impairment, and early Alzheimer's disease. *The Neurologist.* 1995;*(in press),* vol 1, pp 326–344, 1995.
9. Geschwind N. Organic problems in the aged: brain syndromes and alcoholism. *J Geriatr Psychiatry* 1978;11: 161–166.
10. Becker JT, Lopez OL, Wess J. Material-specific memory loss in probable Alzheimer's disease. *J Neurol Neurosurg Psychiatry* 1992;55:1177–1181.
11. Benson DF, Davis RJ, Snyder BD. Posterior cortical atrophy. *Arch Neurol* 1988;45:789–793.
12. Cogan DG. Visual disturbances with focal progressive dementing disease. *Am J Ophthalmol* 1985;100:68–72.
13. Crystal HA, Horoupian DS, Katzman R, Jotkowitz S. Biopsy-proved Alzheimer disease presenting as a right parietal lobe syndrome. *Ann Neurol* 1982;12:186–188.
14. Hof PR, Bouras C, Constantinidis J, Morrison JH. Balint's syndrome in Alzheimer's disease: specific disruption of the occipito-parietal visual pathway. *Brain Res* 1989;493(2):368–375.
15. Jagust J, Davies P, Tiller-Borich JK, Redd B. Focal Alzheimer's disease. *Neurology* 1990;40:14–19.
16. Kirshner HS, Webb WG, Kelly MP, Wells CE. Language disturbance: an initial symptom of cortical degenerations and dementia. *Arch Neurol* 1984;41:491–496.
17. Martin A, Brouwers P, Lalonde F, et al. Towards a behavioral typology of Alzheimer's patients. *J Clin Exp Neuropsychol* 1986;8:594–610.
18. Mesulam M-M, Geschwind N. Disordered mental states in the postoperative period. In: *Symposium of medical aspects of genitourinary surgery.* 1976:199–215.
19. Olson D, Auchus A, Green R. Dementia. In: Lubin M, Walker H, Smith R, eds. *Medical management of the surgical patient.* Philadelphia: JB Lippincott, 1995:361–367.
20. Green RC, Goldstein FC, Mirra SS, Alazraki NP, Baxt JL, Bakay RAE. Slowly progressive apraxia in Alzheimer's disease. *J Neurol Neurosurg Psychiatry* 1995;59:312–315.
21. Mesulam M-M. Slowly progressive aphasia without generalized dementia. *Ann Neurol* 1982;11:592–598.
22. Damasio A, Tranel D. Nouns and verbs are retrieved with differently distributed neural systems. *Proc Natl Acad Sci USA* 1993;90(11):4957–4960.
23. Mesulam M-M. Large-scale neurocognitive networks and distributed processing for attention, language, and memory. *Ann Neurol* 1990;28:597–613.
24. Knapp MJ, Knopman DS, Solomon PR, Pendlebury WW, Davis CS, Gracon SI. A 30-week randomized controlled trial of high-dose tacrine in patients with Alzheimer's disease. *JAMA* 1994;271:985–991.
25. Rogers SL, Friedhoff LT. E2020 improves cognition and quality of life in patients with mild-to-moderate Alzheimer's disease: results of a Phase-II trial. *Neurology* 1994;44(suppl l2):165.
26. Hulette CM, Earl NL, Crain BJ. Evaluation of cerebral biopsies for the diagnosis of dementia. *Arch Neurol* 1992; 49:28–31.
27. Olson D, Green R, Bakay R, Auchus A, Mirra S. Diagnostic biopsy in atypical dementia. *J Neuropsychiatry Clin Neurosci* 1995;7(3):406.
28. Waltregny A, Maula A, Brucher JM. Contribution of stereotactic brain biopsies to the diagnosis in several cases of dementia. *Acta Neurol Psychiatr Belg* 1989;89:161–167.
29. Hyman BT, Van Hoesen GW, Damasio AR. Memory-related neural systems in Alzheimer's disease: an anatomic study. *Neurology* 1990;40:1721–1730.

30. Hyman BT, Van Hoesen GW, Damasio AR, Barnes CL. Alzheimer's disease: cell-specific pathology isolates the hippocampal formation. *Science* 1984;225:1168–1170.
31. Geschwind N. The apraxias: neural mechanisms of disorders of learned movement. *Am Sci* 1975;63:188–195.
32. Geschwind N, Damasio AR. Apraxia. In: Frederiks JAM, ed. *Handbook of clinical neurology.* B.V.: Elsevier Science, 1985:423–432.
33. Rapesak SZ, Croswell SC, Rubens AB. Apraxia in Alzheimer's disease. *Neurology* 1989;39:664–668.
34. Sala S, Lucchelli F, Spinnler H. Ideomotor apraxia in patients with dementia of Alzheimer type. *J Neurol* 1987;234:91–93.
35. Travniczek-Marterer A, Danielcyzk W, Simanyi M, Fischer P. Ideomotor apraxia in Alzheimer's disease. *Acta Neurol Scand* 1993;88:1–4.
36. Benson DF. The history of behavioral neurology. *Neurol Clin* 1993;11(1):1–8.
37. Cummings JL, Hegarty A. Neurology, psychiatry, and neuropsychiatry. *Neurology* 1994;44:209–213.
38. Green RC, Benjamin S, Cummings JL. Fellowship programs in behavioral neurology. *Neurology* 1995;45:412–415.
39. Ross ED. Intellectual origins and theoretical framework of behavioral neurology. *Neuropsychiatry Neuropsychol Behav Neurol* 1995;6(1):65–67.
40. Reyes PF, Deems DA, Suarez MG. Olfactory-related changes in Alzheimer's disease: a quantitative neuropathologic study. *Brain Res Bull* 1993;32:1–5.
41. Tabaton M, Cammarata S, Mancardi GL, Cordone G, Perry G, Loeb C. Abnormal tau-reactive filaments in olfactory mucosa in biopsy specimens of patients with probable Alzheimer's disease. *Neurology* 1991;41:391–394.
42. Talamo BR, Rudel RA, Kosik KS, et al. Pathological changes in olfactory neurons in patients with Alzheimer's disease. *Nature* 1989;337:736–739.
43. Koss E, Weiffenbach JM, Haxby JV, Friedland RP. Olfactory detection and identification performance are dissociated in early Alzheimer's disease. *Neurology* 1988;38(8):1228–1232.
44. Serby M, Larson P, Kalkstein D. The nature and course of olfactory deficits in Alzheimer's disease. *Am J Psychiatry* 1991;148:357–360.

Behavioral Neurology and
the Legacy of Norman Geschwind,
edited by S. C. Schachter and O. Devinsky,
Lippincott-Raven Publishers, Philadelphia © 1997.

22

Apraxia

Kenneth M. Heilman, Leslie J. Gonzalez Rothi, and Robert T. Watson

University of Florida, Department of Neurology, Gainesville, Florida 32610-0236.

Apraxia was one of Norman Geschwind's major interests. In the 1960s, when virtually no one else was interested in apraxia, he renewed interest in the subject. He resurrected Liepmann's contributions and defined apraxia in a manner similar to that of Liepmann: "the incapacity for purposive movement of the limbs despite retained mobility." He thought that the apraxias represented a "group of disorders of higher functions which are best understood anatomically." Although Geschwind was interested in both limb and buccofacial apraxia, the discussion in this chapter will be limited to limb apraxia. When investigating or discussing almost any topic, Norman Geschwind took a historic approach and, in general, that is the approach used in this chapter.

Finkelnburg (1) noted that the abilities to gesture and to think are impaired in aphasics and that the core deficit in aphasia is the inability to comprehend or express symbols. He reasoned that whereas aphasia is the inability to express symbols verbally, an aphasic's inability to gesture is the inability to produce symbols nonverbally. He therefore attributed both aphasia and apraxia to what he termed *asymbolia*. Steinthal (2), according to Hecaen and Rondot (3), was the first to use the term *apraxia* for a loss of motor skills. Steinthal used this term for defects in "the relationship between movements and the objects with which the movements were concerned."

Despite these 19th century descriptions of apraxia, not many important advances were made until the beginning of the 20th century and the work of Hugo Liepmann. Liepmann was a student of Karl Wernicke, who was responsible not only for describing new types of aphasia (e.g., Wernicke's aphasia) but also for introducing explanations of these aphasia syndromes in what are now termed *information-processing systems*. In these systems, specific areas of the brain (modules) store knowledge. Each module may contain unique types of information that are now called *representations*. These information-processing models have heuristic value. For example, they allowed Wernicke to predict what has been called *conduction aphasia*. Liepmann (4) was the first to apply this form of cognitive neuropsychologic analysis to the behavioral disorder of apraxia. He described three forms of apraxia: limb-kinetic, ideomotor, and ideational. In this chapter, we will discuss these three forms of apraxia as well as other forms, and the information-processing models of praxis.

LIMB-KINETIC APRAXIA

Limb-kinetic apraxia is an inability to make fine, precise, independent finger movements of the hand contralateral to a cerebral lesion. Kuypers (5) ablated the corticospinal system in monkeys and found that the monkeys were not weak but had lost the ability to make precise, independent finger movements. Geschwind thought that what Liepmann had termed limb-kinetic apraxia was probably related to injury to the corticospinal neurons or their projections to the spinal cord. Although one needs to be able to make precise, independent finger movements to perform skilled acts, limb-kinetic apraxia is not so much a disorder of learned skilled movements as an elemental motor disorder. Therefore, Geschwind did not like the term *limb-kinetic apraxia* because it did not refer to true apraxia. Limb-kinetic apraxia will not be discussed further in this chapter.

IDEOMOTOR APRAXIA

Liepmann's first major manuscript (6) attempted to demonstrate that apraxia was not a disorder of symbolic behavior (as suggested by Finkelnburg in 1876), an elemental motor disorder, or a disorder of recognition (agnosia). The patient he described (M.T.) was apraxic with his right arm only; when forced to use his left arm, the patient was not apraxic. Liepmann argued that if the core defect was that of asymbolia or agnosia, the patient should have made the same errors with both arms. Liepmann demonstrated that apraxia may occur in the absence of aphasia and that aphasia may occur in the absence of apraxia. In addition, Goodglass and Kaplan (7) demonstrated that when apraxia and aphasia occur together, the severity of the aphasia does not predict the severity of the apraxia, or vice versa. All these observations refute Finkelnburg's asymbolia hypothesis of apraxia.

Kimura and Archibald (8) once again raised the possibility of a unitary mechanism for both aphasia and apraxia associated with left hemisphere lesions. They studied right-hemisphere- and left-hemisphere-damaged subjects by having them perform simple or complex hand gestures. When compared with the right-hemisphere-damaged control subjects, those with left hemisphere damage were impaired on complex gestures that required sequences. Kimura and Archibald (8) proposed that the sequencing defect found in apraxia might also be found in aphasia and suggested that left hemisphere dominance for sequencing might account for its ability to mediate both praxis and speech-language. Although sequencing is important in both speaking and gesturing, apraxia is also associated with spatial errors and other types of temporal errors (9,10). In addition, not only can apraxia occur in the absence of aphasia, and aphasia in the absence of apraxia, but praxis and speech may be mediated by different hemispheres. For example, together with Norman Geschwind, we (11) reported on a left-handed patient who had a large right hemisphere cerebral infarction. Although this patient was severely apraxic, he was not aphasic, suggesting that normally while his right hemisphere was mediating praxis, his left hemisphere was mediating speech and language. These observations refute a unitary hemispheric hypothesis for aphasia and apraxia.

Although the case reported by Liepmann in 1900 (6) demonstrated that asymbolia could not account for apraxia, this patient was not an ideal one for the study of apraxia. The patient's hand preference was not clearly defined, and he had syphilis with multifocal brain disease. Liepmann and Maas (12) described another patient (Ochs) who had right arm and hand weakness and who could not correctly carry out commands with his left hand. On postmortem examination, Ochs was found to have a lesion of his left basis pontis that accounted for his right hemiparesis. Ochs also had a lesion of his corpus callosum that Liepmann and Maas thought accounted for the patient's ideomotor apraxia of the left hand. Liepmann was aware of Broca's and Wernicke's reports demonstrating that, in right-handers, language is mediated by the left hemisphere. Liepmann and Maas could have explained their patient's left-hand apraxia by suggesting that the callosal lesion caused the left hemisphere's language comprehension systems to be disconnected from the right hemisphere's motor systems that control the left hand. Unlike verbal commands, gesture imitation and the use of actual tools or objects do not require language. The right hemisphere's visual, somesthetic, and motor systems were all intact, and if the patient's callosal apraxia was the result of a language–motor disconnection, the right hemisphere should have been able to mediate both gesture imitation and actual tool use, because neither act requires language. Therefore, Liepmann and Maas did not think that their patient's left arm apraxia could be explained by a disconnection between the left hemisphere, which mediates language, and the right hemisphere, which controls movements of the left hand.

The fact that a callosal disconnection impaired these praxic functions suggested to Liepmann and Maas that the left hemisphere of this patient stored some other form of nonlanguage knowledge, and that this store of knowledge was critical for the performance of learned skilled movements. Liepmann and Maas posited that the left hemisphere of right-handers not only mediates language but also contains movement formulas that store the spatial and temporal knowledge of purposeful skilled movements.

Liepmann also recognized that in right-handers apraxia may be associated with left hemispheric lesions that do not directly involve the corpus callosum. In 1905 Liepmann (13) reported a study of 83 right-handed patients with either a right or left hemiplegia. He tested praxis in these patients by asking them to pantomime to command, to imitate both transitive and intransitive gestures, and to work with actual tools and objects. Liepmann reported that none of his patients with left hemiplegia (right hemisphere lesions) were apraxic, but that about one half of the subjects with right hemiplegia (left hemisphere lesions) were apraxic even when using their nonparetic left arm and hand. Based on this study, Liepmann concluded that the left sensory motor cortex is dominant for control of movement of both hands and that the left hemisphere controls the ipsilateral left hand by means of the corpus callosum.

In addition to suggesting that the left hemisphere of right-handers plays a dominant role in the mediation of skilled movements independent of the hand used to carry out these skilled movements, Liepmann also suggested that the left hemisphere of right-handers contains an action system with several distinct components. These components include the movement formula and a mechanism that allows these movement representations to be coded onto innervatory patterns. In contrast to the movement formula that contains information about the spatial loci and temporal patterns of learned skilled movements, the parts of the brain that mediate innervatory patterns transform the movement representations, which are primarily represented in multimodal sensory association cortex, into motor patterns. However, Liepmann recognized that correct use of a limb required other interactions as well as "co-operation of innervatory and extra-innervatory areas" of the brain. Liepmann did not state the location of this innervatory system in the brain, but he implied that it might be in the frontal lobes.

From the time Liepmann published his last paper on apraxia until about three decades ago, there was little or no interest in Liepmann's seminal work or in the general topic of apraxia. In the introduction to his classic paper "Disconnexions in Animals and Man," published in *Brain* in 1965, Geschwind (14) attributed this loss of interest to the growth of "holistically oriented" neurologists such as Head, Marie, and von Monakow and to "holistically oriented" psychologists such as Lashley and the Gestalt school. In addition, many of Liepmann's theories were based on the callosal lesion case that he reported on with Maas. Unfortunately, when Akelaitis (15) studied patients with callosal disconnections for intractable epilepsy, he could not replicate Liepmann's findings. Therefore, Liepmann's seminal observations fell into disrepute.

Norman Geschwind, together with his friend and colleague Edith Kaplan, rekindled interest in apraxia when they reported on a patient with a callosal disconnection (16). Geschwind and Kaplan's patient, like the patient reported by Liepmann, was unable to gesture to command with the left hand. When attempting to write with his left hand, the patient was able to write legible letters but frequently either wrote an incorrect word or misspelled the word. The patient could copy writing and correctly imitate gestures with his left hand. Therefore, Geschwind and Kaplan thought that the patient's defects could not be attributed to an elemental motor deficit. Unlike his inability to correctly pantomime to verbal command when the patient used actual objects or tools with his left hand, his performance was excellent. His right hand praxis was normal in all conditions. Geschwind and Kaplan interpreted these findings as a disconnection of the right motor cortex from the speech areas in the left hemisphere. Furthermore, the preserved ability of the left hand to copy writing, imitate gestures, and use actual objects and tools suggested to Geschwind and Kaplan that the right hemisphere was capable of mediating these activities by itself and without information being transferred from the left hemisphere. Whereas Geschwind and Kaplan's patient could imitate and use actual tools and objects, Liepmann and Maas's patient Ochs could not, suggesting to Geschwind and Kaplan that these two patients with callosal disconnection may have had differences in their brain organization.

Patients with left hemisphere lesions in the region of the inferior parietal lobe may fail to pantomime to command correctly with either hand. Geschwind interpreted Liepmann as suggesting that such lesions disconnect Wernicke's area, important for speech comprehension, from the more anterior left motor association cortex. The motor association cortex on the left side projects to the motor cortex on the left side and to the motor association cortex on the right side, which in turn projects to the motor cortex in the right hemisphere. Therefore, according to Geschwind (14), a left hemisphere supramarginal gyrus lesion that includes the subcortical arcuate fasciculus running beneath this gyrus disconnects Wernicke's area from the motor systems in both hemispheres (Fig. 1). Patients with apraxia from lesions in the region of the supramarginal gyrus are usually also unable to imitate gestures correctly. Geschwind thought that imitation was impaired because the lesions extend deep and interrupt visuomotor connections that also run in the subcortical white matter. Although Geschwind considered the postulate that the left supramarginal gyrus of right handers may contain the "memories for movement," he rejected this hypothesis because these representations should be able to cross the callosum and gain access to the right hemisphere's motor systems. If these movement memories are represented in the supramarginal gyrus of the left hemisphere and are able to reach the right hemisphere, that could not account for why patients with more anterior left hemisphere lesions are apraxic when using their left hand (sympathetic apraxia).

In 1983, Watson and Heilman (17) reported on a woman with a spontaneously occurring callosal lesion that did not appear to involve either hemisphere. Unlike Liepmann's patient, the woman was not hemiparetic. She could gesture to command flawlessly with her right hand but was unable to do so with her left hand. Unlike the patients with callosal disconnection reported by Geschwind and Kaplan (16), Akelaitis (15), and Gazzaniga and his coworkers (18), Watson and Heilman's patient was unable to either imitate or use correctly actual objects with her left arm and hand. Graff-Radford et al. (19) reported a similar case of callosal disconnection. In both of these cases, the right hemisphere of these patients was uninjured and had intact visuomotor and tactile-motor connections. Unlike pantomiming to command, neither imitating nor using actual tools or objects requires input from the speech-language areas. The observation that a callosal

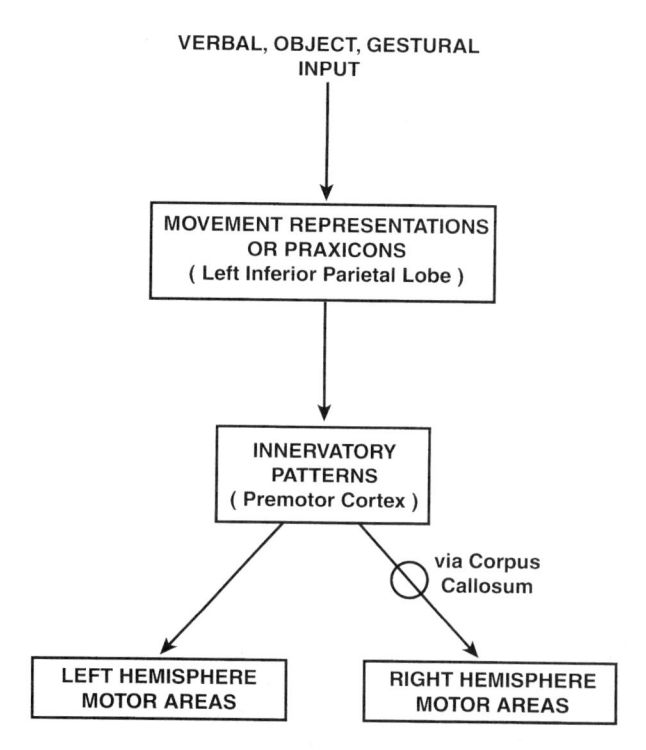

```
        VERBAL, OBJECT, GESTURAL
                INPUT
                  │
                  ▼
      ┌──────────────────────────┐
      │  MOVEMENT REPRESENTATIONS │
      │       OR PRAXICONS        │
      │  ( Left Inferior Parietal │
      │           Lobe )          │
      └──────────────────────────┘
                  │
                  ▼
         ┌──────────────────┐
         │   INNERVATORY    │
         │     PATTERNS     │
         │ ( Premotor Cortex)│
         └──────────────────┘
              ╱       ╲  ○ via Corpus
             ╱         ╲    Callosum
            ▼           ▼
   ┌──────────────┐  ┌───────────────┐
   │ LEFT HEMISPHERE│  │RIGHT HEMISPHERE│
   │  MOTOR AREAS │  │  MOTOR AREAS  │
   └──────────────┘  └───────────────┘
```

FIG. 1. Geschwind's schema of a lateral view of the left side of the brain demonstrating the arcuate fasciculus (AF) that connects Wernicke's area (W) to the motor association cortex (MAC), as well as the visual association cortex (VAC) to the MAC.

disconnection in these patients induced behavioral deficits that could not be accounted for by a language–motor disconnection suggests that Liepmann's original postulate of movement formula could be correct and that in some right-handers movement representations are lateralized to the left hemisphere. In these patients, a callosal disconnection deprives the right hemisphere not only of verbal information from the left hemisphere but also of the temporal and spatial knowledge—also stored in the left hemisphere—needed to perform learned skilled movements with the left hand.

It is not clear, however, why some patients with callosal disconnection can imitate and use actual tools or objects with their left hand and others cannot. Callosal section is often used to treat intractable seizures, and intractable seizures may be associated with anomalies of brain organization. However, Geschwind and Kaplan's patient could imitate and use actual tools or objects and did not have intractable seizures. In addition, one of us (KMH) examined a patient with a surgical disconnection for intractable seizures who was unable to imitate or use correctly actual tools or objects with her left hand. These observations and the knowledge that there are many right-handed patients who, in spite of sustaining large left cerebral infarctions in the distribution of the middle cerebral artery, are not apraxic suggest that in some right-handers these movement representations are bilaterally represented.

As previously mentioned, Geschwind thought that lesions in the region of the left supramarginal gyrus induced apraxia because they involved the arcuate fasciculus that lies in the white matter below the cortex and therefore disconnect both Wernicke's area and visual associations cortex from premotor cortex. However, Geschwind was aware, as was Liepmann, that there were patients who made apraxic errors even when using actual objects or tools. To resolve this dilemma, Geschwind reported that Liepmann had asserted that even the actual handling of tools and objects was frequently learned "visually." However, Geschwind did not specify where this learned visual praxis information was stored. If one presumes that it is stored in the visual cortex, why, then, does one not see apraxia from occipital lesions? Geschwind could also not account for why the visuomotor pathways of the left hemisphere would be dominant.

As an alternative explanation to Geschwind's disconnection hypothesis of apraxia, Heilman et al. (20) and Rothi et al. (21) proposed a representational hypothesis. This hypothesis suggests that right-handed apraxic patients with left parietal lesions cannot correctly gesture to command, imitate, or use actual objects and tools because they have either destroyed the movement representations stored in the left inferior parietal lobule or disconnected them from premotor or motor areas. When one is asked to pantomime a gesture, imitate a gesture, or actually work with an object or tool, one must activate these learned representations. When activated, these stored representations provide the premotor areas with the spatial and temporal information needed to correctly activate the motor systems. To test this representational hypothesis, Heilman et al. (20) and Rothi et al. (21) tested the ability of apraxic subjects and controls to discriminate correctly performed from poorly performed pantomimes as well as their ability to comprehend viewed gestures. If the movement representations are destroyed, then the apraxic subjects should perform these tasks poorly. However, if these representations are intact but have been disconnected from motor areas, then the apraxic subjects should be able to perform these discrimination and comprehension tasks. Heilman et al. (20) and Rothi et al. (21) found that apraxic patients with posterior lesions that involved the left inferior parietal lobule had discrimination and comprehension deficits, but that apraxic patients with anterior lesions were able to discriminate and comprehend gestures. These studies provided evidence that movement representations are stored in the parietal lobe contralateral to the preferred hand. These activated movement representations help program the motor association or premotor cortex that, in turn, selectively activates the motor cortex.

As discussed, lesions anterior to the left parietal lobe can also induce apraxia. If movement representations are stored in the inferior parietal lobe, why would anterior left hemisphere lesions also be associated with apraxia of the left as well as the right hand? Liepmann suggested that before these representations could activate the motor cortex, they had to be transformed into innervatory patterns (12). However, Liepmann never specified exactly where he thought the transformation from a movement representation to a motor pattern took place. Geschwind thought that the convexity premotor cortex was important for praxis. Whereas lesions in this region may be associated with apraxia, these lesions often involve other areas as well as subcortical gray and white matter. Although the convexity premotor cortex may be important in adapting the motor program to environmental perturbations, there is little evidence that innervatory patterns can develop in the convexity premotor cortex.

The premotor cortex (Brodmann's area 6) in the medial portion of the frontal lobe is called the supplementary motor area (SMA). Stimulation of this area produces complex movements that include the fingers, hand, and arm. In contrast, stimulation of the primary motor cortex (Brodmann's area 4) produces simple single movements (22). The SMA receives projections from the parietal lobe and projects to the primary motor cortex. Electrophysiologic studies have revealed that SMA neurons discharge before neurons in the primary motor cortex do (23). Imaging studies of cerebral blood flow demonstrate that when one makes simple finger movements, the contralateral primary motor cortex

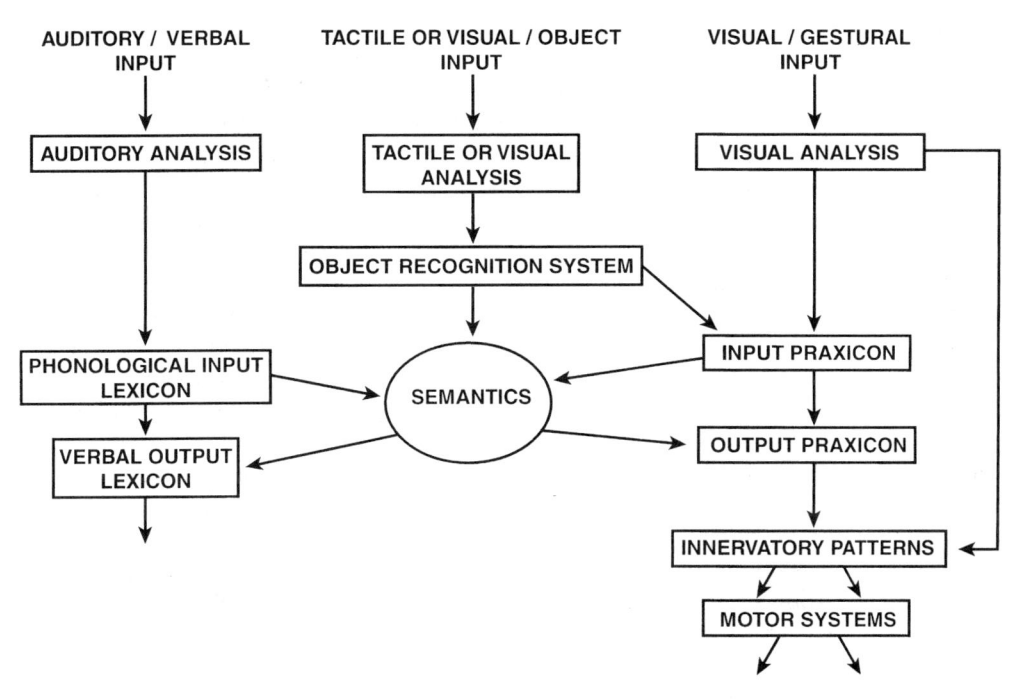

FIG. 2. Diagrammatic model of modules important in the production of learned skilled movements.

becomes activated, but when one makes complex movements, not only is the primary cortex activated but also the SMA. When a person thinks about making a complex movement but does not actually do so, the SMA also becomes activated but the motor cortex does not. These anatomic, physiological, and imaging studies suggest that the SMA would be an ideal area for movement representations to be transcoded to innervatory patterns. In 1986, Watson et al. (24) reported several right-handed patients who had infarcts that destroyed portions of the left medial frontal lobe that included the SMA. These patients demonstrated an ideomotor apraxia of both hands. However, unlike patients with posterior lesions, they were able to discriminate correctly from incorrectly performed movements and could comprehend gestures. Based on the experimental evidence that the parietal lobe may store movement representations and that the SMA may transcode these time-space or visuokinesthetic representations into innervatory patterns, Rothi et al. (25) have proposed a modular system that medicates learned skilled movements (Fig. 2).

CONDUCTION APRAXIA

Ochipa et al. (26) reported on a patient who, like patients with ideomotor apraxia, had an impaired ability to gesture to command. The patient could, however, comprehend gestures, suggesting that his movement representations were intact. Unlike patients with ideomotor apraxia, who typically perform better with imitation than they do in response to command, this patient's imitation was worse than his performance to command. If this patient's deficit was being induced by an inability of the movement representations to gain access to the areas of the brain that generate the innervatory patterns, gesture to imitation should be no worse than gesture to command. Therefore, Ochipa et al. (26) postulated that there may be two stores of movement representations, one more involved in the comprehension and discrimination of gestures (input praxicon) and the other more involved in providing movement instructions (output praxicon). Although gesturing to command requires accessing the output praxicon, it does not require access to and activation of input praxicons. In contrast, imitation does require access to and activation of the input praxicons. However, because the patient could comprehend and discriminate viewed gestures, this patient's failure to imitate could not be accounted for by a defect in the input praxicon. The most parsimonious explanation of his failure to imitate gestures correctly is that his left parietal lesion caused a disassociation between the input and output praxicons (Fig. 3).

According to Rothi et al. (25), because normal people can imitate even nonsense gestures, there should be a means of imitating that does not require movement representations (input and output praxicons). Therefore, there may be a direct connection between the portions of the brain that perform visual analysis of gesture and the premotor cortex that programs innervatory patterns (see Fig. 3). Patients with ideomotor apraxia, in whom these movement representations have been destroyed, may improve on imitation because they are able to use this nonrepresentational means of imitating. Mehler (27) reported on two patients who could normally pantomime to command but who could not imitate nonsense gestures. Rothi et al. (25) posited that this nonrepresentational imitation system may have been selectively damaged in the patients. Theoretically, patients who are unable to imitate meaningful gestures must have impairment of both the representational and nonrepresentational systems.

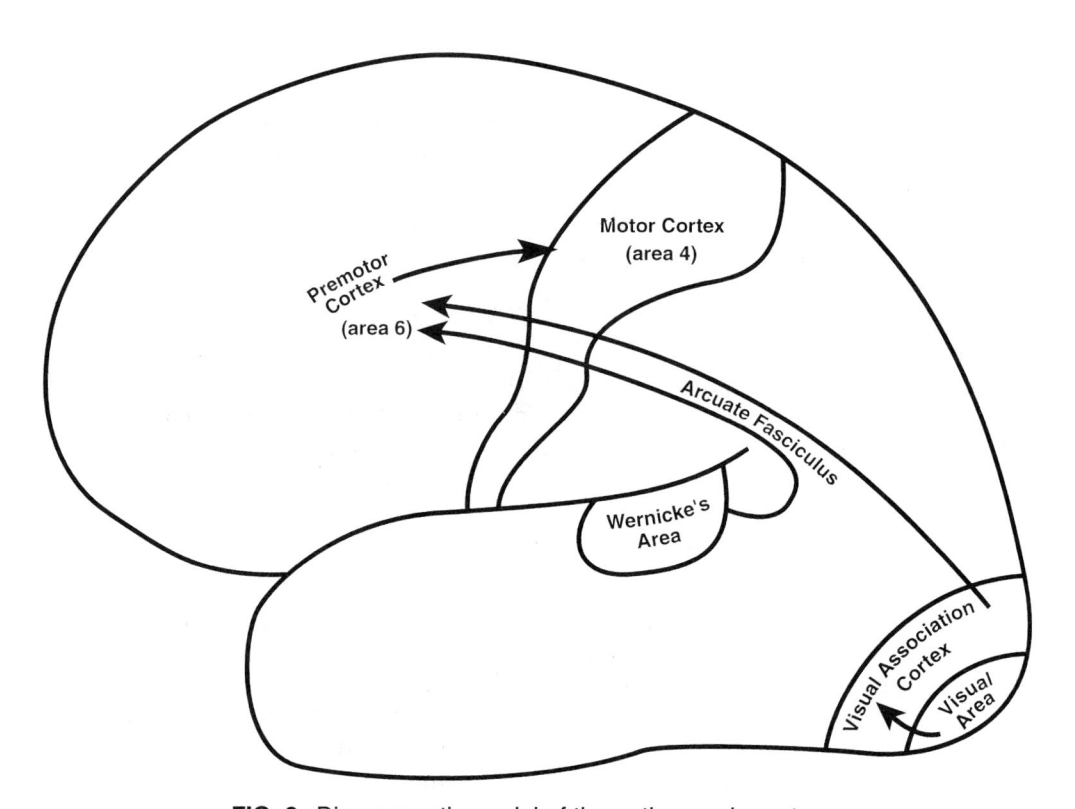

FIG. 3. Diagrammatic model of the entire praxis system.

The patient of Ochipa et al. (26) also had a conduction aphasia, and the impairment of verbal repetition in conduction aphasia has been explained by mechanisms similar to that which we propose for gesture imitation.

DISASSOCIATION APRAXIA

Heilman (28) reported on several patients who were unable to pantomime to command. Unlike patients with ideomotor apraxia, who primarily make spatial and temporal errors (9,10) when given a verbal command, these patients would hesitate to make any meaningful movement. In addition, unlike patients with ideomotor apraxia, when these patients were shown the tool or object that they were asked to pantomime, they were able to pantomime flawlessly. Unlike patients with ideomotor apraxia, they were also able to imitate flawlessly. The article reporting on these patients called their disorder *ideational apraxia* (28), an unfortunate choice of terms for several reasons. First, this term had been used to denote other types of behavioral disorders that will be discussed in a subsequent section. Second, the article stated that the probable mechanism accounting for this disorder was a disassociation between the movement representations discussed previously and the verbal system that interprets the command (see Fig. 3).

The disassociation apraxia described by Heilman (28) is similar to the callosal disconnection described by Geschwind and Kaplan (16) and Gazzaniga et al. (18). However, whereas the inability to gesture to verbal command was restricted to the left hand in the patients with callosal disconnection, the apraxia affected both hands in the patients with disassociation apraxia from intrahemispheric lesions. Unfortunately, these cases were initially described before computer tomography scanning was available. Although the exact loci of lesions that induce disassociation apraxia remain unknown, based on the clinical presentation, Heilman suggested that the lesions were deep under the cortex in the region of the left inferior parietal lobe.

De Renzi et al. (29) replicated Heilman's observations on disassociation apraxia and also described persons who had other forms of disassociation apraxia. They reported on patients who could not correctly gesture to visual stimuli but could correctly gesture to verbal commands. They even described two patients who performed better to verbal commands and visual stimuli than they did when they were blindfolded and holding the tool or object.

IDEATIONAL APRAXIA

Pick (30) described a patient with an aphasia who had some preserved verbal comprehension. However, this patient was unable to use actual tools or objects correctly and had difficulty sequencing a series of acts, using tools or objects, that lead to an action goal. Although failure to recognize a tool or an object (an agnosia) may interfere with a person's ability to use tools or objects correctly, Pick thought that his patient's errors were not related to an agnosia because the patient could name the tools and objects that were incorrectly used. From the time of Pick's description, there has been some conflict as to what actually constitutes ideational apraxia. Is ideational apraxia a defect in using actual tools or is it an inability to perform a sequence of acts that lead to a goal? Liepmann (4) defined ideational apraxia as impaired ability to perform tasks that require a sequence of serial acts using objects or tools, and modern investigators such as Poeck (31) have continued to adhere to this definition.

APRAXIA

Some clinicians and investigators thought that the deficits in patients with ideomotor apraxia were limited to those revealed by tests of pantomime and imitation, but that, when using real tools in the natural environment, these patients did not make errors. De Renzi and Lucchelli (32), therefore, defined *ideational apraxia* as the failure to use actual tools and objects correctly, and they viewed these errors as distinct from those made by patients with ideomotor apraxia, who use actual tools and objects correctly. However, Zangwell (33) noted that the failure even to use actual tools properly may be related to a severe production disorder (ideomotor apraxia) rather than an ideational disorder. Subsequently, using quantitative methods, Clark et al. (34) demonstrated that when patients with ideomotor apraxia do use actual tools or objects, they may make timing and spatial errors. These investigators' research suggested that although the errors made by patients with ideomotor apraxia may be less severe when they are using actual tools or objects than when they are pantomiming, the natures of the errors were similar.

CONCEPTUAL APRAXIA

Roy and Square (35) proposed that physical interactions between an organism and the world may involve the operation of two independent systems: conceptual and production. Whereas patients with ideomotor apraxia make production errors (spatial and temporal errors) primarily, patients with what we have termed conceptual apraxia should make content errors. Ochipa et al. (36) reported on a patient who used actual tools inappropriately in a natural environment. For example, in the bathroom he used a tube of toothpaste to brush his teeth. On another occasion he used a comb to brush his teeth and a toothbrush to pick up his food. One may expect such errors from a patient with visual and tactile agnosia, but this patient was able to name correctly the items he misused. Although a patient with ideomotor apraxia may make production errors with actual tools, the patient reported by Ochipa et al. selected the incorrect tool for a specified action.

In a subsequent study, Ochipa et al. (37) posited that there are four types of conceptual knowledge needed to interact correctly with objects and tools in the environment. These include: (a) tool–action associations, or knowledge of the types of actions that are associated with using specific tools (e.g., the twisting motion that is associated with using a screwdriver); (b) tool–object associations, or knowledge of the types of tools that work on specific objects (e.g., hammers are used to hit nails); (c) the mechanical advantage afforded by tools or mechanical knowledge (e.g., if a hammer is not available to pound in a nail, a wrench, rather than an ice pick, can be used); and (d) tool fabrication, or the ability to make tools (e.g., the ability to bend and use a coat hanger to open a locked car door).

Ochipa et al. (37) studied patients with probable Alzheimer's disease and compared them with matched controls. They demonstrated that many of the Alzheimer's patients did have a conceptual apraxia and that these patients made all four types of conceptual errors. In some patients, conceptual apraxia was not associated with ideomotor apraxia or a semantic language impairment, suggesting that the systems that mediate conceptual praxis knowledge may be independent of the gesture production system and verbal semantics. More recently, to learn if conceptual apraxia can be associated with focal lesions lateralized to one hemisphere, we studied a population of right-handed patients who had strokes in either their right or left hemisphere (38). Only patients with left hemisphere lesions had conceptual apraxia. Unfortunately, many of our patients had large lesions and we did not find a specific anatomic area within the left hemisphere that, when affected by a lesion, induced conceptual apraxia.

CONCLUSIONS

Norman Geschwind virtually resurrected apraxia as a major topic in behavioral neurology. Based on the material discussed in this chapter, we have developed an information-processing model (see Fig. 3). Movement representations (praxicons) are stored in the left inferior parietal lobe of right-handers. These representations code the spatial and temporal patterns of learned skilled movements. Injury to this portion of the brain induces a production deficit called ideomotor apraxia by Liepmann. Patients with these deficits make spatial and temporal errors. Patients with injury to these representations not only are impaired at pantomiming, imitating, and using actual objects, but they also cannot discriminate between correctly and poorly performed gestures and may not be able to comprehend gestures.

In some patients, the ability to imitate gestures is more impaired than the ability to gesture to command (conduction apraxia), suggesting that movement representations (praxicons) may be divided into input and output subdivisions. There is a disassociation between these input and output praxicons in conduction apraxia. For a person to perform skilled acts, these abstract movement representations have to be transcoded into motor programs. This transcoding appears to be performed by a premotor (supplementary motor area)–basal ganglia (putamen-globus pallidus-thalamus) system. Injuries to the brain that interrupt the connections between the movement representations and the portions of the brain where the innervatory patterns develop or the parts of the brain that allow the innervatory patterns to gain access to the motor system may also produce a praxis production deficit (ideomotor apraxia), but not gesture discrimination and comprehension deficits.

In addition to the spatial and temporal errors just discussed, some patients make content errors. Whereas spatial and temporal errors are related to deficits in the praxis production system, content errors are related to deficits in a hypothetical praxis conceptual system or action semantics. Dysfunction of this system may produce deficits of associative knowledge such as tool-action or tool-object knowledge (e.g., knowing that a hammer is used to pound and that a hammer is associated with a nail). Defects in action semantics may also be associated with deficits in mechanical knowledge (e.g., knowing how to use alternative tools and how to fabricate tools). The action semantic representations gain access to the production system by way of the output praxicons. The information-processing model just described is presented in Figure 3.

REFERENCES

1. Finkelnburg F. Ueber Aphasie und Aysmobolie Nebst Versuch Elmer Theorie der Sprachbildung. *Arch Psychiatr* 1876;6.
2. Steinthal P. Abriss der Sprach wissenschaft. Berlin, Germany, 1871.
3. Hecaen H, Rondot P. Apraxia as a disorder of a system of signs. In: Roy EA, ed. *Studies of apraxia and related disorders.* Amsterdam, The Netherlands: Elsevier, 1985.
4. Liepmann H. Apraxia. *Ergeb Ges Med* 1920;1:516–543.
5. Kuypers HGJM. Anatomy of the descending pathways. In: Brooks VE, ed. *Handbook of physiology: sec 1.* The nervous system, vol 2: *Motor control.* Washington, DC: American Physiological Society, 1981.
6. Liepmann H. Das Krankheitshild der Apraxie (motorischen/Asymbolie). *Monatsschr Psychiatr Neurol* 1900;8: 15–44, 102–132, 182–197.
7. Goodglass H, Kaplan E. Disturbance of gesture and pantomime in aphasia. *Brain* 1963;86:703–720.
8. Kimura D, Archibald Y. Motor function of the left hemisphere. *Brain* 1974;97:337–350.
9. Rothi LJG, Mack L, Verfaellie M, Brown P, Heilman KM. Ideomotor apraxia: error pattern analysis. *Aphasiology* 1988;2:381–387.
10. Poizner H, Mack L, Verfaellie M, Rothi LJG, Heilman KM. Three dimensional computer graphic analysis of apraxia. *Brain* 1990;113:85–101.

11. Heilman KM, Coyle JM, Gonyea EF, Geschwind N. Apraxia and agraphia in a left-hander. *Brain* 1973;96:21–28.
12. Liepmann H, Maas O. Fall von linksseitiger Agraphie und Apraxie bei rechsseitiger Lahmung. *Z Psychol Neurol* 1907;10:214–227.
13. Liepman H. Die linke Hemisphare und das Handeln. *Munch Med Wochenschr* 1905;49:2322–2326, 2375–2378.
14. Geschwind N. Disconnexion syndromes in animals and man. (2 parts). *Brain* 1965;88:237–294, 585–644.
15. Akelaitis AJ. A study of gnosis, praxis, and language following section of the corpus callosum and anterior commissure. *J Neurosurg* 1944;1:94–102.
16. Geschwind N, Kaplan E. A human cerebral disconnection syndrome. *Neurology* 1962;12:675–685.
17. Watson RT, Heilman KM. Callosal apraxia. *Brain* 1983;106:391–403.
18. Gazzaniga M, Bogen J, Sperry R. Dyspraxia following diversion of the cerebral commissures. *Arch Neurol* 1967;16:606–612.
19. Graff-Radford NR, Welsh K, Godersky J. Callosal apraxia. *Neurology* 1987;37:100–105.
20. Heilman KM, Rothi LJ, Valenstein E. Two forms of ideomotor apraxia. *Neurology* 1982;32:342–346.
21. Rothi LJG, Heilman KM, Watson RT. Pantomime comprehension and ideomotor apraxia. *J Neurol Neurosurg Psychiatry* 1985;48:207–210.
22. Penfield W, Welsh K. The supplementary motor area of the cerebral cortex. *Arch Neurol Psychiatry* 1951;66:289–317.
23. Brinkman C, Porter R. Supplementary motor area in the monkey: activity of neurons during performance of a learned motor task. *J Neurophysiol* 1979;42:681–709.
24. Watson RT, Fleet WS, Rothi LJG, Heilman KM. Apraxia and the supplementary motor area. *Arch Neurol* 1986;43:787–792.
25. Rothi LJG, Ochipa C, Heilman KM. A cognitive neuropsychological model of limb praxis. *Cognit Neuropsychol* 1991;8:443–458.
26. Ochipa C, Rothi LJG, Heilman KM. Conduction apraxia. *J Neurol Neurosurg Psychiatry* 1994;57:1241–1244.
27. Mehler MF. Visuo-imitative apraxia. *Neurology* 1987;37:129.
28. Heilman KM. Ideational apraxia—a re-definition. *Brain* 1973;96:861–864.
29. De Renzi E, Faglioni P, Sorgato P. Modality-specific and supramodal mechanisms of apraxia. *Brain* 1982;105:301–312.
30. Pick A. *Sudien uber Motorische Apraxia und ihre Mahestenhende Erscheinungen.* Leipzig, Germany: Deuticke, 1905.
31. Poeck K. Ideational apraxia. *J Neurol* 1983;230:1–5.
32. De Renzi E, Lucchelli F. Ideational apraxia. *Brain* 1988;113:1173–1188.
33. Zangwell OL. L'apraxie ideatorie. *Nerve Neurol* 1960;106:595–603.
34. Clark M, Merians AS, Kothari A, et al. Spatial planning deficits in limb apraxia. *Brain* 1994;117:1093–1106.
35. Roy EA, Square PA. Common considerations in the study of limb, verbal and oral apraxia. In: Roy EA, ed. *Neuropsychological studies of apraxia.* New York: Elsevier, 1985.
36. Ochipa C, Rothi LJG, Heilman KM. Ideational apraxia: a deficit in tool selection and use. *Arch Neurol* 1989;25:190–193.
37. Ochipa C, Rothi LJG, Heilman KM. Conceptual apraxia in Alzheimer's disease. *Brain* 1992;115:1061–1071.
38. Heilman KM, Maher LH, Greenwald ML, Rothi LJG. Conceptual apraxia from lateralized lesions. *Neurology* 1995;45(suppl 4):A266.

23

Right Hemisphere Syndromes and the Neurology of Emotion

Elliott D. Ross

Department of Neurology, University of Oklahoma Health Science Center, Oklahoma City, OK 73190-3048.

Over the last two decades, enormous advances have been made in elucidating the contributions of the right hemisphere to behavior and emotions. Most of this progress can be credited to clinical researchers who either trained under Dr. Geschwind or were strongly influenced by his scholarship. Dr. Geschwind, initially as my teacher and mentor, later as a colleague, and ultimately as a friend, was essential in developing my interest in the right hemisphere, because he was intrigued by it. During rounds, he often commented on his inability to examine in detail the functions of the right hemisphere in contrast to the left hemisphere. Although at that time the right hemisphere as considered "minor" or "nondominant" (1) and thus expendable during neurosurgical procedures, Dr. Geschwind always felt uneasy about this cavalier attitude, which unfortunately still persists. He frequently remarked that developmentally the right hemisphere was not a vestigial structure and that its cytoarchitectonics and connectivity were as complex as the left. He was also aware that right-brain-damaged patients often did very poorly in rehabilitation and were more likely to die from their strokes than aphasic left-brain-damaged patients. He did not believe that the long-term effects of right brain damage were necessarily caused by neglect or anosognosia, because these spectacular syndromes were usually transient. Although Dr. Geschwind did not directly discover the secrets of the right hemisphere, he instilled in us a respect for the right hemisphere that led three of his residents—Ken Heilman, Marsel Mesulam, and me—to focus part of our clinical investigations on elucidating its hidden functions. His influence may also have been instrumental for investigators at the Boston Veterans Administration (VA) Aphasia Unit when conducting some of their neuropsychological research exploring the right hemisphere's role in both the verbal (2–4) and nonverbal (5,6) aspects of language and communication.

AFFECTIVE PROSODY, EMOTIONAL EXPERIENCE, DEPRESSION, AND THE RIGHT HEMISPHERE

In 1977, while ward attending, I took care of an unfortunate middle-aged woman who had sustained an ischemic infarction of the right hemisphere. Computed tomography (CT) revealed that the infarction involved mostly the right suprasylvian region, sparing the temporal and posterior parietal lobes. The patient had a severe left hemiplegia with sensory loss and transient left-sided neglect with anosognosia. During the second week of her infirmity, I found her in bed embracing a young man sporting a ponytail. I was astonished because the patient had been married for 20 years to an apparently devoted husband and had two grown children. The young man was clearly embarrassed but the patient seemed unconcerned. In a very dry and nonchalant manner, she introduced him as her boyfriend and college English professor whom she was planning to marry after she divorced her husband. Over the next few days, I encouraged her to postpone any decisions about divorce, because right hemisphere strokes were thought to possibly alter emotions and insight. I always left her room feeling frustrated because her social interactions were always without any enthusiasm. I finally gave up counseling her and decided that she was probably just a typical neurasthenic bored housewife.

One month after discharge she called my office and requested to see me as soon as possible. When she entered my office the next day she sat down and, speaking in a monotone without gestures, confided that "something terrible is wrong with me." She had returned to teaching grade school and discovered that she could no longer maintain control of her classroom because she could not put anger into her voice or actions to signal the students that "I meant business." She then related that at home things were better. If she became angry she would curse. Because it was not her custom to curse, her family instantly recognized that she was angry. However, she felt that it would be unprofessional and unethical to curse in the classroom and refrained from doing so despite her increasing frustration. Feeling emotions or detecting emotions in others was not a problem for her. I rapidly realized that my prior antipathy when interacting with her in the hospital caused by her absolute lack of affect when discussing emotional issues, and that her affectless behavior was a result of her stroke, not of her being a neurasthenic, bored housewife. I was also convinced from her verbal descriptions of current life events, including the untimely death of her father, that she could experience emotions inwardly and could comprehend emotions conveyed by prosody and gestures.

On searching the literature, I found the seminal articles written by Monrad-Krohn (7,8) describing disturbed prosody following brain lesions. Although he had set the clinical foundation for the neurology of prosody, he had not linked the right hemisphere to any particular aspect of prosody. I then rediscovered the remarkable paper written in 1975 by Ken Heilman, Robert Scholes, and Bob Watson (9), entitled "Auditory Affective Agnosia: Disturbed Comprehension of Affective Speech," which described a series of patients with right posterior sylvian infarctions who could no longer comprehend affect in taped sentences conveyed by nonverbal (prosodic) means. Yet their left-brain-damaged patients with mild aphasias performed the task nearly flawlessly. In 1977, Tucker, Watson, and Heilman published a follow-up article (10) that showed that patients with right parietal disease had marked difficulty in evoking affectively toned speech on a repetition task. In the spring of 1978, I discussed the behavioral problems of my patient with Marsel Mesulam. He, too, had recently encountered a patient with the same symptoms after a right-sided suprasylvian infarction. We then wrote a paper in 1979 (1), in which we hypothesized that affective prosody and gestures were a dominant function of the right hemisphere and that the anatomic areas subserving the affective components of language in the right hemisphere were similar to those subserving propositional language in the left hemisphere.

In December of 1978, Niels Lassen visited Dallas and presented studies using a single-photon emission scanning technique (SPECT) that measured focal changes in cerebral blood flow during behavioral activation (11). Toward the end of the lecture, he presented data on speech activation, inasmuch he and his colleagues had wanted to study a highly lateralized brain function with their new technique (12). They chose a simple task of having subjects repetitively count from 1 to 20 during the 4-minute scan, because "everyone knows that language is a dominant function of the left hemisphere." To their surprise, they found that both hemispheres became active during the task with relatively homologous increases in blood flow in the inferior frontal, posterior sylvian, and supplementary motor areas; locations that, when disturbed in the left hemisphere, are associated with aphasic syndromes. Niels ended his lecture by stating that neither he nor his colleagues had any ready explanation for this totally unexpected finding. However, their SPECT data appeared to strongly support the hypotheses that Marsel and I proposed in our paper, which was then in press (1).

The next logical step was to collect a series of patients with right hemisphere infarctions and test their ability to process affective prosody and gestures, using a method similar to that used to test propositional language at the bedside—by assessing spontaneous production of affective prosody and comprehension of gestures. With the help of residents, I rapidly collected 10 right-handed patients with right hemisphere infarctions documented by CT scan. Depending on the location of the infarction, different combinations of affective processing deficits occurred that were analogous to the aphasic syndromes caused by left hemisphere infarction. Thus, I called these syndromes *aprosodias* and used modifiers to classify them in a similar manner to the aphasias (e.g., motor, sensory, global, transcortical motor, transcortical sensory) (13). Two patients had lesions restricted to the basal ganglia and had recovery patterns similar to the aphasias. Although patients with motor types of aprosodias had a flat affect during discourse, they were still capable of feeling emotions inwardly and could laugh or cry in the extreme when recalling emotional life events. One of the patients verbally complained of being suicidally depressed even though he did not project any affective clues of his inner turmoil.

During this period, I had the good fortune to meet John Rush, who had joined the psychiatry department at Southwestern Medical Center in late 1978. John focused on the affective disorders and was the first to publish controlled data showing the efficacy of cognitive (talk) therapy in the treatment of depression (14). Because I was interested in disorders of affect induced by brain lesions, we rapidly became close friends and colleagues. From this relationship and a series of serendipitous observations in stroke patients with preexisting depression, we began to study how focal brain lesions alter the clinical features of depression, in order to infer what areas in the brain modulate depression. We rapidly discovered that disentangling the contribution of depression and brain damage to aberrant behaviors was difficult because depression could alter the signs and symptoms caused by a stroke, and a stroke could dramatically alter the signs and symptoms caused by depression (15,16). Our observations eventually led to a publication in 1981 in which we outlined a neurology for depression and clinical methods for diagnosing depression in the presence of a brain lesion (15). We also proposed that nonendogenous (cognitive) depressions were left hemisphere generated, whereas endogenous (melancholic) depressions were right hemisphere generated, a hypothesis that has received partial support from a SPECT scan study carried out by John Rush and colleagues (17).

ACOUSTICAL STUDIES AND HEMISPHERIC LATERALIZATION OF AFFECTIVE PROSODY

In the early 1980s, with the support of David Rosenfield's Stuttering Foundation at Baylor Medical College and the encouragement of Frances Freeman, a speech pathologist at Callier Institute in Dallas, I purchased a digital computer and other equipment to establish an acoustics laboratory. With various colleagues, residents, and students, a series of quantitative investigations of affective prosody in normal and brain-damaged subjects whose native language was either English, which is a nontone language, or Taiwanese, Mandarin Chinese, or Thai, which are tone languages, were initiated (18–25). These studies helped to establish that regardless of the language one speaks, the verbal/linguistic features and their acoustical underpinnings are dominantly modulated by the left hemisphere, whereas the nonverbal/affective features and their acoustical underpinnings are dominantly modulated by the right hemisphere.

Although I had been aware of a number of publications that reported that left hemisphere lesions that caused aphasias could also disrupt affective prosody (26–28), I had assumed (29) that the presence of nonfluent speech or comprehension deficits interfered with the ability of the researchers to adequately test affective prosody. This seemed to be consistent with the observation that the severity of aphasic deficits correlated with the severity of affective prosodic deficits (27,28). In 1987, when I was helping Wayne Gordon and Len Diller at the Rusk Rehabilitation Institute in New York develop a grant to study depression in brain-damaged patients, my assumptions were proven erroneous. Mary Hibbard and Susan Egelko, who were postdoctoral fellows at Rusk, had made a tape of various brain-damaged patients undergoing affective prosody testing. They made the tape so that I could help them develop a semiquantitative judgmental rating system of the patients' performance. Because none of the patients were overtly aphasic, I assumed that the tape included only subjects with right brain damage, some of whom were mildly dysarthric. I also thought that English was not the patients' first language in all cases, because some seemed to have foreign accents and word finding difficulties. Many of the patients had affective flattening of spontaneous speech and made poor attempts at affective repetition. To my surprise, about one quarter of the patients I had identified as aprosodic had left brain lesions. After reviewing the tapes and discussing possible reasons for this unexpected finding, I developed potential strategies for exploring this phenomenon, which I eventually pursued after assuming a position at the University of North Dakota School of Medicine in 1988.

The basic premise of the research was that affective prosody is a highly lateralized and dominant function of the right hemisphere and that any deficits in affective prosody after left hemisphere damage could be accounted for by either nonfluency, poor comprehension, or disruption of the interhemispheric integration of the affective and propositional aspects of language via the corpus callosum (30,31). An aprosodia battery was developed that tested repetition and comprehension of affective prosody by progressively reducing the verbal/articulatory demands by using "sentences" composed of word constituents [monosyllabic (ba ba ba ba ba ba) or asyllabic (aaahhhhhhhh)] portraying different emotions through prosodic variation. We found that reducing the verbal/articulatory demands robustly improved the performance of left-brain-damaged patients to near normal levels, but this either did not improve or, in some instances, worsened the performance of right-brain-damaged patients (31). However, the performance of the left-brain-damaged patients on the word repetition and comprehension tasks of the aprosodia battery did not correlate with any aphasic deficits as measured by the Western Aphasia Battery. In exploring the reason for this unexpected finding, we noted that some left-brain-damaged patients had deep white matter lesions adjacent to the corpus callosum on magnetic resonance imaging (MRI) scan but were not aphasic. For affective repetition to be disrupted, the critical location for a lesion seemed to involve the white matter just below the supplementary motor area (SMA), a region through which connections from both SMAs course to innervate the contralateral primary and premotor areas and striatum. These data, therefore, helped to validate the hypothesis that affective prosody is both a dominant and a lateralized function of the right hemisphere, as originally suggested by Marsel Mesulam and me in 1979 (1). It also gives strong support to the recent findings by Dawn Bowers, Lee Blonder, Russ Bauer, Branch Coslett, Lynn Speedie, and Ken Heilman (32–34), which suggest that right brain damage causes loss of affective-communicative representations (34) as the theoretical basis for the aprosodias, similar to left brain damage causing loss of verbal/syntactic representations as the theoretical basis for the aphasias.

DIFFERENTIAL HEMISPHERIC PROCESSING OF DISPLAY BEHAVIOR AND PRIMARY AND SOCIAL EMOTIONS

In 1991, I was fortunate to meet Ross Buck at a symposium. He is a social psychologist who is best known for his highly regarded textbook, *Human Motivation and Emotion* (35). Ross had spent a year on sabbatical at the Boston VA Aphasia Unit in the early 1980s, where he met and interacted with Dr. Geschwind, Edith Kaplan, Harold Goodglass, Joan Borod, Elissa Koff, and others. Before his sabbatical, he had developed a nonverbal method of assessing emotional display behaviors in brain-damaged patients and, with Robert Duffy, had tested patients with right and left focal strokes and Parkinson's disease and compared their performance to that of normal adults and preschool children (36). The investigators found that normal subjects sculpted their facial displays according to the emotional valence of the stimulus. Highly positive emotional stimuli produce expansive and easily identifiable facial displays, highly negative stimuli produce minimal and unidentifiable displays, and intermediate stimuli produce partial but reasonably identifiable displays. These findings conformed to the concept of social display rules initially formulated by Ekman et al. (37). Although the right-brain-damaged and Parkinson's disease patients showed significantly diminished expressivity, they still maintained a normally differentiated profile of emotional reactivity. However, the left-brain-damaged patients showed equally substantial and identifiable responses for all stimuli regardless of valence. These data suggested that the development of display rules was a function of the left hemisphere, that the left hemisphere was biased towards positive displays because of display rules, and that the right hemisphere was equally adept at displaying both positive and negative emotions but, because of display rules, was inhibited by the left hemisphere to exhibit negative displays. Although this schema is complex, it reconciles two currently accepted but competing hypotheses concerning the hemispheric lateralization of primary emotions and their displays. The right hemisphere hypothesis (38–40) claims that all emotions are modulated predominantly by the right hemisphere, whereas the valence hypothesis (41–43) claims that positive emotions and their display are modulated predominantly by the left hemisphere, whereas negative emotions and their display are modulated predominantly by the right hemisphere.

When Ross Buck visited Fargo, we reviewed some data that Dick Homan and I had collected between 1983 and 1987 when we were both in Dallas evaluating patients with epilepsy using the Wada test (amytal injections into the right or left internal carotid arteries, causing a reversible neurological deficit). I prevailed upon Dick to allow me to test his patients' production, repetition, and comprehension of affective prosody before, during, and after the right-sided Wada test so that I could acoustically analyze their performance (21). In order to obtain a good sample of spontaneous affective prosody, I usually interviewed the patients the night before the Wada procedure and asked them to recall various emotional experiences. The recall that produced the best affective responses in both voice and gestures was chosen, and during the right-sided Wada test, the patient was asked to recall that experience. The very first patient we tested had a remarkable change in the emotional content of his story. Instead of recalling how "scared" and "frightened to death" he was after a car accident, he stated that he had felt "silly" and "stupid" for getting himself in such a predicament and denied feeling "scared." In subsequent patients, similar changes in emotional recall occurred. For example, one patient who was "mad and angry" about being teased as a child because of her epilepsy recalled, during the right-sided Wada, feeling "embarrassed" and denied feeling either mad or angry when questioned. Of the ten patients studied, eight had dramatic changes in their emotional recall. Although these observations were very interesting, Dick and I sat on the data for more than 5 years, mainly because we could not figure out exactly what the data meant in terms of the neurology of emotions. The observations did not support either the right hemisphere hypothesis or the valence hypothesis. If the right hemisphere hypothesis was correct, then the patients should have lost their emotional recall. If the valence hypothesis was correct, the patients should have recalled a positive emotion; instead, they usually recalled having experienced a different, negative-type emotion.

After pouring over transcriptions of the tape recordings for about a half hour and constructing a chart, Ross suddenly blurted out "social emotions!" and explained very excitedly that what the patients did was shift their recall from a primary to a social emotion. My immediate response was, "What in the world is a social emotion?" Ross briefly explained the concept and furnished appropriate references. After a week of digesting Ross's insight and reading the literature on social emotions and display rules, we decided to write a triauthored paper (44).

The concept of primary emotions evolved from the initial work of Darwin (45), who had suggested that certain emotions had as their substrate an innate neural basis and were, thus, universally expressed and understood across cultures (35,37,46). Primary emotions and their displays include anger, fear, panic, sadness, surprise, interest, happiness (ecstasy), and disgust and have been linked anatomically to the limbic regions of the brain, in particular the medial temporal lobe (44,47–49). Social emotions (35,50–52) are thought to derive from the biological drive of attachment and are based on two distinct social motives: (a) to gain approval by meeting or exceeding the expectations of others, and (b) to gain affection from others. Success (or failure) in meeting social expectations may result in a person experiencing pride (or embarrassment or guilt), whereas success (or failure) in gaining affection may result in joy or euphoria (or shame). If a peer or comparison person succeeds (or fails) in meeting social expectations or gaining affection, emotions such as envy (or pity), or jealousy (or scorn) may be experienced. Both primary and social emotions have positive and negative valences. Primary emotions, however, have a predominantly negative bias. Although social emotions have a more balanced distribution of valence, most formal situations require positive emotional expressions, such as cheerfulness or attentiveness, in keeping with social display rules (37,53–55). Our observations during the Wada test coupled with relevant literature suggest that primary emotions and their displays are modulated by the right hemisphere in support of the right hemisphere hypothesis, whereas social emotions and social display rules are modulated by the left hemisphere in support of the valence hypothesis. Thus, both competing hypotheses could now be incorporated into a new hypothesis of emotional lateralization, which also provides for a potential neurological explanation for the psychiatric constructs of repression and the subconscious and the cognitive aspects of emotions (Table 1) (44). The hypothesis is also consistent with the idea John Rush and I published in 1981 (15), that depression (endogenous/melancholic, as opposed to nonendogenous/cognitive) might be associated with a specific hemisphere.

TABLE 1. *Hypothesized holes of left and right hemispheres in the modulation of emotional behaviors*

Left hemisphere	Right hemisphere
Temporal limbic system (amygdala) Modulates experiential aspects and noncognitive display behaviors associated with *social emotions*. Modulates experiential aspects and non-cognitive display behaviors associated with *primary emotions*. Biased towards *positive emotional* displays because of *social display rules* (see below). Biased towards *negative emotional* displays because most *primary emotions* are negative. Neocortex Stores and elaborates cognitions concerning *social emotional* life experiences of a person. Stores and elaborates cognitions concerning *primary emotional* life experiences of a person.	Able to repress recall of the *primary emotional* experience of a life event stored in the right hemisphere. Able to repress recall of the *social emotional* experiences of a life event stored in the left hemisphere. Modulates *social display rules* by enhancing socially inappropriate *primary emotional* displays generated by the right amygdala and *social emotional* displays generated by the left amygdala. Modulates *graded emotional* behaviors associated with language and communication through affective prosody and gestures. May be able to modulate *social emotional* displays generated by the left amygdala.

Adapted from ref. 44.

CONCLUSION

Norman Geschwind's contributions to the neurology of emotion were enormous. But even more considerable was his influence on others to pursue this fascinating aspect of human behavior. His insistence on scholarship, coupled with Wernicke's concept that information is processed and stored in the brain by parallel distributed networks (56,57), has served as my Rosetta stone by providing me the essential tools for engaging in inductive types of research involving brain/behavioral relationships (1,13,15,16,22,44,58–64).

Acknowledgments

This work was supported, in part, by grants from the Neuropsychiatric Research Institute, Fargo, North Dakota, the Merit Review Board, Department of Veterans Affairs, Washington, D.C., and the EJLB Foundation, Montreal, Canada. I am indebted to my wife, Stephanie, for critiquing the manuscript and helping me reminisce about the wonderful time we spent in Boston during my neurology residency. We both deeply miss Norman's presence.

REFERENCES

1. Ross ED, Mesulam M-M. Dominant language functions of the right hemisphere? Prosody and emotional gesturing. *Arch Neurol* 1979;36:144–148.
2. Winner E, Gardner H. The comprehension of metaphor in brain-damaged patients. *Brain* 1977;100:717–729.
3. Wapner W, Hamby S, Gardner H. The role of the right hemisphere in the apprehension of complex linguistic materials. *Brain Lang* 1981;14:15–33.
4. Brownell HH, Potter HH, Michelow D, Gardner H. Sensitivity to lexical denotation and connotation in brain-damaged patients: a double dissociation? *Brain Lang* 1984;22:253–265.
5. Shapiro B, Danly M. The role of the right hemisphere in the control of speech prosody in propositional and affective contexts. *Brain Lang* 1985;25:19–36.
6. Borod JC, Koff E, Lorch MP, Nichols M. Channels of emotional expression in patients with unilateral brain disease. *Arch Neurol* 1985;42:345–348.

7. Monrad-Krohn GH. Dysprosody or altered "melody of language." *Brain* 1947;70:405–415.
8. Monrad-Krohn GH. The third element of speech: prosody and its disorders. In: Halpern L, ed. *Problems of dynamic neurology.* Jerusalem, Israel: Hebrew University Press, 1963;101–118.
9. Heilman KM, Scholes R, Watson RT. Auditory affective agnosia: disturbed comprehension of affective speech. *J Neurol Neurosurg Psychiatry* 1975;38:69–72.
10. Tucker DM, Watson RT, Heilman KM. Discrimination and evocation of affectively intoned speech in patients with right parietal disease. *Neurology* 1977;27:947–950.
11. Lassen NA, Ingvar DH, Skinhoj E. Brain function and blood flow. *Sci Am* 1978;239(4):62–71.
12. Larsen B, Skinhoj E, Lassen NA. Variations in regional cortical blood flow in the right and left hemispheres during automatic speech. *Brain* 1978;101:193–209.
13. Ross ED. The aprosodias: functional-anatomic organization of the affective components of language in the right hemisphere. *Arch Neurol* 1981;38:561–569.
14. Rush AJ, Khatami N, Beck AT. Cognitive and behavior therapy in chronic depression. *Behav Ther* 1975;6:398–404.
15. Ross ED, Rush AJ. Diagnostic issues and neuroanatomical correlates of depression in brain damaged patients: implications for a neurology of depression. *Arch Gen Psychiatry* 1981;38:1344–1354.
16. Ross ED, Stewart R. Pathological display of affect in patients with depression and right focal brain damage: an alternative mechanism. *J Nerv Mental Dis* 1987;175:165–172.
17. Rush AJ, Schlesser MA, Stokely E, Bonte FR, Altschuler KZ. Cerebral blood flow in depression and mania. *Psychopharmacol Bull* 1982;18:6–8.
18. Gorelick PB, Ross ED. The aprosodias: further functional-anatomic evidence for the organization of affective language in the right hemisphere. *J Neurol Neurosurg Psychiatry* 1987;50:553–560.
19. Ross ED, Edmondson JA, Seibert GB. The effect of affect on various acoustic measures of prosody in tone and non-tone languages: a comparison based on computer analysis. *J Phonetics* 1986;14:283–302.
20. Edmondson JA, Ross ED, Chan JL, Seibert GB. The effect of right-brain damage on acoustical measures of affective prosody in Taiwanese patients. *J Phonetics* 1987;15:219–233.
21. Ross ED, Edmondson JA, Seibert GB, Homan RW. Acoustic analysis of affective prosody during right-sided Wada test: a within-subjects verification of the right hemisphere's role in language. *Brain Lang* 1987;33:128–145.
22. Wolfe GI, Ross ED. Sensory aprosodia with left hemiparesis from subcortical infarction: right hemisphere analogue of sensory-type aphasia with right hemiparesis? *Arch Neurol* 1987;44:661–671.
23. Bell WL, Davis DL, Morgan-Fisher A, Ross ED. Acquired aprosodias in children. *J Child Neurol* 1989;5:19–26.
24. Ross ED, Anderson B, Morgan-Fisher A. Crossed aprosodia in strongly dextral patients. *Arch Neurol* 1989;46:206–209.
25. Ross ED. Non-verbal aspects of language. *Neurol Clin* 1993;11:9–23.
26. Schlanger BB, Schlanger P, Gerstmann LJ. The perception of emotionally toned sentences by right hemisphere-damaged and aphasic subjects. *Brain Lang* 1976;3:396–403.
27. Seron X, van der Kaa MA, van der Linden M, Remits A, Feyereisen P. Decoding paralinguistic signals: effect of semantic and prosodic cues on aphasic comprehension. *J Commun Disord* 1982;15:223–231.
28. de Bleser R, Poeck K. Analysis of prosody in the spontaneous speech of patients with CV-recurring utterances. *Cortex* 1985;21:405–416.
29. Ross ED. Prosody and brain lateralization: fact vs fancy or is it all just semantics? *Arch Neurol* 1988;45:338–339.
30. Ross ED. Lateralization of affective prosody in brain. *Neurology* 1992;42(suppl 3):411.
31. Ross ED, Stark RD, Yenkosky JP. Lateralization of affective prosody in brain and the callosal integration of hemispheric language functions. *Brain Lang* 1996; (in press).
32. Bowers D, Coslett HB, Bauer RM, Speedie LJ, Heilman KM. Comprehension of emotional prosody following unilateral hemispheric lesions: processing defect versus distraction defect. *Neuropsychologia* 1987;25:317–328.
33. Blonder LX, Bowers D, Heilman KM. The role of the right hemisphere in emotional communication. *Brain* 1991;114:1115–1127.
34. Bowers D, Bauer RM, Heilman KM. The nonverbal affect lexicon: theoretical perspectives from neuropsychological studies of affect perception. *Neuropsychology* 1993;7:433–444.
35. Buck R. *Human motivation and emotion.* New York: Wiley, 1988.
36. Buck R, Duffy R. Nonverbal communication of affect in brain-damaged patients. *Cortex* 1980;16:351–362.
37. Ekman P, Friesen WV, Ellsworth P. *Emotion in the human face.* Elmsford, NY: Pergamon, 1972.
38. Schwartz GE, Davidson RJ, Maer F. Right hemisphere lateralization for emotions in the human brain: interactions with cognition. *Science* 1975;190:286–288.
39. Dimond SJ, Farrington L, Johnson P. Differing emotional response from right and left hemispheres. *Nature* 1976;261:690–692.
40. Borod JC, Andelman F, Obler LK, Tweedy JR, Welkowitz J. Right hemisphere specialization for the identification of emotional words and sentences: evidence from stroke patients. *Neuropsychologia* 1992;30:827–844.
41. Gainotti G. Emotional behavior and hemispheric side of the lesion. *Cortex* 1972;8:41–55.
42. Sackeim HA, Greenberg MS, Weiman AL, Gur RC, Hungerbuhler JP, Geschwind N. Hemispheric asymmetry in the expression of positive and negative emotions: neurologic evidence. *Arch Neurol* 1982;39:210–218.
43. Ahern GL, Schwartz GE. Differential lateralization for positive and negative emotion in the human brain: EEG spectral analysis. *Neuropsychologia* 1985;23:745–756.
44. Ross ED, Homan RW, Buck R. Differential hemispheric lateralization of primary and social emotions: implica-

tions for developing a comprehensive neurology for emotions, repression and the subconscious. *Neuropsychiatr Neuropsychol Behav Neurol* 1994;7:1–19.
45. Darwin C. *The expression of the emotions in man and animals.* London: John Murray, 1872. (Reprinted Chicago, Ill: University of Chicago Press, 1965.)
46. Izard CE. *Human emotions.* New York: Plenum, 1977.
47. Papez JW. A proposed mechanism for emotions. *Arch Neurol Psychiatry* 1937;38:725–743.
48. Gloor P, Olivier A, Quesney LF, Andermann F, Horowitz S. The role of the limbic system in experiential phenomena of temporal lobe epilepsy. *Ann Neurol* 1982;12:129–144.
49. Halgren E, Walter RD, Cherlow DG, Crandall PE. Mental phenomena evoked by electrical stimulation of the human hippocampal formation and amygdala. *Brain* 1978;101:83–117.
50. Lewis M, Michalson L. *Children's emotions and moods: developmental theory and measurement.* New York: Plenum, 1983.
51. Panksepp J. Toward a general psychobiological theory of emotions. *Behav Brain Sci* 1982;5:407–467.
52. Kraemer GW. A psychobiological theory of attatchment. *Behav Brain Sci* 1992;15:493–541.
53. Kleck RE, Vaughan RC, Cartwright-Smith J, Vaughan KB, Colby C, Lanzetta J. Effects of being observed on expressive, subjective, and physiological reactions to painful stimuli. *J Pers Soc Psychol* 1976;34:1211–1218.
54. Wagner HL, Smith J. Facial expression in the presence of friends and strangers. *J Nonverbal Behav* 1991;15:201–214.
55. Buck R, Losow JI, Murphy MM, Costanzo P. Social facilitation and inhibition of emotional expression and communication. *J Pers Soc Psychol* 1992;63:962–968.
56. Eggert GH. *Wernicke's works on aphasia: a sourcebook and review.* New York: Mouton Publishers, 1977.
57. Ross ED. Intellectual origins and theoretical framework of behavioral neurology: a response to Dr. Trimble. *Neuropsychiatr Neuropsychol Behav Neurol* 1993;6:65–67.
58. Ross ED. Sensory-specific and fractional disorders of recent memory in man: I. Isolated loss of visual recent memory. *Arch Neurol* 1980;37:193–200.
59. Ross ED. Sensory-specific and fractional disorders of recent memory in man: II. Unilateral loss of tactile recent memory. *Arch Neurol* 1980;37:267–272.
60. Ross ED, Harney J, deLacoste-Utamsing C, Purdy P. How the brain integrates affective and propositional language into a unified behavioral function: hypothesis based on clinicoanatomical evidence. *Arch Neurol* 1981;38:745–748.
61. Ross ED, Stewart RM. Akinetic mutism from hypothalamic damage: successful treatment with dopamine agonists. *Neurology* 1981;31:1435–1439.
62. Chan J-L, Ross ED. Left-hand mirror writing following right anterior cerebral artery infarction: evidence for non-mirror transformation of motor programs by right supplementary motor area. *Neurology* 1988;38:59–63.
63. Ross ED. Acute agitation and other behaviors associated with Wernicke aphasia and their possible neurological bases. *Neuropsychiaty Neuropsychol Behav Neurol* 1993;6:9–18.
64. Ross ED. Cortical representation of the emotions. In: Trimble M, Cummings J, eds. *Behavioural neurology.* Oxford, England: Butterworth-Heineman. 1996; (in press).

Epilepsy

ured during
*Behavioral Neurology and
the Legacy of Norman Geschwind,*
edited by S. C. Schachter and O. Devinsky,
Lippincott-Raven Publishers, Philadelphia © 1997.

24

Behavioral Aspects of Temporal Lobe Epilepsy

Donald L. Schomer

Beth Israel Hospital, Department of Neurology, Boston, Massachusetts 02215.

I came to know Dr. Norman Geschwind personally in late 1979 and early 1980. Of course, I knew of him earlier through his writings, particularly his series of papers on the disconnection syndromes (1,2). I was recruited to develop the laboratory of clinical neurophysiology at Beth Israel Hospital and to establish a program for the diagnosis and management of adults with epilepsy. During the 4-plus years that I worked closely with Dr. Geschwind and was in his department, I came to rely on his counsel on many issues. He was a man of tremendous intellect, but he was also humble and very human. This chapter focuses on various lessons that I learned in my own field from this multitalented man. I was told recently that he was also a decent badminton player!

LESSONS FROM THE EXAMINATION OF PATIENTS WITH TEMPORAL LOBE EPILEPSY

I found it delightful to see any patient referred by Dr. Geschwind, because the highly detailed history that he had already obtained often gave me some insight into the way he thought. Many patients commented that they had been to see him several times before he finished taking their histories and gave them their initial neurological examinations. He paid particular attention to detailing the sequence of symptoms surrounding patients' complaints and the evolution of those symptoms over time.

This attention to detail often resulted in information of enormous clinical importance being uncovered. For example, Dr. Geschwind referred a middle-aged woman to me who had suffered multiple prolonged psychiatric hospitalizations for paranoid/delusional behavior associated with complex visual hallucinations. Over a period of more than 25 years, she had tried numerous antipsychotic medications with only minimal effect. Dr. Geschwind's review of her history included carefully reading more than 15 years of notes covering many admissions and consulting with her referring psychiatrist, also a most dedicated and thoughtful physician. Dr. Geschwind interviewed several of the patient's children and telephoned her estranged husband to obtain from him his remembrances of her early years with the disorder. He learned from this investigation that the patient had suffered only two types of hallucinations, which had been stable over the many years. They had started in late adolescence about a year after the onset of her menses. These hallucinations were either of six German-style soldiers dressed in uniforms worn during the time of Kaiser Wilhelm and lined up one on top of two on top of three, or of an elderly woman sitting in a rocking chair, reminiscent of the painting by Grandma Moses except that the elderly woman reminded the patient of herself and there were small rat-like animals on the floor chewing on the woman's fingers. Years after the patient began to hallucinate, which initially occurred infrequently, her visions were often accompanied by intense fear. This fear was not associated with one of these hallucinations more often than the other. Dr. Geschwind learned from the patient directly that the hallucinations occurred only in the left hemifield. She had sought professional help as a young woman and was admitted to a psychiatric hospital because gradually these events seemed to become more frequent up to the time of her first pregnancy. During one of her hospitalizations, she was assaulted by another patient, who struck her on the head with a hard object. The blow left her unconscious for several days. When she awoke, she had a terrible headache, which she still could recall vividly many years later. She also had a stiff neck, which cleared slowly over several weeks. No additional studies were done during that time. After the assault, however, the patient had loss-of-consciousness episodes, which often followed the hallucinations.

Geschwind theorized that the patient had a structural lesion such as an arteriovenous malformation (AVM) in the nondominant hemisphere, probably at or near the junction of the parietal-temporal-occipital lobes. For years she had simple partial seizures, which were made worse by the trauma. The blow probably caused the AVM to bleed. After I had prescribed various anticonvulsants to no avail, she had a surgical evaluation and subsequently underwent a craniotomy to remove portions of her right temporal lobe. During the procedure, she had a seizure. We were able to capture the event with electrocorticography and acute depth electrodes placed into portions of the patient's right temporal lobe. The onset of her hallucination was associated with sustained electrical activity in the inferior parietal and adjacent posterior superior temporal gyrus. She experienced a sense of fear when the electrical activity spread from the surface contacts to the right hippocampus, right amygdala, and right parahippocampal gyrus. Atrophic cortex stained with hemosiderin was found in the region of seizure initiation, and what the surgeon felt was probably a bed for an old but obliterated AVM. Geschwind just smiled a broad grin when I told him about our intraoperative findings.

Dr. Geschwind was quite interested in understanding the mechanisms behind the seizure triggers that some people described. He had already convinced Dr. Andrew Herzog, the head of our Neuroendocrinology Division, to pursue the relationship of the menstrual cycle to seizure initiation. Geschwind was well aware of the literature that discussed the way some women with temporal lobe epilepsy (TLE) seemed to have a worsening of their seizures premenstrually and for the first few days of their cycle, and some women with absence epilepsy would have a worsening of their seizures during the first 2 weeks of their cycles and improvement in the luteal phase of their cycles and premenstrually. All of us had noted that this relationship in patients with TLE occurred much more often than the literature suggested. However, as Dr. Herzog details in Chapter 27, it was he who pursued this area of research with Dr. Geschwind's strong support and intellectually challenging critiques.

Geschwind made me aware of the utility of formalized cognitive testing in this patient population. I have subsequently adopted the approach that neuropsychologic testing, when done properly, is as helpful as most dynamic imaging studies. Of course, I was fortunate in having available to me the services of people like Sandra Weintraub, Ph.D., former head of the Neuropsychology Division of the Behavioral Neurology Unit at Beth Israel Hospital, and Dr. Marsel Mesulam, former director of that unit and now at Northwestern University. Through them and with the encouragement of Dr. Geschwind, I became aware of how often neuropsychological/cognitive deficits were reversible and how rapidly some difficulties could develop at times when seizure frequency increased. During those years, Drs. Mesulam and Geschwind were pursuing work on specific memory disorders related to epilepsy. I learned of the effects of medication on attentional neural networks before such concepts were fashionable. I observed how medications affected sleep and how disturbances of sleep cycling altered cognitive functioning. We were studying the localizing significance of other types of memory dysfunction, and we were starting to investigate the unusual behavior of enhanced forgetting that some of our patients seemed to manifest although they did not have progressive disorders that would account for it. Most of these areas of interest are still being actively pursued in our unit today in collaboration with the Behavioral Neurology Unit.

Geschwind taught that the role of the physician should be to listen to the patient and obtain as much historical information as possible and then to think about the patient's problem in the context of our understanding of the principles of medicine and our knowledge of the nature of the disease process. He believed that most patients were willing to tell their physicians about their problems as long as the physicians remained nonjudgmental. As soon as patients felt they were being judged, their stories became more contrived. Geschwind would often preface a clinical discussion with a patient, particularly one with epilepsy, by saying that we were all interested in the patient's story and that if he interrupted the patient during the telling of it, it was to make a point for teaching purposes. The patient was always asked at the end of such a presentation if he or she had any questions. The patient was often encouraged to stay for the discussion to help clarify any clinical questions that remained. Geschwind was genuinely interested in how each patient perceived his or her own problem and equally interested in how the patient's family reacted to the disorder and to the patient's disabilities. He often repeated his view that patients usually did not have very good insight into the nature of their disorder from pathological and physiological perspectives. However, he was always interested in their views. One of the many interesting articles he left unwritten was one on patients' theories about their disease processes, theories he had laboriously collected.

Geschwind was a master of the neurological examination. He was quite aware of the classic syndrome of congenital hemihypoplasia associated with contralateral smallness of the skull and face as described by Dyke and colleagues (3). He was forever looking not only for these signs and for more subtle variations of this syndrome, but also for additional features, such as focal areas of alopecia, patches of gray hair, or a quadrant of discoloration in the iris. He would often point out such findings as mild scoliosis, which he explained was the precursor to a herniated lumbar disc. When challenged about what would certainly be considered microneurological signs and pure clinical speculation, he would frequently retort that the good neurologist looks for and finds subtle signs that are often overlooked by the not-so-specialized or less sophisticated physician. He liked to tell the story of the patient who had epilepsy associated with a hamartoma of the temporal lobe. He was examining this patient in front of students and residents one day and was explaining to them that there were signs of growth asymmetry which, when coupled with the patient's history of longstanding and poorly responsive epilepsy but normal cognitive development, pointed to a congenital lesion. The signs were indeed subtle, which explained why many general physicians and even many neurologists had missed the diagnosis. The patient interrupted Geschwind and told him that about a month earlier he had hired a new housekeeper. This woman was with him when she observed him having a very minor seizure, after which he had a slight limp. She asked her new employer if he had epilepsy and a brain tumor. Geschwind's point was that even the untrained can be attentive to the subtle signs that people exhibit neurologically, and we need to constantly look for and find these signs or else we offer little more and maybe even less than the untrained but attentive person.

Geschwind loved to tell the following story, mainly because of his interest in how disease affected patients and their families. He was asked to render an opinion on a patient who, many years earlier, had almost died after suffering a serious subarachnoid hemorrhage from a deep right temporal lobe AVM. Before that event, the man had been a high school gym teacher with a normal family life. After he recovered, the man felt an overwhelming, almost compulsive need to write poetry. His began to view his job as unoriginal and boring. Geschwind learned that he had changed religions several times and had even explored several of the Eastern religions. His family and friends noted that he had great difficulty ending conversations with them, and several confessed that this was so bothersome that they often avoided him so as to not become entangled. His wife observed that he was no longer interested in sexual matters and stated that although she was quite disturbed about this change in his behavior, she was afraid to discuss it openly with him because he tended to have episodes of easily provoked rage. Most important, Geschwind learned that the patient was probably having simple partial seizures and perhaps also complex partial seizures. The patient was only partially aware of how his new-found behavior affected those who cared deeply about him. The family, the patient to some extent, and most of the patient's treating physicians attributed these behavioral changes to his having recovered from a serious, life-threatening disorder that had struck him down without warning. Although he had recovered physically from this insult, the emotional trauma had left him severely impaired psychologically. Geschwind viewed the difficulty quite differently. He explained his more biologically oriented view to the patient and his family. They were all relieved to learn that the patient's disordered behavior could have a physical cause. Even though treatment helped control only some of the epileptic phenomena, the family and patient remain grateful to this day to Geschwind for his openness and for his reformulation of the problem.

Geschwind's open, frank approach has been one that I have emulated with most of my patients with this disorder. I will frequently discuss my view that the behavioral characteristics of the patient's problems may have physical causes similar to the more overt and discrete epileptic events. Treatment is still often empiric for behavioral disorders. Patients are usually relieved to know that someone believes there may be physical reasons why they have only minimal control over their thoughts and behavior. The conventional view, particularly in the United States, is that patients with epilepsy are no different from anyone else. For the most part this is true. However, patients with behavioral sequelae to their epilepsy are often grateful just to know that someone is willing to listen. This is perhaps one of the greatest lessons that I learned from Geschwind.

Another of Geschwind's special interests related to TLE was autonomic dysfunction. He believed that the autonomic systems of patients with epilepsy functioned fairly normally at baseline. When patients were stressed, however, disordered function was evident if one looked carefully for it. Stress could come from overt seizures but also from daily emotional provocations. Geschwind often said to me that he thought that the mechanism was mediated through temporal lobe structures, particularly the amygdala, to the hypothalamus, in a manner similar to that of the endocrinologic abnormalities that Dr. Herzog was demonstrating. Geschwind pointed out some early work in this area, as noted in Chapter 26 (4). Geschwind also convinced Roy Freeman to make a career of studying the disorders of autonomic function. We, too, have pursued many of the studies that we started in the early 1980s. Specifically, my Cognitive Evoked Potential Lab is actively studying the differences between patients with TLE and controls in distinguishing pictures of pleasing, neutral, and disgusting objects. This work is similar to that of Bear and Geschwind, but we are studying physiological aspects of specific regions of the brain. In addition, we are examining the effects of temporal lobectomy on those responses. We are also studying right versus left temporal lobe asymmetries in the auditory long latency evoked potentials (EPs) in matched groups of men and women controlled for right- versus left-handedness and schizophrenia. Our work in linking functional magnetic resonance imaging (fMRI) to neurophysiological data, particularly live events recorded on an electroencephalogram (EEG), continues (5). Much of this later activity is a result of Geschwind's emphasis on the importance of excellent engineering to our research. He became a strong supporter of my recruitment of Mr. John Ives to my unit to head technologic development.

Finally, I could not conclude this section on Geschwind's clinical lessons without mentioning his theories about brain plasticity (6,7). He was always careful to make a semantic distinction between plasticity and late changes. He preferred to use the latter term because plasticity seemed to suggest to most people changes that were "good." The behavioral changes that occur with epilepsy are often detrimental to the patient. Geschwind believed that these changes were probably mediated by the same forces that mediated such functions as long-term memory, but that they reflected something gone awry. I remember his commenting that he liked David Bear's term *pathological hyperconnectivity*. In January 1978, he wrote to Dr. Schneider at the Massachusetts Institute of Technology about how minor congenital lesions could cause a compensatory sprouting of various pathways, such as the dopaminergic pathways, to frontal structures or the noradrenergic pathways to the occipital cortex. Geschwind noted that when that happened, the functional aspects of those projections produced very different functional correlates. Therefore, an external force had altered the development of a specific aspect of neurological function. To those of us in his department, Geschwind used to paraphrase his theory as: "We are what our dead brains have determined us to be." Although he did not believe that people do not have any influence over their own development and he believed that there is tremendous brain plasticity, he did mean to suggest that many of our more basic capabilities are determined very early in life and without our conscious involvement.

LESSONS ABOUT THE ASSOCIATION BETWEEN BEHAVIORAL ALTERATIONS AND TLE

Geschwind's formal lectures about behavioral neurology were legendary. His impromptu discussions were even more exciting because of the give and take that was always part of such interactions. When I arrived, I was intrigued by the work that Drs. Geschwind, Bear, and Mesulam had already done on behavioral disorders and TLE. This work was the primary reason that I joined Dr. Geschwind and Dr. Marc Dichter at Beth Israel Hospital in Boston. My training in epilepsy and clinical neurophysiology was firmly based in traditional and classic teaching through my work with Drs. Fred Andermann and Pierre Gloor at the Montreal Neurological Institute. I had been well taught in epilepsy semiology, medical management principles, and presurgical evaluation of patients with medically resistant forms of epilepsy. I still think that Geschwind hired me because I was a traditional epileptologist yet was in the "Montreal school" image, because Geschwind had great respect for the neurologists and neurosurgeons at McGill and admiration for their pioneering work on epilepsy surgery. However, perhaps his most admiring comments were made about Dr. Brenda Milner for her work on cerebral localization. Because of my tendencies and Geschwind's feelings for my teachers, I found an immediate home with him at Beth Israel Hospital. Little did he know that I was a closet behavioral neurologist.

I will not repeat Dr. Bear's discussion in this book on the TLE inventory and personality disorder. But I would like to present my observations on this topic and the issue of schizophreniform behavior in light of my clinical experience with patients and my exposure to Geschwind's teachings. Perhaps one of the most intriguing aspects of the TLE personality is that its major features tend to all be present in the same person. Why should compulsive writing in journals or of poetry be associated with an overwhelming interest in matters "cosmic," including multiple religious conversions? Additionally, why should those two aspects of one personality be associated with altered sexual interests, most commonly a lack of interest in sexual matters? Further, why should patients all manifest the trait of finding it difficult to end conversations (i.e., of becoming socially viscous)? Because these behaviors clustered, they were judged by Geschwind to represent a syndrome (8). He often explained his reasoning using this analogy: "Why should large red blood cells and polymorphonuclear white blood cells be associated with premature gray hair, achlorhydria, and degeneration of the posterior columns of the spinal cord?" We all know now that these signs are due to an absence of vitamin B12. However, in the early years of medicine, clinicians knew about this syndrome but had no plausible explanation. Although each aspect of either syndrome may have, on its own, multiple etiologies, when they all cluster it seems more likely that there is a single common explanation. In the one case, the explanation is a deficiency of vitamin B12, and in the other it's the presence of abnormal temporal-limbic function.

The lessons to be learned from patients with schizophreniform personality disorder, as noted by Dr. Bear (9), continue to evolve. Geschwind taught that this disorder seemed to occur only after the seizure disorder had been identified and was present for many years. It also tended to occur much more frequently in females, particularly left-handed females with left TLE. Curiously, there was often an identifiable lesion present, such as a hamartoma. In these cases, the personality disorder developed slowly over many years, the average interval from the onset of epilepsy to the development of the personality trait being 12 to 15 years. What I have learned from this group of patients is that paranoia, in general, is much more common in patients of both sexes when they have longstanding left temporal lobe seizures. This paranoia may not be restricted to patients with temporal lobe seizures, but it seems to be more common when seizures are of left hemisphere origin. In addition, our surgical experience with this population is similar to that with other groups in that the disordered thinking is not improved by successfully controlling the seizure disorder by means of temporal lobectomy (10).

I have also found that patients with left hemisphere seizure foci tend to have more frequent and more severe agitation and irritability either just before a seizure or immediately after one. In a few families in my practice, the family members can tell, days before, that their member with epilepsy is going to have a seizure, because the person changes from being calm and pleasant to angry and irritable. In all these cases, the patients have either left frontal or temporal seizure foci.

Geschwind's interest in aggression and disorders that predisposed people to "limbic dyscontrol" had become publicly muted by the time I knew him. Many of his early views had been publicly misinterpreted. He remained genuinely interested in obtaining help for patients with these types of problems, but he did not make any public displays or pronouncements about them. He no longer had any interest in the development of a public policy or in public debate about the issues. On several occasions, however, I became involved with him in specific cases. I remember one such case quite well. Geschwind had referred a young woman to me shortly after I arrived. She was mildly retarded, but with the help of dedicated parents she had developed reasonably well until puberty. At that time, she became overwhelmingly interested in writing in her diary, moderately obsessed with religious matters that in most respects were beyond her mental limits, and profoundly sexually promiscuous, to the point that she had made, on occasion, life-threatening choices of sexual partners. She also experienced periods of uncontrolled rage, usually provoked by some minor irritant in her life. She was no longer able to live in the community alone because of these aggressive outbursts. She did not have "events" that suggested she had epilepsy or "ictal" behavior. Geschwind convinced me to obtain an EEG using sphenoidal electrodes because the patient's routine EEGs were always normal. I did so and found profound bilateral but strikingly left-side-predominate high-voltage spike-and-wave discharges in both the awake and sleep states. Perhaps he did not want to push me beyond my set of beliefs at the time, but Geschwind told me that he was going to refer the woman to Dr. Vaernet in Copenhagen, who was a stereotactic neurosurgeon and close personal friend. There, the patient would have electrodes placed into various limbic sites and EEG recordings would be taken for several days while her physicians decided whether to perform a unilateral or a bilateral amygdalotomy. A left-sided amygdalotomy was performed, and the patient returned to a fairly normal life. This was a lesson I'll remember.

Like the association between schizophreniform personality traits and longstanding epilepsy, depression appears to be related but without such a clear side predominance. Geschwind pointed out to me that the person with an impulsive personality who also had depression often turned out to have a lethal disorder: these were the people who committed suicide. Whether their impulsiveness was related to their primary problem or secondary to their medication was not important. Geschwind had known a number of such patients who were successful at committing suicide. He convinced me that to properly care for this group of patients, other professionals needed to be readily available. I again had the services of the Behavioral Neurology Unit available to me. As time has gone on, I've become convinced that a dedicated multidisciplinary group is essential to the management of patients with poorly responsive epilepsy, whether they are surgical candidates or not. As a result, I established the Comprehensive Epilepsy Program for adults—the first of its kind in the Boston area. I modeled it on the Children's Hospital program that had been started by Dr. Lennox and continued under Dr. Lombroso, for they, too, had recognized the importance of a team approach to such a complex disorder that affects so many aspects of a person's life.

Geschwind seemed to have had the rather unusual ability to compartmentalize his views about both subjects and people. I recall my introduction to the topic of the relationship of TLE to multiple phobias. He had just finished speaking to me about why he felt that Dr. Bruce Herman, a noted neuropsychologist who was also interested in behavioral disorders and epilepsy, had completely misunderstood his view on the relationship of TLE to the personality disorder. He then stopped and turned back to me after he had started to leave and said, "His [Herman's] views on the relationship of partial epilepsy to phobia development are right on." It was as if he wanted to end the discussion on a positive rather than a negative note. Herman's view was that patients who experienced fear along with their seizures were the ones who went on to develop multiple phobias. This turned out to be, in Herman's experience, patients who were more likely to have right-sided seizures. We spoke about phobias as learned experiences. Patients have an event, during which they experience an intense feeling of fear or doom. They "learn" or match what is happening in their environment to this intense emotion and then avoid similar situations in a rather classic avoidance-learning paradigm. In practical terms, this learned behavior can be helpful for many patients because what is learned can, with effort, be unlearned. Several of my patients have worked successfully with therapists to accomplish just that.

Geschwind was always fascinated by rare and unusual disorders. When seeing or discussing patients with such disorders, he always tried to make sure that he gave credit where it was due. While I was reading through some of his office notes recently, I was reminded of such a situation. He had told me about a patient with TLE whom he had seen. She experienced, as part of her aura, a sense of a presence behind her and to the left side. During our conversation, he asked me what I thought of Dr. Guy Remillard from the Montreal Neurological Institute, whom he had just recently met on one of his several trips to Montreal. He went on to tell me that Dr. Remillard had seen cases of ictal and postictal water-drinking behavior and was in the process of writing an article about this observation. Several weeks later, he referred a patient to me who had been followed closely by Dr. Bear. The patient was a young girl about 16 years old at the time. She had been well until about 3 years of age, when a severe febrile disorder developed that was associated with aseptic meningitis. Within a few months, she began to have complex partial seizures. She experienced fear as part of the seizures and, consequently, multiple phobias developed. I admitted the patient to the hospital for a presurgical EEG evaluation, and only after several weeks of my talking with her daily did she tell me that she felt an evil presence over her left shoulder as part of the aura. She even had a name for this "person." I spoke with Geschwind about this part of the girl's history. He was so taken by the history that he came and visited with her many times during the remainder of her stay. He always came alone and spoke with her alone, sensitive to the fact that she was very shy and would talk only in strict confidence. I was reminded of this story when I came across a letter from Geschwind to Remillard thanking him for showing Geschwind, when he was in Montreal, the very patient whom he had spoken to me about. In the letter, Geschwind also thanked Remillard for telling him about the cases of water-drinking behavior.

This last case also reminds me about the great respect that Geschwind's patients had for him. Many of his former patients are now my patients. Whenever his name comes up in conversation, invariably patients will speak lovingly and fondly about just how unusual his interest in them was. He was interested in them as human beings, not just as patients with fascinating disorders. He was interested not only in them but also in their families, their jobs, and their lifestyles. He was always trying to make their lives easier and more comfortable. He succeeded to a large degree by just being there for them. There were very few evenings when, as I left work feeling exhausted and overwhelmed, I did not see Geschwind still in his office talking with one of his patients or on the telephone with one of his patient's physicians. This is further amplified in Chapter 11.

LESSONS ABOUT TREATMENT OF PATIENTS WITH TLE

Patient care at McGill was primarily given, at least by the resident staff, on the inpatient unit. Although we did participate in outpatient clinics, we did not follow patients over a long enough interval to know how they reacted to their illnesses and dealt with the many problems that their disorders created for them. We did have their written records, but we had no real opportunity to personally watch and be a part of the evolution of events. When I came to Boston, one of my only requirements was that I be allowed to follow patients for the long term. I did not want to establish just a surgical service in which patients would be evaluated and, if they were not suitable for surgical intervention, dismissed. I found Geschwind and the Beth Israel Hospital a good match, for both Geschwind's policy and the hospital's policy, as outlined by its president, Dr. Mitchell Rabkin, was that all patients admitted to Beth Israel were treated as private patients. Even if a patient was admitted through the emergency room, he or she was assigned to a senior staff physician, who then became that patient's permanent physician.

I quickly learned that the day-to-day management of patients with poorly controlled epilepsy was demanding beyond reasonable limits. Geschwind, as I mentioned, supported the establishment of a Comprehensive Epilepsy Service modeled after the design he had for his own unit headed by Dr. Mesulam. When my program finally took hold, I had time to reflect on a number of matters clinically. Closely linked to the time demands of these patients was their apparently very high incidence of drug intolerance in the form of overt drug allergies, drug sensitivities, and paradoxical drug reactions.

Geschwind and I spoke several times about this observation. We never developed a uniform theory to explain it, but several therapeutically important observations resulted. First, the fewer drugs the better. Although monotherapy and rational polypharmacy are common practice now, Geschwind was promoting these ideas in the 1970s. In notes to referring physicians, he frequently stated that, in his experience, when the number of anticonvulsants given to patients with pharmacologically resistant epilepsy was reduced, they improved cognitively and, paradoxically, often seemed to have better seizure control. If the patient had a major psychiatric disorder, that condition would probably require medical treatment. However, psychotropic drugs could often be given at considerably lower doses than the doses that patients without seizures required. These doses were often in the homeopathic range. One explanation for the higher-than-expected rate of adverse drug reactions in this group of patients could be that these reactions represent a mechanism similar to that of phobia production; that is, during the introduction of a drug, patients have events that they then associate with the most recent change (i.e., the new drug). Certainly, another explanation is the common experience that polypharmacy causes multiple drug-drug interactions, many of which are associated with subjective complaints.

One of Geschwind's greatest talents was his ability to synthesize large volumes of data and see relationships that were not apparent to most of us. Some of those fresh insights into diseases are the subjects of many of the chapters in this book. One of these insights is the relationship of autoimmune disorders to migraine, handedness, and learning disorders. His interest in the endocrine system became for him almost a cause unto itself. My involvement was primarily with Dr. Herzog, who was already actively pursuing this field when I arrived. My real introduction to the whole area came quickly. Geschwind referred a patient to me with an unusually brief clinical note. He asked if I would help him work up a patient referred to him by another prominent Boston neurologist. The patient, who was about 35 years old when I met her, was exceptionally talented and played the violin professionally. Her husband was a noted Boston intellectual. She had a history of intermittent psychotic episodes over more than 20 years. She had a strong family history of various autoimmune diseases, migraine, and anomalous handedness. Her neurologist had noted that during one of her recent psychotic episodes, her right hand became quite clumsy. He ruled out a structural lesion and prescribed phenytoin after an abnormal but nonspecific EEG. Within a few days, the clumsiness went away and the psychosis improved a little. I learned from the patient's history that since adolescence she had experienced episodes of unprovoked fear. These episodes started within 6 months of the onset of her menses and occurred only premenstrually until about 10 years ago, when they began to happen at any time. When they clustered, she would become confused and often sexually aggressive. She would leave the house if left unattended or not restrained. She would wake up several days later, usually in a psychiatric institution, and improve over the next few days. She had experienced two periods during her adult life when these episodes went away for extended intervals. Both episode-free periods surrounded her two pregnancies. After the first pregnancy, she breast-fed her baby for about 6 months, and when she stopped, she had a recurrence within 2 weeks. After the second child's birth, she took the baby on tour with her so that she could continue to breast-feed him until she returned. Again, within a few weeks of stopping, she had a recurrence. I discussed these historical notes with Geschwind, who simply commented that he had obtained similar details but wanted to see if someone else was as impressed by the associations as he was. We discussed the case with Herzog and decided to suggest a trial of progesterone. We reasoned that the woman was always in a state of relative estrogen excess when she was symptomatic and relative progesterone excess when she was well. Her referring neurologist agreed to the trial. She has been symptom free since the trial started more than 14 years ago, and I occasionally still hear from her husband.

This next story about Geschwind demonstrates for me, unlike any other story I know, the true nature of the man. In 1983, he called me to ask my opinion about a man whom he had not seen but to whom he had spoken over the telephone. The man was in his early twenties, a law student at Harvard. Starting 3 years earlier, he had experienced about four episodes during which he would become mentally cloudy for a day or two. During these episodes, his feelings were very distinct, and he experienced a loss of depth perception and a graying of his vision followed by confusion. He would have an overwhelming desire to sleep. He would go to bed and sleep for 24 or more hours, only to awaken and still feel tired. When awake, he would eat voraciously and somewhat indiscriminately. He would also have unusually strong sexual urges. He became aggressive with his girlfriend and would masturbate several times in a row. The symptoms would last for 1 to 2 weeks and clear like "the fog rolling out." He wanted to know if I thought that he could have epilepsy. I told him that I had seen several patients with similar symptoms on Dr. Fred Andermann's service in Montreal. He and Dr. Joseph Martin, then the director of the institute and neurologist-in-chief, were interested in this disorder of unknown etiology, called the Kleine-Levin syndrome. Geschwind told me that he had never heard of this disorder and asked if I was sure I had the right name. I was impressed, for two reasons. First, I knew of a neurological disorder that he didn't; second, although he was perhaps the premier American neurologist of his time, he casually admitted to me that he had not heard of the syndrome. The story does not end here. Geschwind called back later that same day to give me the patient's telephone number and to ask me to consult. After I was done seeing the patient, he wanted me to call him so we could discuss strategy. I saw the patient about a week later. I was greatly impressed by his knowledge of the literature about this obscure disorder. He told me that Geschwind had told him that he wanted me to see him and that I had mentioned to Geschwind that I thought that he had Kleine-Levin. The patient had gone immediately to the Countway Library and looked up all the references he could find on the disease. He said that during several days of reference work, he kept running into a very distinguished, older, professorial-looking man in a velour shirt who seemed to be seeking all the same journals. Finally, after having to ask the man if he could borrow one of the books that he had put in his carrel, the patient introduced himself. He then learned that the man was Dr. Geschwind, who had canceled all his appointments for that week so that he could dedicate himself to learning about this disorder in preparation for our discussion. During his research, Geschwind had come across some obscure journal of neuroanatomy, in which someone had reported on some work done with juvenile monkeys. The investigator had placed lesions in the raphe nuclei of immature male and female monkeys. When the female monkeys became sexually active, an anorexia-nervosa-like condition developed in some of them, and a condition similar to the Kleine-Levin syndrome developed in a few of the males. He was fascinated by this obscure reference and promised to get it for me. He went on to reason that perhaps if we could give this man 5-hydroxy tryptophan, a precursor of serotonin, it would have a beneficial effect. He had already telephoned Dr. Mark Hallett, who was then the head of the EEG lab at Brigham Hospital and was experimenting with serotonin precursors in the treatment of myoclonus. Mark told Geschwind that clonazepam was just as effective in elevating brain serotonin as any of his precursor drugs. Because Institutional Review Board approval was not required for its use, prescribing clonazepam was probably the easiest way to accomplish what he wanted to do. We met with the patient, and he decided to try this approach. About 4 or 5 months later, the patient had another attack and was admitted to the hospital. Within 2 or 3 days of starting the drug, he was well again. We kept him on the medication for the next few months and then tapered him off. He had a recurrence very quickly, which was aborted by reintroducing the drug. The patient graduated from law school and moved to New York City. Over the years, he has tried to discontinue the drug, only to experience recurrences. I still hear from him occasionally, and he continues to do well when he is taking the drug. I have not had the opportunity to try this treatment in any other cases since then. I have not written this case up for journal publication because I have never been successful in finding that reference. This case demonstrates for me all the finest attributes of this great man: his humility, his dedication to knowledge, his ability to find important links that have eluded others, his dedication to his patients' welfare, and his willingness to explore and try new therapies.

My last memory of Geschwind pertains to our discussion after radiology rounds on the Friday before he died. He had just finished leaving everyone on Dr. Jon Kleefield's neuroradiology rounds in stitches. I approached him about an article in the current issue of *Epilepsia* that described the relationship between Flaubert's epilepsy and his writing. Geschwind had become an expert on the relationship of epilepsy to the accomplishments of many great people, including Van Gogh and Dostoyevsky (11). We would speculate about whether Martin Luther had epilepsy or whether the writings of Lewis Carroll were influenced by epilepsy rather than by drugs or migraines. Geschwind said that he did not know that Flaubert had had a form of epilepsy but quipped that the length of his work should have made him suspicious. He took the article and said that he would read it over the weekend. Mrs. Geschwind returned the journal to me about 6 months later, having just come across it on Norman's desk.

REFERENCES

1. Geschwind N. Disconnexion syndromes in animals and man. I. *Brain* 1965;88(2):237–294.
2. Geschwind N. Disconnexion syndromes in animals and man. II. *Brain* 1965;88(3):584–644.
3. Dyke CG, Davidoff LM, Masson CB. Cerebral hemiatrophy and homolateral hypertrophy of the skull and sinuses. *Surg Gynecol Obstet* 1933;57:588.
4. Bear DM, Shenk L, Benson H. Increased autonomic responses to neutral and emotional stimuli in temporal lobe epilepsy. *Am J Psychiatry* 1981;138:6–7.
5. Warach S, Ives JR, Schlaug G, Patel MR, Darby DG, Thangaraj V, Edelman RR, Schomer DL, EEG-triggered echo-planar functional MRI in epilepsy. *Neurology* 1996;47:89–93

6. Geschwind N. Late changes in the nervous system. In: Stein D, Rosen J, eds. *Plasticity and recovery of function in the central nervous system.* New York: Academic Press, 1974;467–508.
7. Geschwind N. Mechanisms of changes after brain lesions. *Ann NY Acad Sci* 1985;457:13–18.
8. Waxman SG, Geschwind N. The interictal behavior syndrome of temporal lobe epilepsy. *Arch Gen Psychiatry* 1975;32:580–586.
9. Slater E, Beard AW. Schizophrenia-like psychosis of epilepsy. *Br J Psychiatry* 1963;109:95–150.
10. Geschwind N. Effects of temporal lobe surgery on behavior. *N Engl J Med* 1973;289(9):480–481.
11. Geschwind N. Dostoyevsky's epilepsy. In: Blumer D, ed. *Psychiatric aspects of epilepsy.*, Washington, DC: American Psychiatric Press, 1984;325–334.

25
Other Forms of Epilepsy

Orrin Devinsky

Department of Neurology, NYU School of Medicine, Hospital for Joint Diseases, New York, New York 10003.

Norman Geschwind was the attending physician during my neurology rotation in medical school. A patient was presented who had a brain tumor and a post-ictal Todd's paralysis. Geschwind asked me to describe the mechanism underlying Todd's paralysis. I readily volunteered the exhaustion hypothesis—that the electrical discharge depletes energy or neurotransmitter stores from involved neurons, causing a post-ictal deficit. Raising his eyebrows slightly and displaying his characteristic wry look of pleasure as he engaged in a point of intellectual interest, Geschwind responded that I was right, but only partly. He then moved on to recount some of the historic descriptions of Todd's paralysis. Todd had observed that the hemiplegia was usually more prominent on the side with more intense muscular contraction. However, Todd also noted that there may be a hemiplegia when both sides are "equally convulsed."

Continuing, Geschwind came to Hughlings Jackson, who essentially adopted Todd's concept of exhaustion. Paraphrasing from Geschwind's discussion:

> Now Jackson made some important observations, although he may not have been the first to do so. He knew that patients with focal motor seizures could arrest a fit by placing a ligature above the level of the convulsing area (1). However, in many cases, when the fit was aborted in this manner, the post-ictal weakness was, curiously, more severe or prolonged. Jackson, whose name was given to focal motor and sensory seizures with spread, was, in the history of neurology, the neurologist with the best press secretary—for the theory of exhaustion remained unscathed for the next 80 years, although Gowers, a clinician and empiricist of unmatched skills, gave us more penetrating thoughts on the matter. One of Gowers' patients was a young man with longstanding epilepsy (2). His seizures began with pain in the right arm—not associated with convulsive movements of the arm but with weakness of the arm and twitching of the corner of the mouth. His tongue swelled and his speech became slurred. When his mouth began to twitch, the pain resolved. His arm, curiously enough, never twitched, but it was weak for about 15 minutes. Gowers also observed another man whose seizures caused disordered speech and right upper extremity weakness. Gowers correctly reasoned that exhaustion, although it might account for some cases of Todd's paralysis, couldn't account for these cases. Rather, these were cases in which there must be active inhibition. Furthermore, Gowers used Jackson's own observations of the ligature to seal the fate of the exhaustion theory as an exclusive explanation. Gowers reckoned that the ligature must act on sensory cortex, increasing inhibition on the sensorimotor cortex. This observation was incompatible with exhaustion as the sole mechanism.
>
> Gowers' ideas were ignored for almost a century. Jackson's press secretary was much more effective. Bob Efron [who was best man at Geschwind's wedding] observed a remarkable man, whose case was similar to the one that helped establish Gowers' concept of inhibition in Todd's paralysis (3). This young man had posttraumatic seizures beginning as paresthesia in the foot. The paresthesia spread upwards over a minute or so, and when it reached the shoulder, he convulsed.

Efron told the man that, as soon as the tingling began, he should vigorously rub his leg, using a stiff brush, above the level of the tingling. By doing so, he was able to block most grand mal seizures. However, these aborted seizures were associated with greater weakness in the man's left arm and leg. The most interesting feature was that the weakness in his arm developed even if the seizure was aborted below the level of the knee. Inhibition is the only explanation, for the motor centers of the arm surely could not be exhausted. Also, if exhaustion was the only mechanism, how could you explain that one man has a severe grand mal seizure lasting several minutes and then 5 minutes later gets up and walks away, whereas another man has a slight motor seizure in an arm and is weak in that arm for an hour afterwards? Active inhibition must be important. This is not to say that exhaustion can't occur, but inhibition is more intriguing.

Geschwind's training at Queen Square undoubtedly stimulated much of his interest in epilepsy and, specifically, temporal lobe epilepsy. Charles Symonds was one of the first physicians to stress the importance of localizing the lesion before specifying the disease process in neurological diagnosis. Symonds was interested in many clinical areas, with epilepsy high on his list. The interest in anatomy was the central issue in Geschwind's neurological thinking. Anatomy was more than location: it helped specify mechanism.

EPILEPSY AND LANGUAGE

Every spring semester at Harvard Medical School, Geschwind gave a no-credit seminar on the neurology of behavior. This series of evening lectures nearly filled the largest lecture hall at the medical school by the time of my arrival in 1977. By then, one of his lectures on epilepsy and disorders of language had given way to other topics that had captured his interest. I recently acquired a copy of the transcript of his 1976 lecture on epilepsy and language (4).

Geschwind's lecture on epilepsy and language began with a discussion of the effects of electrical stimulation of language areas. Stimulating perisylvian frontal, parietal, or temporal language cortex did not evoke verbal or even vocal output but, rather, caused speech arrest or, if a mild current was applied, anomia. In contrast, after a person has a seizure, one observes deficits typical of aphasias corresponding to the area from which the seizure arose. Geschwind then focused on the supplementary motor cortex. Stimulation in this area also caused speech arrest, which was not anticipated. Further, Brickner (5) observed that this is the only area from which stimulation can cause the patient to say or repeat a syllable, word, or phrase. Seizures cause the same effects as electrical stimulation in these perisylvian and supplementary motor areas. Some patients' vocalizations with supplementary motor seizures are stereotypic. One French patient always repeated (in French), "Slap me, slap me." In contrast to these examples, if a patient produces comprehensive language during a seizure, the seizure most often arises from the right hemisphere.

What then of lesions of the dominant supplementary motor cortex? Do such lesions cause language impairment? In the 1920s, Godfried Pershin removed this area in some patients and found that on the third postoperative day (when edema may be maximal), the patients stopped speaking. Later examination of these patients would reveal that their spontaneous speech was lacking but their repetition was preserved; that is, they had transcortical motor aphasia. The stimulation results were confirmed by Penfield and Welch (6) and the lesion effects confirmed by observations in stroke patients. The language deficits after destruction or removal of the supplementary motor cortex improved over several weeks, without permanent language impairment. Similarly, stimulation of the pulvinar nucleus of the thalamus can cause speech arrest or naming difficulties (7). Also, thalamic lesions can cause a transient anomic aphasia. Geschwind argued that language deficits after supplementary motor and thalamic lesions were transient. He was perplexed by how these areas fit into the language circuitry. In a lecture at Harvard in 1974 he said: "The fact that the syndrome is transient doesn't remove the fact that there is a syndrome. . . . The area somehow must be implicated in the activities of language, but I certainly have no idea how it fits in. . . ."

Geschwind turned to the relationship of aphasia, the loss of language, and seizures. He found that in adults, long-term language impairment after seizures was rare. In contrast, "There's a group of children in whom after seizures there may be very prolonged difficulty with language" that may last for several weeks. It can occur after each seizure in this selected group of children. Why this occurs in children and not adults is "a great mystery." Yet in his later lecture on memory, Geschwind provided a simple yet eloquent answer to this problem. For adults, language requires no learning. For children, language must be learned. Thus, medial temporal lobe structures that subserve memory functions are probably much more critical to language acquisition and development in children. In contrast, because adults already have learned language, the use of well-known language is disrupted little by mesial temporal lesions or physiological dysfunction (4).

LANGUAGE-INDUCED EPILEPSY

In 1965 and 1967, Geschwind and Ira Sherwin published a unique case, that of a 47-year-old man with language-induced epilepsy (8,9). Although cases of reading epilepsy were well described (10–13) and a single case of graphomotor epilepsy was reported (14), Geschwind and Sherwin's patient had seizures induced by three language modalities: reading, writing, and speaking. That case exemplified several characteristic features of Geschwind's contributions to neurology: Geschwind would take a single patient and, through careful testing, identify unique features of the case, thereby making original contributions to areas that appeared peripheral to his main interests but were nevertheless related to behavioral neurology; in so doing, he would challenge the prevailing wisdom and reinforce his central theme of the relationship between behavior and anatomy.

The patient was admitted to the Boston Veterans Administration Hospital's neurology service. He had had blackouts since his early thirties and academic problems relating to stuttering since early childhood. His spells occurred without any warning. He first noted jerking of his jaw followed by tremulousness of his hands, speech arrest, and, on occasion, loss of consciousness without convulsive movements. There were no post-ictal deficits. His wife noted that many but not all of these episodes occurred while he was reading.

The results of the patient's examination were normal except for the stuttering. When the patient was not taking antiepileptic medications, he had frequent "clinical seizures precipitated by certain language stimuli. These included reading (aloud or to himself), speaking (aloud or whispered), and writing" (9). The seizure began with speech arrest and, in some episodes, guttural sounds. He was able to respond to verbal commands throughout the typical seizure. Hyperventilation, intermittent photic stimulation, and optokinetic stimulation failed to provoke seizures. Similarly, repetitive lip, tongue, and jaw movements and humming a tune without words were ineffective stimuli. Although writing language was an effective stimulus, drawing geometric forms was ineffective.

Seizures were most easily provoked in the patient when he read. The material could be quite simple; for example, a Mickey Mouse comic book. Geschwind and Sherwin made another unique observation in this case: that reading often sensitized the patient to have seizures when speaking or writing. The EEG revealed generalized spike-and-wave discharges during seizures, although there was no one-to-one correlation of electroencephalographic spikes and palatal electromyographic activity. The administration of ethosuximide and phenobarbital markedly improved both his seizures and spontaneous stuttering.

Geschwind and Sherwin had taken an extra step in evaluating their patient and helped to settle an ongoing controversy over specificity of the stimulus and underlying mechanism. The prevailing view had been that it was necessary to look beyond reading and assume a more basic mechanism such as proprioceptive jaw input from mouth movements, scanning eye movements, concentration, and affective state. In his 1976 lecture, Geschwind encouraged the audience to read the original paper by Bickford et al. (10). Although they had found that the only stimulus that induced the seizures was reading, this seemed so unlikely that they went to a fair amount of trouble to try to show why this was not really a case of reading-induced epilepsy. However, they failed in this attempt. In discussing this case at the American Neurological Association meeting in 1965, Geschwind noted that:

> There has been a very strong tendency to feel that we have to find another explanation for these cases. In the end we will really have simply to accept the fact that highly specific stimuli can be epileptogenic. This need not surprise us; the normal process of learning which we carry on all the time consists in forming linkages between different parts of the nervous system, in combining highly specific stimuli to other highly specific stimuli. In fact, since this is probably one of the most common activities of the brain, it is astonishing that stimulus-specific epilepsy is not more common.

Geschwind observed that there were no known cases of reflex epilepsy precipitated by hearing spoken language. However, he noted that if such a case did occur, "it would be very easy to misinterpret it" (4). Similarly, when the house officer saw the patient described by Geschwind and Sherwin, the patient was thought to be in spontaneous status epilepticus, because, every time he tried to speak, he had a seizure. In the speculative case of spoken language provoking seizures, "people would come up [to the patient] and say 'How do you feel?' and every time the patient would start to speak he would trip a seizure off.... It would probably be exceedingly difficult to have him in an environment in which he didn't hear the speech" (4).

The anatomy of language-induced epilepsy was a mystery. As with other cases of reading-induced epilepsy, the EEG discharge was bilateral and generalized, not arising in or restricted to the left hemisphere. Geschwind distinguished two types of reflex epilepsies: in one type, seizures were provoked by a very specific stimulus, such as viewing a safety pin [as in the classic case of Mitchell and colleagues (15), which Geschwind frequently mentioned] or hearing a particular group of church bells [as in the case described by Poskanzer et al. (16)]. Both patients had temporal lobe epilepsy, which usually has a cortical origin. In the other type of reflex epilepsies, a highly specific class of stimuli, such as language stimuli, could provoke a seizure (thus any word, but not humming or whistling). However, this type of discharge reflected subcortical activation (i.e., generalized epilepsy). "This distinction may well point to some highly significant factors in physiological organization, but it is not possible even to speculate about these at this time" (2).

Before concluding his 1976 lecture on epilepsy and language, in which he strongly argued for relating behavior to anatomy, Geschwind made one additional appeal to students of behavioral neurology:

> The stimulus which comes in this area is from the clinic.... I mean the bird-watching aspects of the clinic,... that patient who appears randomly, presents himself to your eyes unexpectedly and has some feature which has not previously been observed. And that is quite different from what a lot of people would regard as clinical observation—which is taking 30 people with gout and

studying them. . . . I'm talking about . . . the fact that you are prepared for something unexpected to appear. I happen to think that this is so important that it really can't get enough stress, because it's a very common notion that clinical observation is dead—so that there's very little future in it. . . . In fact it may be true in all of internal medicine for all I could care, but it's not true in neurology. . . . The neurology of behavior is going to be in a terrible way if this kind of bird-watching activity is removed or diminished. . . . When I first became interested in this field, I was astonished to find that many of the people in [it] already regarded it as unnecessary to carry out what they called contemptuously "bird-watching activity" because it was felt that all of the clinical observation that had ever been done would be done, and from here on . . . study things methodologically. . . . The only difficulty . . . was that much of the methodological studies consisted of lumping together things which should have been separated, and you had no way of separating them except by realizing on the basis of observation that you were seeing something new. . . . A lot of journals won't accept reports of patients now. . . . If you weighed something, you can trust the numbers, but not if someone described something that he saw. I think it's nonsensical, and I think what you obviously do is to start publishing many very boring papers and you omit all sorts of terribly interesting observations.

MYOCLONIC EPILEPSY

Geschwind's professional correspondence and office notes reveal that although non-temporal-lobe epilepsy was at best a peripheral interest, his knowledge and insights were remarkable. In 1981, Dr. Walter Levitsky referred a woman to Geschwind who had a form of myoclonic epilepsy (probably juvenile myoclonic epilepsy, which was not recognized by Geschwind) that treatment with phenytoin made worse. Geschwind related his own personal experience that Baltic myoclonus may be made "distinctly worse by Dilantin, but is improved by valproic acid. The fact that drugs which might damage the cerebellum [referring to large doses of phenytoin] could lead to myoclonus, rather than a straightforward cerebellar syndrome, is, however, not too surprising. . . . There are a number of conditions characterized by myoclonus in which cerebellar lesions are prominent, such as the well-known Lafora form of myoclonus. I have personally seen the same effect in a patient who was toxic on phenobarbital. In those patients in whom neurologic symptomatology develops on Dilantin it is not at all unusual for this to occur even with a single dose, just as it did in your patient. I have recently seen a patient who developed attacks of cerebellar dysarthria. Thinking that this might be like some attacks of multiple sclerosis which get better on Dilantin, she was put on this drug but would develop an attack within 40 minutes of even a single dose." In other cases, Geschwind specifically mentions that absence of myoclonus—an important historical point that continues to be regularly missed despite the attention to juvenile myoclonic epilepsy.

In another woman, who had aphasia after a cerebral abscess, Geschwind observed in his correspondence that "brain abscesses are intensely epileptogenic," and he recommended maintaining antiepileptic drugs for at least several years. He also noted that, at her young age:

> . . . [the] firing . . . does not occur more often than once every twenty minutes. This even raises a possibility of one disadvantage, i.e., that the medication might reduce the number of attacks to only a few a day, which might in fact increase the risks of kindling. All in all, both Dr. Sherwin and I would favor the use of anticonvulsant medication, probably Dilantin, which has less effect on cognitive function than phenobarbital.
>
> I would add only one further recommendation. . . . It might be quite useful to test the patient with singing while she was in a position which would usually induce a seizure (i.e., standing), but at the same time one could simply place a finger on the side of the child's head. It would be interesting to see if such an extraneous stimulus would, in fact, inhibit the attacks. If this were the case, one could conceive that she could even wear some simple sort of head band, since if this maneu-

ver unexpectedly did work one might be able to control the seizures in a very simple fashion. It would also be interesting to see if there is a difference between an external touch and one coming from her own hand. Thus some patients with dystonia will inhibit their movements by touch with the patient's own hand but not in response to a touch by someone else. (17)

Geschwind ended his lecture on "Epilepsy and Language" where he often began: anatomy.

One of the things that I wanted to stress was the particular usefulness of understanding the anatomy of behavior. I certainly don't think that anatomy is the only approach to the understanding of brain–behavior relationships. . . . However, I also happen to believe that it is uniquely important and the fact of the matter is, it is the one that has been most neglected. In an odd way, the kind of anatomical analysis that has been common, let's say the physiological psychology for the last 30 years, has been the curious result that in order to avoid talking about localization, they have become extreme localizationists. Because you don't want to talk about connections and analyze things that way . . . dealing with a series of mysteries each of which has a localization . . . but these are areas which are in a certain sense floating. . . . I think the approach of anatomy in terms of connections, in terms of the attempt to look at how different areas are related is the kind of analysis that was extremely common in the 1920s and then essentially disappeared almost entirely from neurology . . . one of the great advantages of the anatomical analysis leads to showing you where it's inadequate. Because you're on very concrete grounds and you can immediately say it predicts this but it doesn't explain that, and at that point you know that you have to modify it. I don't think this is a disadvantage, I think this is an advantage, because I think this is the way that any useful scientific method works. And if I have left you with an appreciation for the importance of anatomy, I will have succeeded.

REFERENCES

1. Jackson JH. *Selected writings*. Taylor J, ed. New York: Basic Books, 1958;6,15,16,34.
2. Gowers WR. *Epilepsy and other chronic convulsive diseases: their causes, symptoms and treatment*. London, England: JA Churchill, 1881.
3. Efron R. Post-epileptic paralysis: theoretical critique and report of a case. *Brain* 1961;84:380–394.
4. Geschwind N. *Epilepsy and disorders of language*. Unpublished lecture at Harvard Medical School, May 28, 1976.
5. Brickner RM. A human cortical area producing repetitive phenomena when stimulated. *J Neurophysiol* 1940;3:128–130.
6. Penfield W, Welch K. The supplementary motor area of the cerebral cortex. *Arch Neurol Psychiatry* 1951;66:289–317.
7. Ojemann G. Language and the thalamus: object naming and recall during and after thalamic stimulation. *Brain Lang* 1975;2:101–120.
8. Sherwin I, Geschwind N, Abramowicz A. Language-induced epilepsy. *Trans Am Neurol Assoc* 1965;90:183–188.
9. Geschwind N, Sherwin I. Language-induced epilepsy. *Arch Neurol* 1967;16:25–31.
10. Bickford RG, Whelan JL, Klass DW, et al. Reading epilepsy. *Trans Am Neurol Assoc* 1956;81:100–102.
11. Critchley N, Cobb W, Sears TA. On reading epilepsy. *Epilepsia* 1959/1960;1:403–417.
12. Baxter DW, Bailey AA. Primary reading epilepsy. *Neurology* 1961;11:445–449.
13. Stevens H. Reading epilepsy. *N Engl J Med* 1957;257:165–170.
14. Asbury AK, Prensky AL. Graphogenic epilepsy. *Trans Am Neurol Assoc* 1965;88:193–194.
15. Mitchell W, Falconer MA, Hill D. Epilepsy with fetishism relieved by temporal lobectomy. *Lancet* 1954;2:626–630.
16. Poskanzer DC, Brown AE, Miller E. Musicogenic epilepsy caused by a discrete frequency band of church bells. *Brain* 1962;85:77–92.
17. Geschwind, N. Correspondence to Walter Levitsky, MD, July 16, 1981.

26

Interictal Behavior in Temporal Lobe Epilepsy

David M. Bear

Department of Psychiatry, University of Massachusetts Medical Center, Worcester, Massachusetts 01655.

A PERSONALIZED INTRODUCTION TO BEHAVIOR AND EPILEPSY

My first encounter with behavioral symptoms of patients with temporal lobe epilepsy (TLE) predated my introduction to Norman Geschwind. During a Harvard undergraduate rotation at Massachusetts General Hospital (MGH), I had first met a series of patients who were under the care of Drs. Vernon Mark and Frank Ervin and who experienced complex partial seizures and had histories of extreme aggression. As related in their controversial monograph, *Violence and the Brain* (1), these investigators were testing a dramatic hypothesis: that epileptic discharges, conducted to emotion-controlling structures within the temporal lobe, could trigger unintended, automatic acts of aggression.

The concept of a "violent automatism" as a form of psychomotor seizure had significant implications. As dramatized by Michael Crichton in *The Terminal Man* (2), it raised the possibility that patients with TLE, with otherwise normal personalities, might abruptly lose control of behavior and commit primitive sexual or aggressive assaults. Legally, such patients might not be held responsible for their automatisms.

Since TLE was then (in the early 1970s) and, indeed, is now a difficult condition to confirm by electroencephalography (3), the "ictal aggression" hypothesis raised the possibility that many violent persons might suffer from a subtle form of temporal lobe dysfunction. Investigations at MGH involved recordings from the depth of the temporal lobe, particularly the amygdaloid complex, in violence-prone persons. If abnormal discharges were detected, the experimental intervention was to induce a radiofrequency (burn) lesion adjacent to the discharging area, with the hope of destroying an epileptic focus and modifying behavior.

As I learned during my freshman year at Harvard Medical School, Norman Geschwind endorsed the concept of a linkage between TLE and behavioral changes. Despite a general lack of therapeutic success in the MGH program, Geschwind remained a strong supporter of the investigative efforts of the neurosurgeons William Sweet and Vernon Mark, and the psychiatrist Frank Ervin.

In fact, the technique of producing stereotactic radiofrequency lesions proved relatively ineffective in seizure control or behavioral amelioration. Among other difficulties, epileptic foci were often multiple and not accurately localized in three-dimensional space by the indwelling electrode arrays. More fundamentally, as I later appreciated, Dr. Geschwind did not share the MGH clinicians' major hypothesis about epilepsy and behavior.

Attending my first lecture on TLE from Geschwind, I felt well prepared to field his frequent questions, an unmistakable aspect of the Socratic method that he employed extensively. I thought I knew the basic facts about psychomotor seizures, emotional behavior, and the amygdala. Armed with the first-year medical student's neuroanatomic vocabulary, I pointed confidently to major connections that linked the amygdala within the temporal lobe to the hypothalamus, a structure mediating sexual arousal, fear, and aggressive responses. It was "not surprising," I suggested, "that temporal lobe seizures could lead to dramatic, emotionally driven behaviors."

As Dr. Geschwind pondered my confident analysis, he smiled slowly yet began to shake his head in a clearly negative fashion. "In my experience, patients rarely, if ever, engage in a violent or sexual, or, indeed, any emotionally motivated act during their seizures; in the great majority of spells, patients smack their lips, fumble with objects, or repeat insignificant, stereotyped phrases without memory of their behavior."

Norman Geschwind's generalization about complex partial seizures, which was repeated to me in somewhat different terms by John Van Buren, the former Chief of Neurosurgery at the National Institutes of Health, has proven clinically accurate. But, as a medical student, I was both deflated and puzzled. I muttered, "But what about the limbic system—the amygdala and the hypothalamus—what, then, is the link between temporal lobe epilepsy and behavior?" Norman Geschwind opened his eyes widely and paused, preparing a careful answer. Like a Zen master, he had first shaken the false belief of his student and now a new idea, which he believed was subtler and closer to the truth, might find its place in a receptive mind.

SCHIZOPHRENIA-LIKE PSYCHOSIS OF EPILEPSY

Geschwind's emphasis then, often repeated during my year of neurology internship under his tutelage at Boston City Hospital, was that the major changes in behavior of TLE patients were not paroxysmal, episodic events; they were not "seizure equivalents." Rather, the relevant changes in behavior developed gradually, over months or years, after the formation of a TLE focus. The behavioral features became pervasive, interictal aspects of the patient's personality, often at a time when the person's seizures were infrequent.

In promoting this point of view, Geschwind was drawing attention to studies that were well known and extensively published in the English neurological and psychiatric literature, but largely neglected, especially by American psychiatrists. In 1963, Elliot Slater and Alfred Beard (4) had described a series of patients with TLE who, on an average of 14 years after the appearance of seizures, acquired a "schizophrenia-like psychosis." In many of these patients, strong religious ideation, paranoid delusions, and intense emotions suggestive of the positive symptoms of schizophrenia developed; a contemporary diagnostician might characterize the symptoms as closer to schizoaffective psychosis. However, in patients with the "schizophrenia-like psychosis of epilepsy," other thought disorders such as clang associations or blocking, or negative symptoms such as alogia, neglect of hygiene, blunted emotions, or social withdrawal, rarely developed.

In the mid 1970s, Norman Geschwind conducted evening lectures, frequently on the subject of behavior and TLE, which drew such large crowds of physicians, and especially psychiatrists, that fire marshals were summoned to clear the aisles of the major lecture hall at Harvard Medical School. With somewhat uncharacteristic reserve, Geschwind usually announced that he had not written a single paper on TLE but felt confident in stressing two fundamental points: (a) the importance of interictal behavior observations as opposed to preoccupation with events during individual complex partial seizures, and (b) the development of a paranoid, schizophrenia-like psychosis among a significant number of patients with TLE.

Geschwind's views were most compelling in the setting of frequent case conferences, both at Boston City Hospital and at the Aphasia Research Unit of the Boston Veterans Administration Hospital. Norman's penetrating yet invariably entertaining interviews focused on the stereotyped, unemotional nature of most patients' seizures, in contrast to the depth of their interictal emotions, paranoid ideation, and relatively preserved interpersonal relationships.

INTERICTAL BEHAVIOR CHANGES—THE GESCHWIND SYNDROME

However, by the late 1970s, it became clear to his close students that Dr. Geschwind's characterization of interictal behavior had evolved beyond the concept of schizophrenia-like psychosis. In a consultation to the chairman of Neurosurgery at MGH, he wrote:

> I saw a patient at the Massachusetts General Hospital at the request of Dr. William Sweet. I would like to mention that the diagnosis was made for me even before I had seen the patient, since, when I opened up the record, a large number of yellow sheets were seen which contained extensive writing of a strongly religious and cosmic nature in the handwriting of the patient. This phenomenon of hypergraphia, i.e., a tendency to produce extensive writing, particularly of a religious or cosmic nature, is extremely characteristic of patients with temporal lobe epilepsy.
>
> I was struck by certain features of his personality. Although he was unusual in many ways, it was obvious that one had no trouble at all making verbal contact with him. I wish to stress that point because the literature often speaks about the schizophreniform psychosis of temporal lobe epilepsy. This phrase gives the impression that in many patients with temporal lobe epilepsy there is a behavior disorder which resembles schizophrenia. In fact, however, patients with temporal lobe epilepsy, even the most bizarre ones, usually differ in very important ways from the typical schizophrenic.
>
> In particular, the patients with temporal lobe epilepsy are very rarely (emotionally) flat and make contact easily with the examiner. Indeed, they commonly show a feature which is quite different from that of typical schizophrenia, i.e., stickiness, a strong tendency to make excessive and prolonged contact with the examiner. It is unusual for these patients to show blocking or to turn away from the examiner or to fail to answer.
>
> The patient was talkative, especially about his religious views. At the same time, he expressed a great deal of hostile ideation. He admitted he had very little sexual activity, and no social life with women in recent years. His aggressiveness is very well documented. His mother told me that he had been so aggressive that the other siblings in the family had refused to come home.
>
> Thus the patient had features of the *interictal personality disorder* of TLE—hypergraphia, religiosity, hyposexuality, aggressiveness, and stickiness.

The concept of a syndromic change in behavior, including the novel observation of hypergraphia, was introduced by Steven Waxman and Norman Geschwind in publications in *Neurology* (5) and the *Archives of General Psychiatry* (6). His observations were regarded as clinically astute and accurate by some observers, but they elicited extremely emotional, negative responses from other quarters.

I remember well a clinical conference at MGH at which Dr. Geschwind's first mention of interictal behavior changes was greeted by a round of obviously rehearsed hisses from a group associated with a visiting epileptologist. This well-known neurologist, who rarely attended Geschwind's case conferences, believed that the proposal of specific behavior changes in TLE could only add to the stigma borne by epileptic patients. Although the concerns were understandable, I have always found this reasoning on the subject most unconvincing, tending to establish either that in some patients with generalized epilepsies behavior changes may also develop, or that a selected psychiatric population could manifest some of the behavioral symptoms to a more extreme degree. Neither proposition is incompatible with Geschwind's perspective, especially since patients initially thought to have nonfocal, generalized epilepsy are often discovered to harbor temporolimbic abnormalities.

Having witnessed Dr. Geschwind demonstrate behavior changes in clinical interviews, and having then encountered respected neurologists who vehemently challenged the observations, I was unsure about the reality of the "Geschwind syndrome." Perhaps Norman Geschwind had selected atypical patients to demonstrate, or we simply had not seen nonepileptic patients who would show similar interests in writing, religion, or prolonged interpersonal contact. Despite my confidence in Geschwind's acumen, I tried to remain agnostic. My hope was that, when I went to the National Institute of Neurological Disease and Stroke as a Fellow, it would be possible to investigate the Geschwind syndrome objectively. The problem that Dr. Paul Fedio, a National Institutes of Health (NIH) neuropsychologist, and I faced was to proceed from Geschwind's qualitative picture of a patient, something that came out beautifully in a clinical interview, to a quantitative concept. How can one measure behaviors like hypergraphia or stickiness, or the tendency to dwell on peripheral details?

In fact, observations like hypergraphia had never been part of traditional psychological assessments, and the literature on behavior change in epilepsy, which was conflicted, had relied on standardized tests, such as the Minnesota Multi-Phasic Personality Inventory, that measured psychopathology (7,8). One of Geschwind's caveats was that one should investigate behavioral changes such as hypergraphia in a neutral context and not be limited by psychiatric nosologic systems.

My first year of work at the NIH, therefore, involved constructing straightforward true/false questions about a person's interest in writing or level of sexual desire, trying to choose appropriate wording to bring out qualities of the interictal syndrome. During this time, I often would recall Dr. Geschwind's lectures or his clinical interviews with the thought: How can I capture what he demonstrates so clearly with a live patient?

The laboratory in which I worked at the NIH was not particularly receptive to studies of behavior. My laboratory chief would have preferred that I study basic neurophysiology and concentrate on the behavior of individual neurons within the epileptic focus. Dr. Geschwind's supportive comments on our studies were, therefore, very important.

Dr. Fedio and I appreciated the benefits of obtaining a quantitative measure of the interictal behavior syndrome. An objective measure might establish the prevalence of interictal behavior alterations, opening the door to careful behavioral epidemiology. If we could quantify the interictal behavior syndrome, it would be possible to follow its progress over time to determine, for example, whether the behavior changes are static or progressive. We could look at the effect of particular interventions in terms of behavioral symptoms. However, there were considerable difficulties in achieving meaningful quantitative behavioral assessments. It was a challenge to boil down subtle features of behavior to short true/false questions, and obtaining the appropriate wording was a demanding chore. Because there is extensive variability in the emotions of human beings, any set of questions sensitive to the behavior changes in persons with epilepsy would also reflect intensity of emotions and conflicts in persons without epilepsy.

In testing the first version of the interictal behavior inventory at the NIH, for example, I found that many normal adolescents endorsed a fair number of items, not generally as many as persons with TLE but more than older persons. This finding may well reflect an important biological effect of steroid hormones on temporolimbic structures, so that the search for absolute specificity, in which items are endorsed only by TLE patients, will always be futile. In fact, I assumed that many of the patients with TLE were significantly depressed and that another group of primarily depressed patients, if we had tested them, would have endorsed the mood-sensitive items.

Considering the complexity of such behavioral assessments, we focused on a specific question: Would a significant fraction of patients with unambiguous TLE endorse interictal behavior changes? If the answer to this preliminary question was positive, we could systematically perform comparisons with other groups and examine contributing variables.

The results we obtained, based on testing 27 patients whom neurologists had identified as having TLE, and contrasting them with normal subjects or patients with severe neuromuscular diseases, provided strong evidence for the interictal behavioral syndrome. Based on our 100-item questionnaire, the patients with TLE self-reported specific interictal behaviors; in addition, third-person raters, usually family members, identified these traits. The statistical differences between the TLE groups and the contrast subjects were robust (9).

Our basic question about the reality of the interictal behavior syndrome was, therefore, answered affirmatively. Since these studies, I have never doubted the existence of the Geschwind syndrome. Furthermore, the hundreds of medical students, interns, and residents who have been influenced by Dr. Geschwind and his teachings have no doubt that there is a Geschwind syndrome. Students are most powerfully convinced when they meet individual patients who exemplify the behavior changes. However, I think the weight of quantitative studies, initiated by my work with Fedio, also demonstrates the reality of interictal alterations (10,11).

It may well be that the initial presentation of our data, as a result of overzealous analysis, fed confusion and controversy. We initially measured 18 different characteristics of behavior that had been referenced in the literature on TLE (9). Many of these variables were overlapping. We knew they were redundant and were hoping that a multivariate statistical procedure could reduce these variables to a smaller number.

The problem was that with a small number of patients and a large difference in behavior between epileptic patients and the contrast subjects, the statistic can give a misleading "short list" of behaviors that achieves virtually perfect group assignment. The potential misunderstanding from this study was that the interictal behavior syndrome was an all-or-none phenomenon, that every patient reported identical behaviors, and that we could identify the behavior syndrome with two or three cardinal characteristics such as circumstantiality, religious interest, or hypergraphia.

If one examines the data closely, there was substantial variability among patients, with some having an interest in writing, others more troubled by irritability and anger, others by sexual issues. Indeed, one of the most intriguing aspects of the study was the suggestion that patients with a right temporal lobe focus might have a different quality to their behavioral syndrome compared to those with a left temporal lobe focus. Right-hemisphere patients appeared to express and act on emotion more readily. Left-hemisphere patients tended to think about or verbalize their strong emotions and engage in philosophical or paranoid ideation (9,11).

This work was completed as I was returning to Boston to join Drs. Geschwind and Mesulam at the newly founded Behavioral Neurology Unit of Beth Israel Hospital. Geschwind was excited by the data, believing that they verified his clinical observations. At his suggestion, we submitted the manuscript to a number of prestigious journals. In each case, he wrote an accompanying letter of support. However, we received numerous rejections! At one point, he clearly sensed my disappointment and related that one of his first major papers, a classic description of disconnection of the corpus callosum, was also repeatedly rejected. Eventually, our study was published in the *Archives of Neurology* with a strong editorial endorsing the findings by Dr. Geschwind (9).

One issue that Geschwind, Fedio, and I considered beyond the scope of our initial study was whether the interictal behavior changes resembled specific psychiatric syndromes or whether they were differentiable. This was a problem I later addressed with Dr. Dietrich Blumer at McLean Hospital, where we compared patients with TLE to a number of psychiatric groups—patients with affective disorder, aggressive character disorder, or schizophrenia (12). As observers, we were blinded to diagnosis and had to rate patients on such variables as circumstantiality, sexual interest, and religious preoccupation. These data showed both overlapping symptoms and distinctive features of TLE patients, such as their extreme interest in detail and the frequent combination of social clinging or "stickiness" with a lack of interest in sexual contact. In addition to quantitative differences in behavior, the study also underscored qualitative aspects of particular behaviors such as aggression. Among the TLE patients, we found persons who became incensed by moral transgressions but rarely acted aggressively because of strong ethical prohibitions, and who, on the rare occasions when they did engage in violence, experienced full recall and remorse. On the other hand, patients with aggressive character disorders had little interest in religious or moral values, reported no moral compunction or remorse after their acts, and often claimed amnesia for violent behavior (12).

MECHANISMS OF BEHAVIORAL CHANGE IN EPILEPSY

What most interested Geschwind was the question of underlying mechanism. Why should an epileptic focus in the temporolimbic cortex produce behavior change? In his early papers with Waxman, Geschwind (5,6) drew attention to the role of limbic structures such as the amygdala in regulating sexual, aggressive, or fearful behavior, but to my reading, no particular mechanism was proposed.

As I pondered this issue, I was drawn back to Norman Geschwind's remarkable paper on disconnection syndromes, published in *Brain* in 1965 (13). In this prophetic monograph, Geschwind, utilizing the scanty neuroanatomic information available at the time, proposed that sensory processing—for example, information from the visual system—would be conducted into the temporal lobe, where connections with structures like the amygdala and thus the hypothalamus could take place.

Geschwind's proposal was that the temporal lobe is a critical meeting place for sensory percepts and drive representations concerning hunger, fear, sexual desire, or anger. This analysis provided a powerful understanding of the Kluver-Bucy syndrome in which, after bilateral temporal lobe removals, monkeys could not distinguish food from nonfood objects, identify relevant sexual partners, or experience appropriate fear or aggressive responses. Geschwind described this as "sensory–limbic disconnection" (13). Recalling Sigmund Freud's concept of cathexis as the investment of a percept with emotional valence, I have often thought of the Kluver-Bucy syndrome as "global decathexis" (14).

The French epileptologist Henri Gastaut had pointed out that some behavior changes in epileptic patients, like hyposexuality, were the converse of changes in the Kluver-Bucy syndrome, which produces hypersexuality (15). My hypothesis, as proposed in *Cortex* (14) and the *Archives of Neurology* (9), was more general: that a chronic discharging focus involving the temporal limbic structures might lead to extraneous sensory–emotional connections—"hyperconnections." Thus, the behavioral features of the interictal behavior syndrome, although they vary among different persons, reflect an investment of the world with fortuitous emotional associations—leading some patients to engage in philosophical inquiry, others to manifest religious inspiration, and others to record seemingly incidental details in extensive diaries, as if each item were highly significant.

The concept of hyperconnection has been criticized as untestable. However, I believe recent discoveries in neurophysiology make several mechanisms plausible. For example, studies of excitatory amino acid receptors, such as the class activated by *N*-methyl-D-aspartate (NMDA), have revealed a mechanism for the strengthening of synapses between neurons that fire coincidentally (16). Such Hebbian synapses (17) would be ideal for storing associations between a visual object and a change in the level of hunger, anger, or sexual desire. Both the hippocampus and amygdala are studded with NMDA receptors, and there are now multiple proposals to account for the strengthening of intervening synapses after synchronous neuronal activation (16).

Because the common denominator of all epilepsies is a tendency for neurons to fire adventitiously and hypersynchronously, one can imagine that a fortuitous epileptic discharge could be mistaken for a signal of emotional content, leading to spurious strengthening of associations between a visual, auditory, or somatosensory event and an emotional tag or label (14). This process could produce hyperconnection, although the detailed mechanisms are clearly subject to further research.

Geschwind was strongly supportive of the concept of hyperconnection. He called it an "elegant phrase." When I was working directly with him as the co-director of the Behavioral Neurology Unit at Beth Israel Hospital, we attempted to test the concept of sensory limbic hyperconnection in a preliminary way. If the temporal limbic system of a person with epilepsy were more prone to place emotional weight on a neutral stimulus, perhaps visually elicited autonomic responses of TLE patients, reflecting hypothalamic output, would be enhanced.

With Drs. Herbert Benson and Laura Schenk, we assembled a group of photographs chosen as neutral, emotionally pleasant, or unpleasant. These photos were shown to a

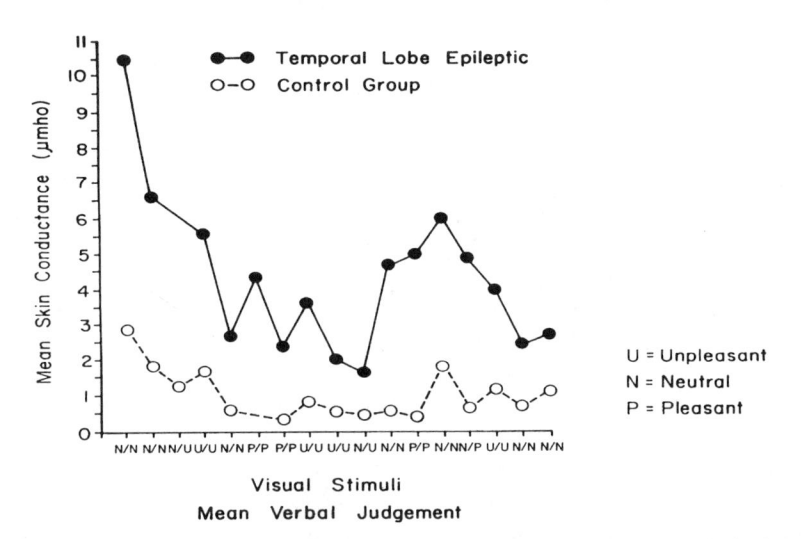

FIG. 1. Galvanic skin conductance responses to visual stimuli, whether verbally labeled neutral, pleasant, or unpleasant, were greater among patients with temporal lobe epilepsy than normal subjects. There was no overlap in means across stimuli, and the overall group difference reached a high level of significance. 2-way Anova, $p < .001$ (18).

group of patients with TLE and to normal subjects. As illustrated in Figure 1, the results were compatible with our hypothesis. For each of the 27 stimuli, the TLE group experienced larger galvanic skin responses than the control subjects; this was true regardless of the pleasant, unpleasant, or neutral nature of the stimulus, which was rated equivalently by the groups. In 24 of the 27 individual stimulus trials, the differences reached statistically significant levels. Across all stimuli, the two groups were powerfully differentiated (18).

None of the epileptic patients experienced a seizure during testing. In fact, during resting periods in which patients were not viewing objects, their autonomic responses were indistinguishable from those of controls. These results are, therefore, consistent with the concept of enhanced interictal emotional associations.

For psychiatric theory, there are few processes more fundamental than the selective association of emotion with a particular stimulus or event. I believe that functional brain imaging, either positron emission tomography or echoplanar magnetic resonance studies, could clarify the role of the limbic system in epilepsy and other psychiatric conditions. As we are now equipped with the functional anatomy of an "object" visual pathway projecting into the temporal lobe, it would be quite feasible, for example, to examine the locus of activation of relevant visual stimuli (e.g., food objects) as a function of hunger level or salient reinforcers.

NORMAN GESCHWIND'S CONTRIBUTIONS TO NEUROPSYCHIATRY

In my opinion, one of Geschwind's fundamental contributions, especially to psychiatry, was to open the window to regions of the brain critically involved in forming emotional associations. Based on his observations, he theorized that the Kluver-Bucy syndrome was an example of structural sensory–limbic disconnection (13), whereas TLE represented physiological sensory–limbic hyperconnection (14).

Catalyzed by Geschwind's insights, the field of behavior and epilepsy has been an area of fertile exploration in the last decade. Certain recent observations might have proven initially surprising but undoubtedly fascinating to him if he were alive today. For example, in large part through the contributions of Geschwind's student Orrin Devinsky, it has become clear that many patients experience multiple simple partial seizures in which they retain consciousness and memory for their experiences and have no ictal EEG changes (3). Geschwind, of course, was familiar with the auras of TLE patients but assumed that these would most often be followed by a complex partial seizure. However, investigators have now encountered patients who repeatedly experience strong emotions such as fear or anger, or dissociative experiences such as autoscopy, which may lead to significant behavioral pathology. We have described one such patient, who experienced a prolonged, frightening auditory hallucination during her simple partial seizures (19).

A major frontier has been opened in the study of frontal lobe epilepsy, including seizures originating from the orbitofrontal cortex or anterior cingulate area, which may produce behavior syndromes distinct from TLE. For example, my colleagues Tisher and Holzer and I described a 64-year-old woman in whom a remarkable pseudomanic syndrome developed in the setting of repeated partial seizures emanating from the right orbitofrontal cortex (19).

This case and others like it led me to reconsider a patient discussed by Geschwind in the *Journal of Clinical Psychiatry* (20). She was thought to have TLE. At the time, we recognized anomalous features of her presentation: a lack of social modesty, extreme hypersexuality rather than hyposexuality, and rapid reversal of symptoms in response to carbamazepine. In retrospect, I believe her picture is more consistent with a cingulate or frontal lobe focus.

One of Dr. Geschwind's most inspiring statements—an overarching consideration in shaping the careers of many of his students—was that the study of neurological effects on human behavior represented basic, not applied, science. He was indicating by this statement that the highest integrative activities of the nervous system are uniquely manifested in the human brain and that fundamental observations with patients might generate novel hypotheses, which could then be tested in animal models. This perspective is even more important to recall today, when the techniques of molecular biology, so impressive in their own right, are sometimes assumed to hold the answer to all questions about the nervous system. Surely, the organization of human behavior will require additional approaches to understand, for example, how we select from the vast universe of stimuli assailing us those that are emotionally pertinent, and how, prompted by our massively parallel nervous system to act in so many disparate ways, we select an appropriate response.

In my view, these integrative processes depend on two great corticolimbic networks regulated at the highest levels by the anterior temporal and orbitofrontal cortices (Fig. 2). The plasticity of limbic cortex makes these areas frequent sites of focal epilepsy in the adult brain. This vulnerability creates an opportunity, through the close study of behavior in epilepsy, to clarify the function of the most advanced stages of processing in the human nervous system.

Before the contributions of Norman Geschwind, emotional behaviors in TLE were typically explained as subcortical "seizure equivalents." His emphasis on interictal behavior change and limbic connections shifted attention to epilepsy as a subtle modulator of the highest levels of integrative cortex. Rather than the "violent automatism," he sought to explain the relentless philosophic and moral ruminations motivating Dostoyevsky's prolific writing or the blinding emotional incandescence leaping from the canvasses of Van Gogh.

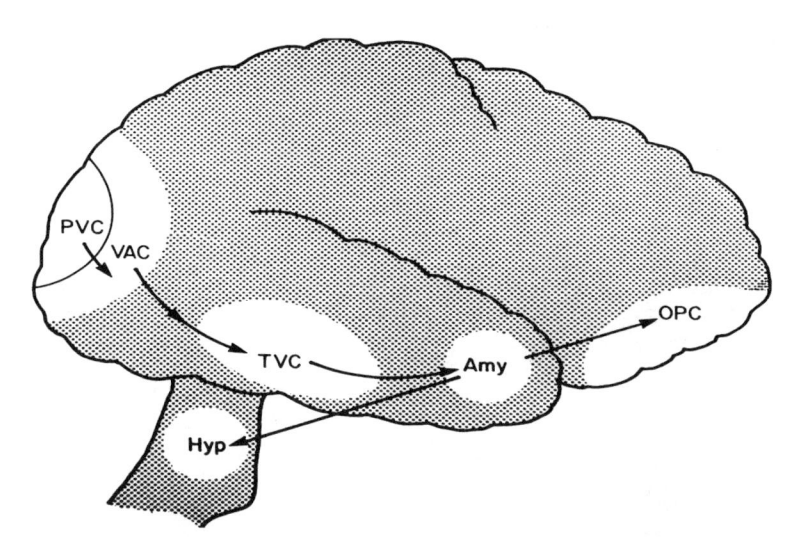

FIG. 2. A major visual pathway, specialized for object detection in central vision, projects to the primate amygdala. Two subsequent streams of processing are indicated: (a) from the amygdala to the hypothalamus and brain stem nuclei, and (b) from the amygdala to the rostral temporal pole and subsequently to the orbital prefrontal cortex. The first pathway may mediate autonomic symptoms and motor automatisms in temporal lobe seizures. Geschwind's observations and theoretical work focused on the cortical components enabling sensory–emotional associations (rostral temporal cortex) and the selection of appropriate emotional responses (orbital prefrontal cortex). PVC, primary visual cortex; VAC, visual association cortex; TVC, temporal visual cortex; HYP, hypothalamus; AMY, amygdala; OPC, orbital prefrontal cortex.

REFERENCES

1. Mark V, Ervin F. *Violence and the brain.* New York: Harper & Row, 1970.
2. Crichton M. *The terminal man.* New York: Knopf, 1972.
3. Devinsky O, Kelley K, Porter RJ, Theodore WH. Clinical and electroencephalographic features of simple partial seizures. *Neurology* 1988;38:1347–1352.
4. Slater E, Beard AW. Schizophrenia-like psychoses of epilepsy. *Br J Psychiatry* 1963;109:95–150.
5. Waxman SG, Geschwind N. Hypergraphia in temporal lobe epilepsy. *Neurology* 1980;30:314–317.
6. Waxman SG, Geschwind N. The interictal behavior syndrome of temporal lobe epilepsy. *Arch Gen Psychiatry* 1975;32:1580–1586.
7. Tizard B. The personality of epileptics: a discussion of the evidence. *Psychol Bull* 1962;59:196–210.
8. Mignone RJ, Donnelly EF, Sadowsky D. Psychological and neurological comparisons of psychomotor and non-psychomotor epileptic patients. *Epilepsia* 1970;11:345–359.
9. Bear DM, Fedio P. Quantitative analysis of interictal behavior in temporal lobe epilepsy. *Arch Neurol* 1977;34:454–467.
10. Benson DF. The Geschwind syndrome. *Adv Neurol* 1991;55:411–421.
11. Bear DM, Freeman R, Greenberg M. Psychiatric aspects of temporal lobe epilepsy. *Ann Rev Psychiatry* 1985;4:190–210.
12. Bear DM, Levin K, Blumer D, Chatham D. Interictal behavior in hospitalized temporal lobe epileptics—relation to other psychiatric syndromes. *J Neurol Neurosurg Psychiatry* 1982;45:481–488.
13. Geschwind N. Disconnexion syndromes in animals and man, Part I. *Brain* 1965;88:237–294.
14. Bear DM. Temporal lobe epilepsy: a syndrome of sensory–limbic hyperconnection. *Cortex* 1979;15:357–384.
15. Gastaut H, Collomb K. Étude du comportement sexuel chez les épileptiques psychomoteurs. *Ann Med Psychol* 1954;112:675–696.
16. Manabe T, Nicoll RA. Long-term potentiation: evidence against an increase in transmitter release probability. *Science* 1994;265:1888–1892.
17. Hebb DO. *The organization of behavior: a neuropsychological theory.* New York: Wiley, 1949.
18. Bear DM, Schenk L, Benson H. Increased autonomic responses to neutral and emotional stimuli in temporal lobe epilepsy. *Am J Psychiatry* 1981;138:6–7.
19. Tisher PW, Holzer JC, Greenberg M, Benjamin J, Devinsky O, Bear D. Psychiatric presentations of epilepsy. *Harvard Rev Psychiatry* 1993;1:219–228.
20. Bear DM, Levin K, North E, Chetham D, Geschwind N. Case report in behavioral neurology. *J Clin Psychiatry* 1980;41:89–95.

27

Neuroendocrinology of Epilepsy

Andrew G. Herzog

Department of Neurology, Beth Israel Hospital, Boston, Massachusetts 02215.

Discovery consists of seeing what everybody has seen and thinking what nobody has thought.
Albert Szent-Gyorgyi, 1962

Late one day in 1980, when the corridors of Beth Israel Hospital in Boston were already deserted, I took my accustomed walk down the hall and stood by Norman Geschwind's open office door on Kirstein 4. Norman was deep in thought as he sat behind his desk, surrounded by piles of correspondence and office notes, his eyeglasses dangling from his neck and pipe in hand. I always felt a little sheepish and had a twinge of guilt about disturbing him when he was so busy. But that was the part of the workday I most cherished. It was the time when I could present to Norman the most challenging clinical case of the day or discuss with him the latest seemingly immovable roadblock to the evolution of neurological theory. Actually, the topic did not have to be neurology. Those priceless minutes, occasionally an hour, could be spent discussing philosophy, Hungarian musicians, or, rarely, sports. No, Norman was not a great sports enthusiast, but he was the only person I knew who could handle almost any topic with equal aplomb and great competence. In response to the inadvertent mention of any sport, therefore, he would draw on his own limited but adventurous athletic experiences in badminton and launch into a conversation about badminton strategies and mechanics and the history of the Harvard Faculty Club, where he played. Indeed, even on the subject of sports, Norman could be dazzling. One Friday, for example, I made the "mistake" of mentioning to him that I had tickets to an afternoon Red Sox game that weekend. In fact, I frivolously added while leaving—I don't remember why—that I hoped to get a great suntan at the ballpark. Norman appeared disturbed and inquired, with a surprising look of consternation, about the location of my seats. Then he began, after quickly puffing on his pipe, "No, no, you see . . . ." These words always served as the introduction to a lengthy treatise on a usually, but not necessarily, related topic. This time, his treatise was both relevant and serious. Indeed, over a span of 15 or 20 minutes, Norman proceeded to lay out the arrangement of Fenway Park according to its compass coordinates and argued unerringly and convincingly, as one might in defense of a doctoral thesis, that at that particular time of year, the sun would dip behind the right field wall before the end of three innings. I did not take any suntan lotion!

On that day in 1980, however, we discussed the progress of our new neuroendocrine project. We were intrigued by the theoretical possibility that temporolimbic epileptiform discharges could produce hormonal changes that might contribute to interictal reproductive, sexual, and behavioral changes in men and women with temporal lobe epilepsy (TLE). After all, there already existed animal experimental findings to show that major direct anatomic pathways connected the amygdala to the ventromedial hypothalamus, which regulated pituitary gonadotropin secretion, and that amygdaloid stimulation and ablation were associated with predictable changes in gonadal steroid secretion. There was, moreover, abundant evidence that hormones play an important role in reproductive functions and sexual behavior. Our own clinical data were showing endocrine changes in men and women with untreated as well as treated epilepsy. A remarkable number of the women had elevated androgen levels, whereas a remarkable number of the men had low biologically active testosterone levels. That day, however, we puzzled over male serum estradiol levels that fell above the control range, and sometimes markedly so. Because estradiol constitutes only about 1% of the total male gonadal steroid, most of our colleagues were prepared to conclude that this observation had no clinical significance. After all, no one in those days spoke about estrogen levels in men. I remember clearly, however, Norman's caution about disregarding that observation. He said, "Who knows, this may be the key to the whole situation." I frequently queried but never disregarded Norman's comments. I continued to measure estradiol levels in men and have come to appreciate the apparently substantial biological significance of our finding. Today, I wish I could tell him, "Norman, I think you were right and I think we can now prove it."

HORMONES AND EPILEPSY IN MEN

Reproductive and Sexual Dysfunction in Men With Epilepsy

Reduced potency and hyposexuality occur in 38% to 71% of men with epilepsy (1–8). The etiology of those conditions is likely multifactorial, including psychosocial, epileptic, medication, and hormonal causes (4). Because androgens are considered to play an important role in the regulation of potency and libido (9,10), measurement of the serum levels of androgen should be a regular part of the medical evaluation. The most important androgen is testosterone. Testosterone exists in the serum in three forms: free, albumin bound, and sex-hormone-binding-globulin (SHBG) bound (11). Approximately 2% occurs in the free form, 53% to 55% is bound to albumin, and 43% to 45% is bound to SHBG (11). The SHBG-bound fraction is not biologically active, but the non-SHBG-bound fraction—that is, the free and albumin-bound steroid—is available to tissues (11–13). Today, there is considerable evidence to suggest that low serum levels of biologically active testosterone may contribute to diminished potency and hyposexuality in men with epilepsy (14–19).

The Causes of Androgen Deficiency

Epilepsy

Our investigations support the notion that the disruption of normal temporolimbic modulation of hypothalamo-pituitary function by epileptiform discharges may promote the development of reproductive endocrine disorders (20). Hypogonadism is unusually common among men with epilepsy. In our own series of 20 men with partial seizures of temporal lobe origin (TLE), 11 (55%) had reproductive dysfunction or hyposexuality (16). Nine of these 11 (45% overall) had reproductive endocrine disorders: hypogonadotropic hypogonadism in 25%, hypergonadotropic hypogonadism in 10%, and functional hyperprolactinemia in 10%. A causal role for epilepsy itself is highlighted by the finding that hypogonadism and abnormal semen analysis are as common among men with untreated epilepsy as among men with treated epilepsy (21). Lateralized cerebral and hypothalamic asymmetries may be responsible for the association of different patterns of reproductive endocrine secretion with left and right TLE (17,22). Paroxysmal unilateral epileptiform discharges and paroxysmal slowing, moreover, may have opposite endocrine effects. Hyposexual men with TLE have a predominance of right-sided foci (17,23) and lower serum levels of biologically active testosterone than sexually asymptomatic counterparts (14–17,24). The findings suggest that the laterality and nature of temporal lobe paroxysmal discharges may be important determinants of reproductive endocrine and sexual function.

Antiseizure Medication

Induction of SHBG synthesis. Several antiseizure medications induce the hepatic synthesis of increased amounts of SHBG (14,18,25–28), which can result in normal or even elevated levels of total testosterone yet reduced concentrations of non-SHBG-bound (that is, biologically active) testosterone (14,18,25–28). This medication effect was frequently cited to explain the commonly reduced levels of biologically active serum testosterone in men with epilepsy. It did not explain, however, why reduced levels of biologically active testosterone were not readily corrected by the usually finely tuned hypothalamo-pituitary-testicular servomechanism. Additional explanations were required.

Suppression of gonadal steroid synthesis. Norman's worldwide following always attracted numerous highly qualified international candidates to our unit for clerkships and fellowships and led to many very interesting and productive collaborations. A case in point was a medical student named Mark Muller who, during his clinical clerkship, introduced me to the technique of using *in vitro* rat Leydig cells to assess the effects of various chemical substances on testicular steroid synthesis. He learned this model from Professor Kuhn-Velten in Germany, who was using it to determine how uremic serum blocks testosterone synthesis. Although I had relatively little interest in the effects of uremic serum, it occurred to me that this model could be used to assess the possibility that antiseizure medications reduce biologically active testosterone by direct inhibition of gonadal steroid synthesis. Using the *in vitro* rat Leydig cell model, we found that carbamazepine exhibited potent inhibitory effects at therapeutic range concentrations. Phenytoin required higher concentrations. Valproate effects were the least. Moreover, the different antiseizure medications acted at different levels of the synthesis cascade to inhibit testosterone synthesis (29). This finding could provide one explanation for the failure of the servomechanism. It could not explain, however, why the majority of our patients with hypogonadism were hypogonadotropic rather than hypergonadotropic.

Enhancement of testosterone conversion to estradiol. As a follow-up to our 1980 conversation, we eventually compared serum reproductive steroid levels in 20 men whose complex partial seizures were treated with phenytoin, 21 men with untreated complex partial seizures, and 20 age-matched normal controls. Total and non-SHBG-bound estradiol levels were found to be significantly higher in the phenytoin group than in either the untreated or normal control groups (30). Serum biologically active estradiol correlated with serum phenytoin levels but not with measures of hepatic dysfunction (31). These findings suggest that some antiseizure medications may lower biologically active testosterone not only by the induction of SHBG synthesis but perhaps also by the induction of aromatase, which converts free testosterone to estradiol. Although estradiol constitutes only 1% of the male gonadal steroid, it exerts almost 50% of the negative feedback on male luteinizing hormone secretion (32,33). Suppression of luteinizing hormone secretion results in hypogonadotropic hypogonadism. Chronically low testosterone leads to testicular failure and hypergonadotropic hypogonadism. This fact may explain the frequent occurrence of both of these reproductive endocrine disorders in men with epilepsy (16). Finally, estradiol has been shown to produce premature aging of the hypothalamic arcuate nucleus, which secretes gonadotropin-releasing hormone (34,35). Murialdo et al. (19) have since confirmed significantly higher serum estradiol levels and significantly lower ratios of free testosterone to estradiol in hyposexual epileptic men than in either normosexual epileptic men or normal controls. They found, moreover, a blunted luteinizing hormone response to gonadotropin-releasing hormone stimulation in the hyposexual men, a finding consistent with hypogonadotropic hypogonadism. Our own more recent

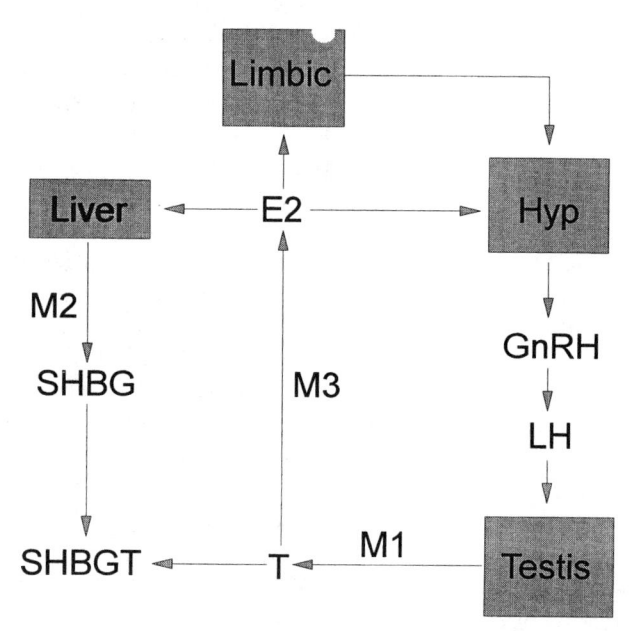

FIG. 1. The hypothalamopituitary axis (Hyp) regulates testosterone secretion by the testis. Hypothalamic gonadotropin-releasing hormone (GnRH) is secreted in a circhoral pulsatile fashion primarily by the arcuate nucleus. It stimulates pituitary luteinizing hormone (LH) release to reflect GnRH pulse parameters. Temporolimbic epileptiform discharges can alter LH secretion. In particular, they produce a significantly wider than normal range of mean baseline and pulse frequency of LH secretion (17). The nature, specific location, and laterality of limbic discharges may be important determinants of specific patterns of LH secretion (17). Some antiseizure medications can inhibit testosterone synthesis by the testis (M1) (29). They can also act on the liver to increase SHBG synthesis (M2), thereby lessening the biologically active portion of testosterone (T) (36). They may also increase the conversion of testosterone to estradiol (E2) by aromatase (M3) (30). This action, too, would lower T. Because E2 stimulates SHBG synthesis and androgens oppose it, the net result may be a progressive increase in E2/T. This effect could produce a premature decline in serum T levels. Increased E2/T may play a role in sexual dysfunction (19). Medication-induced elevations in E2 may act at the limbic level to induce epileptiform discharges. They may act at the hypothalamic level to decrease GnRH secretion and produce hypogonadotropic hypogonadism. They may possibly cause premature aging of the arcuate nucleus, which may also contribute to hypogonadotropic hypogonadism and premature decline of reproductive function.

data extend these findings to show a significant inverse correlation between the ratios of biologically active serum estradiol to biologically active serum testosterone and luteinizing hormone pulse frequency. Indeed, as Norman predicted, estrogen may really be "the key to the whole situation." This possibility is further strengthened by our observations during the use of endocrine therapy (see following discussion). A summary of interactions between epilepsy, antiepileptic drugs, and reproductive hormones in men is presented in Figure 1.

Therapy

Testosterone

Testosterone replacement is the most common therapy for hypogonadism. Its efficacy in men with epilepsy has not been reported. In our own experience with 12 men, intramuscular injections of testosterone enanthate in dosages of 200 to 400 mg every 3 or 4 weeks was associated with normalization of serum free testosterone levels and moderate improvement in sexual interest and potency scores in all 12 men. Seizure frequency showed no significant change.

Testosterone and Aromatase Inhibitor

Testosterone therapy in our experience has been only moderately effective in restoring reproductive and sexual function. Moreover, testosterone has not lessened seizures despite some reports of its anticonvulsant properties in experimental animals (37). One possible explanation is that antiseizure medications that induce increased enzyme synthesis may enhance the conversion of testosterone to estradiol by aromatase (38). Estradiol lowers male sexual interest and function (39) and increases seizure discharges (40,41). The addition of testolactone, an aromatase inhibitor, and testosterone to baseline antiseizure medication therapy has improved sexual-interest-and-function questionnaire measurement scores and decreased the frequency of seizures more than the addition of testosterone alone in a series of men with intractable seizures and hyposexuality (42,43). Of additional interest is a concomitant reduction in anxiety, a finding that will be addressed later.

Clomiphene

Clomiphene, an estrogen analog that binds estradiol receptors but exerts only weak estrogen actions, can act as an estrogen antagonist and stimulate gonadotropin and testosterone secretion. According to a case report, clomiphene dramatically increased sexual interest, potency, and seizure control in a man with complex partial seizures and hypogonadotropic hypogonadism (44). Seizures were eliminated during clomiphene use in another man with epilepsy and oligospermia (45). The drug was of no benefit, however, to a man who had complex partial seizures and hypergonadotropic hypogonadism, that is, gonadal failure (44). Total and free antiseizure medication levels were not affected. The method of clomiphene action on seizure activity is conjectural but may involve either the normalization of the serum testosterone level or direct antiestrogenic effects on epileptogenic limbic structures that have high-density estradiol receptors.

HORMONES AND EPILEPSY IN WOMEN

Reproductive and Sexual Dysfunction in Women With Epilepsy

Reproductive dysfunction is unusually common among women who have epilepsy (1). Some observations suggest that it is more common with TLE than with generalized or focal motor seizure disorders (1). Studies that pertain exclusively or predominantly to women who have TLE reveal that 14% to 20% of these women have amenorrhea and that more than 50% overall have some form of menstrual dysfunction (46–49). Fertility is reduced to 69% to 80% of the expected number of offspring (50,51). More than one-third of women with epilepsy may have reproductive endocrine disorders (47,52). These reproductive endocrine disorders are characterized by anovulatory cycles with an inadequate luteal phase (53). Cummings et al. (53) have found that 35% of cycles among epileptic women have an inadequate luteal phase compared with 7% in age-matched controls. Anovulatory cycles with an inadequate luteal phase are clinically relevant to both epilepsy and reproductive function. They are associated with higher seizure frequency (54,55) and are a probable cause of menstrual disorders and infertility, and, possibly in the case of hypothalamic amenorrhea (hypogonadotropic hypogonadism), hyposexuality (47).

There is also evidence to suggest that paroxysmal electroencephalogram (EEG) disorders are overrepresented among women with reproductive disorders. Sharf et al. (56), for example, found that 56.5% of women with anovulatory cycles or amenorrhea, most of whom also had polycystic ovarian syndrome (PCO), had EEG abnormalities, including, in some cases, focal paroxysmal epileptiform discharges. Treatment with the antiestrogenic agent clomiphene restored EEGs to normal in 54% of these women. There was, moreover, an association between normalization of the EEG and the occurrence of ovulation and pregnancy.

Reproductive Endocrine Disorders in Women with Epilepsy

Temporal lobe epilepsy promotes the development of reproductive endocrine disorders by neuroendocrine mechanisms. Specifically, it disrupts the normal limbic modulation of the hypothalamic regulation of pituitary secretion (Fig. 2). TLE may also promote these disorders by neural mechanisms: that is, by altering the neural influences of limbic structures on the gonads (16,17,20,47,57,60). Among women with TLE, PCO and hypogonadotropic hypogonadism (HH) (also known as hypothalamic amenorrhea) are overrepresented (46). Although medications can certainly affect hormonal levels (47,59,61), PCO is 2.5 times more common in women with untreated than with treated epilepsy (47). Moreover, PCO is significantly associated with left-sided temporal epileptogenic foci, and HH, with right-sided foci (47,60). Hyposexuality tends to occur with right-sided foci in patients with HH and low gonadotropin levels (46). It is unusual with PCO, except in patients with clinically significant depression. Depression intermittently affects up to 75% of women with PCO and is generally improved by treating the PCO (47).

Gonadal Steroid Effects on Seizures

Considerable animal experimental and clinical evidence suggests that gonadal steroids influence the occurrence of seizures (40,62). The reproductive endocrine environment of a woman with epilepsy can undergo physiological, pathological, and pharmacologic

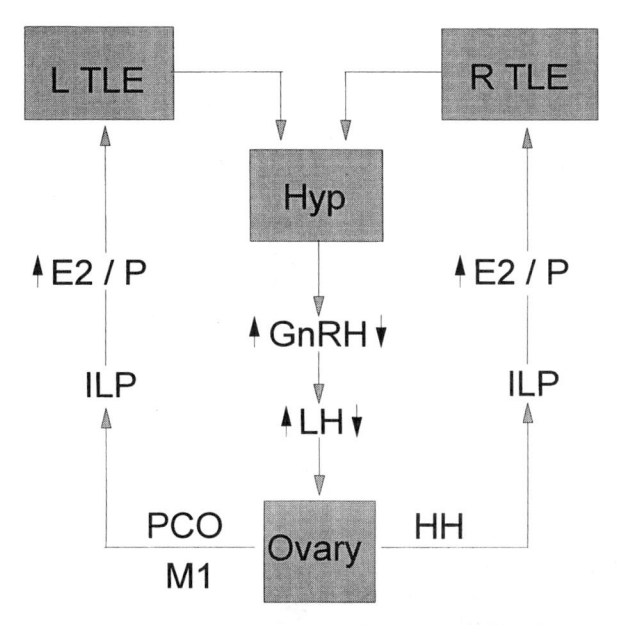

FIG. 2. The ovary secretes estrogen and progesterone under the regulation of pituitary gonadotropins: luteinizing hormone (LH) and follicle-stimulating hormone. Gonadotropin levels are determined by the pattern of hypothalamic (Hyp) gonadotropin-releasing-hormone (GnRH) secretion. The mean baseline and pulse frequency of LH secretion may be determined by the nature, specific location, and laterality of temporolimbic electrical discharges. Specifically, left temporolimbic epilepsy (L TLE) is associated with increased mean baseline and frequency of pulses (57) and the development of PCO (58). Right temporolimbic epilepsy (R TLE) is associated with low baseline and frequency of pulses (57) and the development of hypothalamic amenorrhea (HH) (58). In women with nontemporal epileptiform discharges, it may be right-sided laterality that is associated with the development of PCO (58). Both of these reproductive disorders are characterized by anovulatory cycles with an inadequate luteal phase (ILP) (46), and ILP cycles are unusually common in women with TLE (52). The resultant elevation in estradiol-to-progesterone ratio may exacerbate seizure frequency (53). Certain antiseizure medications may differ in their association with the development of reproductive endocrine disorders. Specifically, valproate use has a strong association with PCO (M1) (59). This association may reflect a specific mechanism by which valproate induces the development of PCO and/or the difference between the effects of valproate and hepatic enzyme inducing medications on the metabolism of testosterone in epilepsy-induced PCO.

changes. Menarche (63,64), menstruation (65,66), pregnancy (67,68), and menopause (64,69) can be associated with altered seizure frequency. Reproductive endocrine disorders are overrepresented among women with epilepsy (47,52). The anovulatory and inadequate luteal phase cycles associated with these disorders often exacerbate seizures (55,70). Oral contraceptives (71) and menopausal hormonal replacement (69) can exacerbate or benefit a seizure disorder, depending on the particular circumstances of the treatment. Knowledge of some of the interactions between hormones, epilepsy, and antiseizure medications, therefore, may provide the clinician with a more comprehensive basis for the effective treatment of epilepsy and related neuroendocrinological disorders in women.

In many experimental animal models, estrogen lowers the thresholds of seizures induced by electroshock, kindling, pentylenetetrazol, kainic acid, ethyl chloride, and other agents and procedures (41,72–75). In fact, topical brain application or intravenous systemic administration of estradiol in rabbits produces a significant increase in spontaneous electrically recorded paroxysmal spike discharges (41). The increase is more dramatic in animals with preexistent cortical lesions (76). Progesterone, on the other hand, lessens spontaneous and induced epileptiform discharges (73,74,77–79). Testosterone raises the electroshock threshold, and orchiectomy lowers it (cf ref. 39).

Hormones also influence human electrical brain wave activity and epilepsy. Logothetis et al. (80) showed that intravenously administered conjugated estrogen clearly activated epileptiform discharges in 11 of 16 women and was associated with clinical seizures in 4. Backstrom et al. (77) found that intravenous infusion of progesterone, sufficient to produce luteal phase serum levels, was associated with a significant decrease in interictal spike frequency in 4 of 7 women with partial epilepsy. Clinical reports of testosterone therapy in women with epilepsy are lacking.

Catamenial Epilepsy

Catamenial epilepsy refers to seizure exacerbation in relation to the menstrual cycle (65). Three patterns exist (Fig. 3) (81): (a) one quarter to three quarters of women with epilepsy describe an increase in seizures during the few days before menstruation and the first 2 or 3 days of menstruation; (b) a predilection for seizure exacerbation may also occur near the middle of the cycle, between days 10 and 14 (before ovulation) (the onset of menstruation is the reference point for day 1); and (c) a more difficult pattern to discern is one in which seizures are frequent between day 10 of one cycle and day 3 of the next, relative to occurrences in the interval between days 3 and 10.

Physiological endocrine secretion during the menstrual cycle influences the occurrence of seizures. In ovulatory cycles, seizure frequency shows a statistically significant positive correlation with the serum estradiol-to-progesterone ratio (54). This ratio is highest during the days before ovulation and menstruation, and lowest during the early luteal and midluteal phase (54). Premenstrual exacerbation of seizures has been attributed to withdrawal of the antiseizure effects of progesterone (65). Midcycle exacerbations may be due to the preovulatory surge of estrogen unaccompanied by any rise in progesterone until ovulation occurs (54). Seizures are least common during the midluteal phase, when progesterone levels are highest (54,55).

The term *inadequate luteal phase* refers to less-than-normal progesterone secretion during the second half of the cycle, regardless of whether or not ovulation occurs (82–84). It can be documented by one or preferably more findings, including (a) a failure of the basal body temperature to rise by 0.7°F for at least 10 days during the second half of the menstrual cycle; (b) a serum progesterone level of less than 5.0 ng/ml during the midluteal phase, generally measured between days 20 and 22 of a 28-day cycle; and (c) a biopsy specimen that shows underdeveloped secretory endometrium 8 to 10 days after ovulation. Serum estradiol-to-progesterone ratios and seizure frequencies tend to be higher than in normal ovulatory cycles during the second half of these cycles (54,55), and seizure exacerbation may extend from day 8 of one cycle to day 2 of the next cycle (81).

The reproductive endocrine disorders associated with TLE are characterized by inadequate luteal phase cycles (47). As noted previously, such cycles expose temporal lobe limbic structures to a continuous estrogen effect without the normal luteal phase elevations of progesterone and thereby tend to heighten interictal epileptiform activity. A summary of interactions between epilepsy, antiepileptic drugs, and reproductive hormones in women is presented in Figure 2.

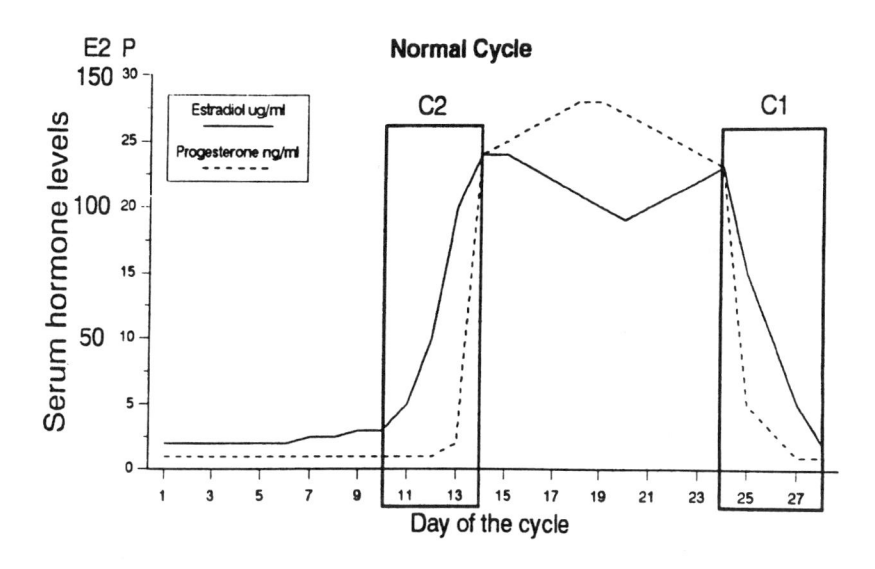

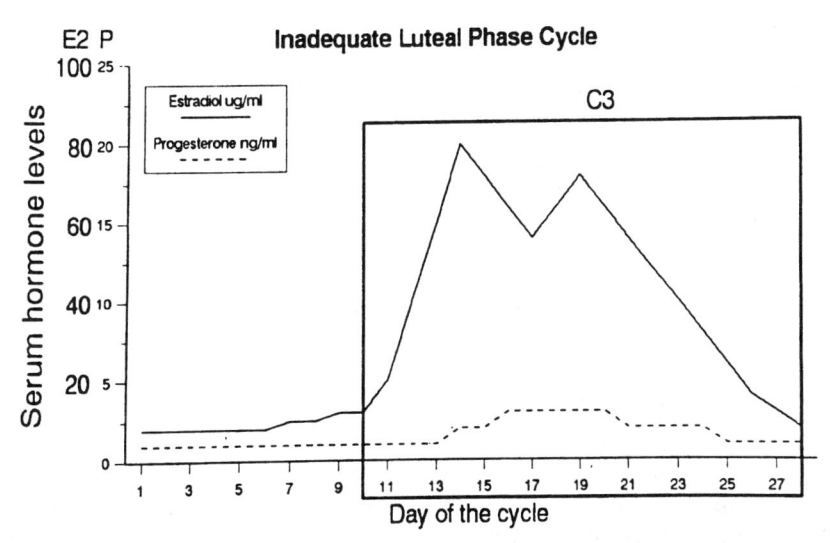

FIG. 3. The three patterns of catamenial exacerbation of epilepsy C1, C2, C3 in relation to serum estradiol and progesterone levels.

Therapy

Progesterone

Natural progesterone therapy benefits women with catamenial epilepsy (78). In one investigation of women who had inadequate luteal phase cycles with catamenial exacerbation of intractable complex partial seizures, 6 of 8 women experienced improved seizure control with a 68% decline in average monthly seizure frequency over 3 months for the whole group (78). In a subsequent similar investigation of 25 women, 19 (72%) experienced fewer seizures, with an overall average monthly decline of 54% for complex partial seizures and 58% for secondary generalized seizures over 3 months (85).

Several mechanisms have been postulated to explain the hypnotic, anesthetic, and antiseizure properties of progesterone that were first described by Hans Selye (86). Here are some of the hypotheses:

1. Progesterone exerts a depressant effect on oxygen and glucose metabolism.
2. Progesterone acts directly on the cortex to suppress epileptiform discharges.
3. Progesterone acts indirectly via metabolites that have potent depressant effects.
4. Progesterone acts indirectly via the potentiation of the inhibitory gamma-aminobutyric acid (GABA) neurotransmitter system.
5. Progesterone acts indirectly through competition with antiseizure medications for sites of hepatic inactivation.
6. Progesterone acts indirectly by potentiating the effects of endogenous anticonvulsants such as adenosine.

Combinations of mechanisms, of course, are not ruled out and appear likely.

Seizure activity depends on increased oxygen and glucose metabolism by the brain (87,88), whereas anesthesia is associated with decreased oxygen and glucose metabolism (89). Progesterone crosses the blood–brain barrier and is concentrated in the brainstem, limbic system, and cerebral cortex of the female monkey (90). Cerebrospinal fluid concentrations of progesterone correlate directly with plasma levels in man (70). Progesterone decreases oxygen utilization by neurons in brain slices (89). This effect may explain the antiseizure as well as anesthetic properties of progesterone (91).

Landgren et al. (79) have raised the possibility that progesterone acts directly at a cortical level. Their thinking was based on their observation that, in the cat, local application of progesterone to the cortical surface inhibited the electrical discharges from a penicillin focus.

Backstrom et al. (77) described a delay of 1 to 2 hours in the antiseizure effect of intravenously administered progesterone on the frequency of EEG epileptiform discharges in women with partial epilepsy. They considered this feature to be consistent with the possibility that progesterone acts through metabolites that have been established to have marked central nervous system depressant effects. For example, one progesterone metabolite, 3-hydroxy-5-dihydroprogesterone, is a potent barbiturate-like ligand of the GABA receptor chloride ion channel complex and potentiates the inhibitory actions of GABA in cultured rat hippocampal neurons (92).

Antiseizure medication serum levels decrease premenstrually in epileptic women, especially those with perimenstrual seizures (93,94). Antiseizure medications and reproductive steroid hormones are degraded by the same hepatic microsomal enzyme system (93). The premenstrual decrease in reproductive steroid serum levels, therefore, may permit increased hepatic metabolism of antiseizure medications (93) and result in elevated seizure frequency. The premenstrual supplementation of progesterone, in contrast, may reduce this effect. This mechanism, however, is unlikely to account for all the antiseizure effects of progesterone, because 2 of the 6 women in our series improved even though they did not receive concomitant antiseizure medications (78).

Finally, Swanson and Phyllis (95) have presented data that suggest that progesterone may potentiate the effects of the endogenous anticonvulsant adenosine.

Another feature of progesterone therapy that may help to elucidate its mechanism of action, and that may also serve as a practical note, is illustrated by the observation that some epileptic women with hormonally treated epilepsy do well each month during the course of therapy but may experience their usual premenstrual exacerbation of seizures after the discontinuation of progesterone. This effect is eliminated or greatly lessened when these patients gradually taper the progesterone over 3 or 4 days rather than discontinue it abruptly.

Synthetic progestin therapy has also benefited some women with epilepsy (96,97). Parenteral depomedroxyprogesterone significantly lessens seizure frequency when the dosage is large enough to induce amenorrhea (96,97). A regimen of approximately 120 to 150 mg given intramuscularly every 6 to 12 weeks generally achieves this goal (96). Side effects include those encountered with natural progesterone. Depomedroxyprogesterone administration, however, is also commonly associated with hot flashes, irregular breakthrough vaginal bleeding, and a lengthy delay of 6 to 12 months in the return of regular ovulatory cycles (96). Long-term hypoestrogenic effects on lipoprotein concentrations and cardiovascular status need to be considered with chronic use. In our own experience, the weekly intramuscular administration of 400 mg of depomedroxyprogesterone to a 44-year-old woman with PCO and intractable complex partial seizures of left temporal and right frontal origin despite extensive antiseizure medication trials, was associated with a reduction in average monthly seizure frequency from 22.5 to 2.4. Lower or less frequent dosages were less effective.

Oral synthetic progestins administered cyclically or continuously have not proved to be an effective therapy for seizures in clinical investigations (96,98), although individual successes with continuous daily oral use of norethindrone and combination pills have been reported (99,100).

Clomiphene

Clomiphene acts as an estrogen antagonist to increase gonadotropin secretion and induce ovulatory cycles in estrogen-secreting anovulatory women who do not have primary pituitary or ovarian failure (101). Normalization of reproductive endocrine functions and menstrual cycles in women who have both partial seizures and menstrual disorders with a documented inadequate luteal phase has been demonstrated to significantly and sometimes dramatically lessen seizure frequency (102,103). In one investigation of 12 women, 10 improved and seizure frequency declined by 87% (102). Clomiphene, however, is a drug with considerable pharmacologic potency and potentially disturbing side effects. Therefore, it should be used only after potential risks and benefits are weighed carefully and treatment with antiseizure medications and progesterone prove inadequate to control seizures.

EPILEPSY, HORMONES, AND EMOTIONS

Hormonal Influences on Emotions

The temporolimbic structures of the brain that are highly epileptogenic are also important in relating emotions to perception and behavior (104). As discussed previously, these structures also play an important role in the modulation of hormonal secretion and mediation of hormonal feedback. Temporolimbic dysfunction can, therefore, influence emotions both directly by neural pathways and indirectly by altering hypothalamopituitary regulation of gonadal steroid secretion, which can lead to abnormal hormonal influences on emotional behavior. Estrogen is highly epileptogenic and exerts energizing and antidepressant effects (105). Excessive estrogen influence produces agitation, irritability, lability, and anxiety. It can promote the development of anxiety manifestations such as panic, phobias, and obsessive–compulsive disorder. Progesterone inhibits kindling and seizure activity. It has mood-stabilizing effects, possibly by virtue of its GABAergic activity. Excessive progesterone influence produces sedation and depression.

Hormones can also have a progressive effect on emotional behavior. When they are secreted continuously and unopposed for days or weeks, their normal physiological effect on the patient's emotions becomes transformed into a pathological one. This effect may reflect progressively increasing neuronal sensitivity and reactivity to continuous hormonal exposure, whether by virtue of changes in hormonal receptor numbers, kindling effect, or both. Finally, there is reason to believe that repeated episodes of psychosocially triggered emotional stress, perhaps especially in persons who are genetically predisposed to epilepsy, may utilize the limbic kindling paradigm to promote more spontaneously occurring recurrent mood and anxiety disorders (106,107). Such an emotionally kindled process could also play an important role in the frequent association of reproductive dysfunction with anxiety and mood disorders in both men and women (Fig. 4).

Role of Anomalous Brain Substrates

Norman Geschwind repeatedly pointed out that drug effects on the brain depended not only on the drug but also on the specific receptors and characteristics of the brain substrates on which it acted. He delighted in telling the story of a left-handed patient with a static encephalopathy and epilepsy who phoned him after trying a minuscule dosage of a prescribed sedative medication to say, "You idiot, are you trying to kill me?" Norman would point out that this person's exaggerated or idiosyncratic drug reaction confirmed that this patient was someone with an anomalous brain substrate, whether manifested as left-handedness, static encephalopathy, epilepsy, or some other brain condition. It follows, therefore, that anomalous substrates such as medial temporal lobe limbic structures in TLE may be responsible for anomalous behavioral responses to hormones. This suspicion was supported by our findings, which showed that markers of anomalous brain substrates, such as paroxysmal EEG abnormalities, left-handedness, neurological findings of hemispheric dysfunction, and major mood disorders, are significantly more common among women who have clinically significant agitated depression in relation to menses or menopause than among unaffected controls (35,37). Paroxysmal EEG abnormalities were present in 27% of women with menstrually related agitated depression and in 36% of women with perimenstrual depression, a striking overrepresentation compared with the expected value, which is on the order of 1% to 2%. Observations suggest that paroxysmal EEG abnormalities may also be overrepresented among women with rapidly cycling depression, anxiety, panic attacks, and possibly obsessive–compulsive disorder (23,108,109). Hormonal effects, therefore, may tend to be exaggerated or idiosyncratic in patients with an abnormal or anomalous temporolimbic substrate, especially TLE.

Neuroendocrine Aspects of the Emotional Disorders Associated with TLE

Agitated depression, anxiety, panic attacks, phobias, and obsessive–compulsive disorders, are frequent concomitants of TLE that often show catamenial patterns of exacerbation and respond favorably to treatment with progesterone or clomiphene (109). The role of brain–hormone interactions in the pathophysiology and treatment of emotional, sexual, and reproductive disorders in TLE is illustrated by a 43-year-old woman who consulted us because of a 22-year history of complex partial seizures and agitated depression, both of which were intractable and showed a type 3 catamenial pattern of exacerbation despite treatments with antiepileptic drugs, tricyclics, monoamine oxidase inhibitors, and electroconvulsive therapy. The patient's agitated depression remained uncontrolled and associated with recurrent suicidal attempts. The onset of the disorder, which occurred when the patient was about 20 years old, closely coincided with that of irregular menses. Her irregular cycles, hirsutism, and reproductive endocrine findings suggested PCO with inadequate luteal phase cycles. Elevated serum androgen levels and low midluteal phase progesterone levels confirmed this diagnosis. Normalization of the patient's serum progesterone levels during the second half of each cycle by the administration of natural progesterone lozenges regulated her cycle interval, stabilized her mood, eliminated her agitation and suicide attempts, and reduced the frequency of her seizures from weekly to monthly.

Hormonally mediated behavioral effects need to be considered not only in terms of quantity of hormonal exposure but also in terms of duration of exposure. The cumulative effects of hormones are readily illustrated in the case of a 36-year-old woman who pre-

Reproductive Endocrine Disorders

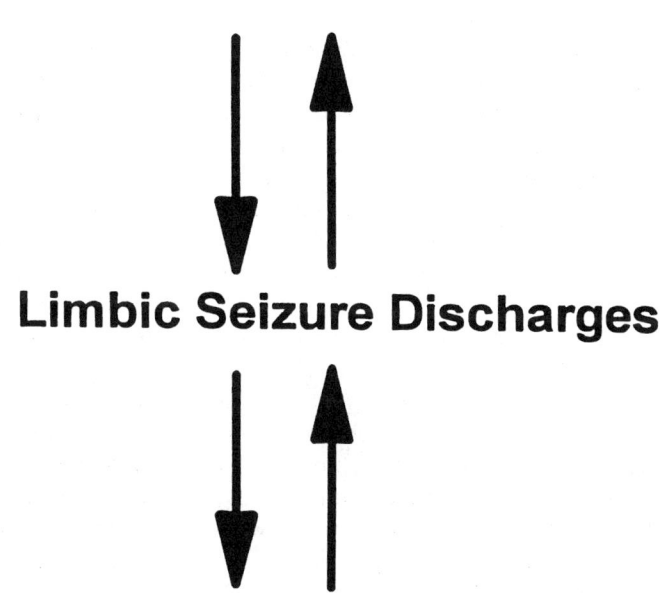

Limbic Seizure Discharges

Emotional Disorders

FIG. 4. Proposed interactions among TLE, hormones, and emotional disorders. 1. Because temporolimbic structures are sites of hormonal regulation and emotional representation, temporolimbic dysfunction, especially in the form of epilepsy, may provide a basis for the development of reproductive endocrine and emotional disorders. 2. Because temporolimbic structures have a high density of hormonal receptors and are highly sensitive to the effects of gonadal steroids, they may serve as important substrates for the mediation of hormonal effects on emotions and epilepsy. 3. Finally, because temporolimbic structures may be susceptible to kindling effects by recurrent emotional stress, they may mediate the frequent occurrence of reproductive and endocrine dysfunction in men and women with emotional disorders.

sented with severe anxiety, widely fluctuating moods, and intermittent psychosis. She had been well until 2 years earlier, when she had a total hysterectomy and bilateral oophorectomy. These procedures were necessitated by an intrauterine infection that developed during a hysterosalpingography, which was performed as part of an infertility evaluation. Postoperatively, she was given a prescription for conjugated estrogen 0.625 mg daily. For 3 months, she did well on estrogen replacement. Subsequently, however, increasing anxiety, agitation, irritability, and mood lability began to develop. At times, her anxiety would become so intense that she would shake, experience palpitations, and become only loosely tied to reality. Over the course of 2 years, she was seen by several psychiatrists and her condition was variably diagnosed as a major mood disorder or anxiety disorder. When she used minor tranquilizers regularly, they produced excessive sedation and depression. Antidepressants increased her agitation. She tolerated major tranquilizers poorly. Discontinuing her estrogen replacement therapy left her depressed and without energy, but increasing her dosage of estrogen aggravated her anxiety. The patient was left-handed and developmentally delayed. She began to walk late, between 2 and 3 years of age, and required elocution lessons in school because of trouble pronouncing some letters, especially "s." She was always very athletic and creative, and she started successful businesses until her emotional difficulties developed. Her neurological evaluation was remarkable for skeletal asymmetry: her left side was larger than her right. An EEG showed bitemporal paroxysmal sharp waves and slowing, especially on the left side. When the woman discontinued estrogen therapy, she at first felt a rapid, dramatic reduction in anxiety and agitation. After 3 days of feeling well while not taking estrogen, however, she experienced rapidly increasing asthenia. She could not get out of bed and felt hopelessly depressed. The reintroduction of conjugated estrogen resulted in a noticeable improvement within hours. She became animated and lively. After 4 days of therapy, however, she became racy, agitated, panicked, disorganized, and very concerned about "losing her mind." Progesterone lozenges, 100 mg three times daily, were added to her regimen. After 1 hour, she became calm and organized. She did very well for 4 days. By the 5th day, however, she once again could not get out of bed and felt asthenic and hopeless. Both hormones were discontinued, leading to improvement for 2 days, followed by a recurrence of low energy and mood. At this point, the woman was placed on a cyclic 10-day regimen of estrogen for 4 days, estrogen plus progesterone for the next 4 days, and then no hormone for 2 days. On this unusual 10-day cycle, she has done very well. She has been able to establish a new business and return to her former community activities.

In summary, hormonal effects on emotional behavior are often exaggerated in the setting of abnormal or anomalous temporolimbic substrates. Hormones can also have a progressive, cumulatively increasing effect on behavior, an extreme example of which is provided by the case just presented. Both responses are especially obvious in patients with temporolimbic epileptiform discharges. An understanding of these relationships and the therapeutic role of reproductive hormones should lead to more effective and comprehensive management of anxiety and mood disorders in men and women who have temporolimbic dysfunction with or without epileptic manifestations.

CONCLUSIONS

Norman Geschwind devoted a great deal of his remarkable academic career to the development of biological models of behavior. His most notable contributions included the description of (a) disconnection syndromes (110,111); (b) left and right hemispheric structural asymmetries, functional specializations, and clinical syndromes (112–114); and (c) the interictal personality features of TLE (115). Dr. Geschwind's legacy lives on vividly in the hearts and minds of the many whom he unselfishly inspired and encouraged to pursue academic careers in the field that he established: behavioral neurology. In his published writings, lectures, and personal correspondence, he made extensive references to the role of reproductive hormones in brain development as well as to the development and ongoing modulation of behavior and emotions. He staunchly supported the evidence for reciprocal relationships between epilepsy, behavior, and reproductive hormones. His remarks were instrumental in launching neuroendocrinology as a clinical discipline. Since then, the emphasis in this field has shifted from pituitary tumors and the basic science of neuropeptides to the role of hormones in behavior, emotions, memory and cognitive functions, epilepsy, movement disorders, sleep disorders, peripheral nervous system disorders, autoimmune diseases, and even oncology. Today, I wonder if Norman, the great master of discovery and creative thinking, would chuckle at our concept that TLE is a neuroendocrine disorder of androgen excess in women and estrogen excess in men, or whether he would say, "No, no, you see . . . ."

REFERENCES

1. Gastaut H, Collomb H. Étude du comportement sexuel chez les epileptiques psychomoteurs. *Ann Med Psychol* 1954;112:657–696.
2. Hierons R, Saunders M. Impotence in patients with temporal lobe lesions. *Lancet* 1966;2:761–764.
3. Kolarsky A, Freund K, Machek J, et al. Association with early temporal lobe damage. *Arch Gen Psychiatry* 1967;17:735–743.
4. Taylor DC. Sexual behavior and temporal lobe epilepsy. *Arch Neurol* 1969;21:510–516.
5. Blumer D. Changes of sexual behavior related to temporal lobe disorders in man. *J Sex Res* 1970;6:173–180.
6. Jensen I, Larsen JK. Mental aspects of temporal lobe epilepsy. *J Neurol Neurosurg Psychiatry* 1979;42:256–265.
7. Shukla GD, Srivastava ON, Katiyar BC. Sexual disturbances in temporal lobe epilepsy: a controlled study. *Br J Psychiatry* 1979;134:288–292.
8. Fenwick PBC, Toone BK, Wheeler MJ, et al. Sexual behavior in a centre for epilepsy. *Acta Neurol Scand* 1985;71:428–435.
9. Davidson JM. Neurohormonal basis of sexual behavior. In: Greep RP, ed. *Reproductive physiology II*. Baltimore, MD: University Park Press, 1977;225.
10. Davidson JM, Camargo CA, Smith ER. Effects of androgen on sexual behavior in hypogonadal men. *J Clin Endocrinol Metab* 1979;48:955–958.
11. Sodergard R, Backstrom T, Shanbhag V, Carstensen H. Calculation of free and bound fractions of testosterone and estradiol-17 beta to plasma proteins at body temperature. *J Steroid Biochem* 1982;16:801–810.
12. Manni A, Partridge WM, Cefalu W, et al. Bioavailability of albumin-bound testosterone. *J Clin Endocrinol Metab* 1985;61:705–710.
13. Cummings DC, Wall SR. Non-sex hormone binding globulin and bound testosterone as a marker for hypogonadism. *J Clin Endocrinol Metab* 1985;61:873–876.
14. Toone BK, Wheeler M, Nanjee M, et al. Sex hormones, sexual activity and plasma anticonvulsant levels in male epileptics. *J Neurol Neurosurg Psychiatry* 1983;46:824–826.
15. Fenwick PBC, Mercer C, Grant R, et al. Nocturnal penile tumescence and serum testosterone levels. *Arch Sex Behav* 1986;15:13–21.
16. Herzog AG, Seibel MM, Schomer DL, Vaitukaitis JL, Geschwind N. Reproductive endocrine disorders in men with partial seizures of temporal lobe origin. *Arch Neurol* 1986;43:347–350.
17. Herzog AG, Drislane FW, Schomer DL, et al. Abnormal pulsatile secretion of luteinizing hormone in men with epilepsy: relationship to laterality and nature of paroxysmal discharges. *Neurology* 1990;40:1557–1561.
18. Isojarvi JIT, Pakarinen AJ, Ylipalosaari PJ, Myllyla VV. Serum hormones in male epileptic patients receiving anticonvulsant medication. *Arch Neurol* 1990;47:670–676.
19. Murialdo G, Galimberti CA, Fonzi S, et al. Sex hormones and pituitary function in male epileptic patients with altered or normal sexuality. *Epilepsia* 1995;36:358–363.
20. Herzog AG. A hypothesis to integrate partial seizures of temporal lobe origin and reproductive endocrine disorders. *Epilepsy Res* 1989;3:151–159.
21. Taneja N, Kucheria K, Jain S, Maheshwari MC. Effect of phenytoin on semen. *Epilepsia* 1994;35:136–140.

22. Herzog AG, Coleman AE, Drislane FW, Schomer DS. Asymmetric temporal lobe modulation of luteinizing hormone secretion. *Neuroendocrinology* 1994;60:35.
23. Bear DM, Fedio P. Quantitative analysis of interictal behavior in temporal lobe epilepsy. *Arch Neurol* 1977;34: 454–467.
24. Herzog AG, Levesque LA. Testosterone, free testosterone, non SHBG-bound testosterone and free androgen index: which testosterone measurement is most relevant to reproductive and sexual function in men with epilepsy? *Arch Neurol* 1992;49:133–134.
25. Barragry JM, Makin HLJ, Trafford DJH, et al. Effect of anticonvulsants on plasma testosterone and sex hormone binding globulin levels. *J Neurol Neurosurg Psychiatry* 1978;41:913–941.
26. Dana-Haeri J, Oxley J, Richens A. Reduction of free testosterone by antiepileptic drugs. *Br Med J* 1982;284: 85–86.
27. Connell JM, Rapeport WG, Beastall GH, Brodie MJ. Changes in circulating androgens during short-term carbamazepine therapy. *Br J Clin Pharmacol* 1984;17:347–351.
28. Macphee GJA, Larkin JG, Butler E, et al. Circulating hormones and pituitary responsiveness in young epileptic men receiving long-term antiepileptic medication. *Epilepsia* 1988;29:468–475.
29. Kuhn-Velten WN, Herzog AG, Muller MR. Acute effects of anticonvulsant drugs on gonadotropin-stimulated and precursor-supported testicular androgen production. *Eur J Pharmacol* 1990;181:151–155.
30. Herzog AG, Levesque LA, Drislane FW, Ronthal M, Schomer DL. Phenytoin-induced elevation of serum estradiol and reproductive dysfunction in men with epilepsy. *Epilepsia* 1991;32:550–553.
31. Herzog AG, Coleman AE. Serum estradiol correlates with phenytoin but not hepatic enzyme and albumin levels in men with epilepsy. *Epilepsia* 1994;35:52.
32. Loriaux D, Vigersky S, Marynick S, et al. Androgen and estrogen effects in the regulation of LH in man. In: Troen P, Nankin H, eds. *The testis in normal and infertile men*. New York: Raven Press, 1977;213.
33. Winters S, Janick J, Loriaux L, Sherine R. Studies on the role of sex steroids in the feedback control of gonadotropin concentrations in men. II. Use of the estrogen antagonist clomiphene citrate. *J Clin Endocrinol Metab* 1979;48:222–227.
34. Finch CE, Felicio LS, Mobbs CV, Nelson JF. Ovarian and steroidal influences on neuroendocrine aging processes in female rodents. *Endocrinol Rev* 1984;5:467–497.
35. Brewer J, Schipper H, Robaire B. Effects of long-term androgen and estradiol exposure on the hypothalamus. *Endocrinology* 1983;112:194–199.
36. Isojarvi JIT, Repo M, Pakarinen AJ, Lukkarinen O, Myllyla VV. Carbamazepine, phenytoin, sex hormones, and sexual function in men with epilepsy. *Epilepsia* 1995;36:364–368.
37. Werboff LH, Havlena J. Audiogenic seizures in adult male rats treated with various hormones. *Gen Comp Endocrinol* 1963;3:389–397.
38. Herzog AG, Hormonal changes in epilepsy. *Epilepsia* 1995;36(4):323–326.
39. Beach FA. *Hormones and behavior: a survey of interrelationships between endocrine secretions and patterns of overt response*. New York: Haber, 1948.
40. Longo LPS, Saldana LEG. Hormones and their influences in epilepsy. *Acta Neurol Latinoam* 1966;12:29–47.
41. Logothetis J, Harner R. Electrocortical activation by estrogens. *Arch Neurol* 1960;3:290–297.
42. Herzog AG. The effects of aromatase inhibitor therapy on sexual function and seizure frequency in a man with epilepsy. *Neurology* 1992;42:400.
43. Klein P, Jacobs AR, Herzog AG. A comparison of testosterone versus testosterone and testolactone in the treatment of reproductive/sexual dysfunction in men with epilepsy and hypogonadism. *Neurology* 1996;46: A177.
44. Herzog AG. Seizure control with clomiphene therapy: a case report. *Arch Neurol* 1988;45:209–210.
45. Check JH, Lublin FD, Mandel MM. Clomiphene as an anticonvulsant drug. *Arch Neurol* 1982;39:784.
46. Cogen PH, Antunes JL, Correl JW. Reproductive function in temporal lobe epilepsy: the effect of temporal lobectomy. *Surg Neurol* 1979;12:243–246.
47. Herzog AG, Seibel MM, Schomer DL, Vaitukaitis JL, Geschwind N. Reproductive endocrine disorders in women with partial seizures of temporal lobe origin. *Arch Neurol* 1986;43:341–346.
48. Jensen I, Vaernet K. Temporal lobe epilepsy: follow-up investigation of 74 temporal lobe resected patients. *Acta Neurochir* 1977;37:173–200.
49. Trampuz V, Dimitrijevic M, Kryanovski J. Ulga epilepsije u patogenezi disfunkeije ovarija. *Neuropsihijatrija* 1975;23:179–183.
50. Dansky LV, Andermann E, Andermann F. Marriage and fertility in epileptic patients. *Epilepsia* 1980;21: 261–271.
51. Webber MP, Hauser WA, Ottman R, Annegers JF. Fertility in persons with epilepsy: 1935–1974. *Epilepsia* 1986; 27:746–752.
52. Bilo L, Meo R, Nappi C, et al. Reproductive endocrine disorders in women with primary generalized epilepsy. *Epilepsia* 1988;29:612–619.
53. Cummings LN, Giudice L, Morrell MJ. Ovulatory function in epilepsy. *Epilepsia* 1995;36:353–357.
54. Backstrom T. Epileptic seizures in women related to plasma estrogen and progesterone during the menstrual cycle. *Acta Neurol Scand* 1976;54:321–347.
55. Mattson RH, Kamer JA, Caldwell BV, Cramer JA. Seizure frequency and the menstrual cycle: a clinical study. *Epilepsia* 1981;22:242.
56. Sharf M, Sharf B, Bental E, et al. The electroencephalogram in the investigation of anovulation and its treatment by clomiphene. *Lancet* 1969;1:750–753.

57. Drislane FW, Coleman AE, Schomer DL, et al. Altered pulsatile secretion of luteinizing hormone in women with epilepsy. *Neurology* 1994;44:306–310.
58. Herzog AG. A relationship between particular reproductive endocrine disorders and the laterality of epileptiform discharges in women with epilepsy. *Neurology* 1993;43:1907–1910.
59. Isojarvi JIT, Laatikainen TJ, Pakarinen AJ, et al. Polycystic ovaries and hyperandrogenism in women taking valproate for epilepsy. *N Engl J Med* 1993;329:1383–1388.
60. Herzog AG. Lateralized asymmetry of the cerebral control of endocrine secretion in women with epilepsy. *Neurology* 1991;41:366.
61. Levesque LA, Herzog AG, Seibel MM. The effect of phenytoin and carbamazepine on serum dehydroepiandrosterone sulfate in men and women who have partial seizures with temporal lobe involvement. *J Clin Endocrinol Metab* 1986;63:243–245.
62. Holmes GL, Donaldson JO. Effects of sexual hormones on the electroencephalogram and seizures. *J Clin Neurophysiol* 1987;4:1–22.
63. Lennox WG, Lennox MA. *Epilepsy and related disorders.* Boston, MA: Little, Brown, 1960;645–650.
64. Turner WA. *Epilepsy: a study of the idiopathic disease.* London, England: MacMillan, 1907;44–46.
65. Laidlaw J. Catamenial epilepsy. *Lancet* 1956;271:1235–1237.
66. Newmark NE, Penry JK. Catamenial epilepsy: a review. *Epilepsia* 1980;21:281–300.
67. Knight AH, Rhind EG. Epilepsy and pregnancy: a study of 153 pregnancies in 59 patients. *Epilepsia* 1975;16:99–110.
68. Schmidt D, Canger R, Avanzini G. Change of seizure frequency in pregnant epileptic women. *J Neurol Neurosurg Psychiatry* 1985;46:751–755.
69. Sallusto L, Pozzi O. Relations between ovarian activity and the occurrence of epileptic seizures: data on a clinical case. *Acta Neurol* 1964;19:673–681.
70. Backstrom T, Carstensen H, Sodergard R. Concentration of estradiol, testosterone and progesterone in cerebrospinal fluid compared to plasma unbound and total concentrations. *J Steroid Biochem* 1976;7:469–472.
71. Mattson RH, Cramer JA. Epilepsy, sex hormones and antiepileptic drugs. *Epilepsia* 1985;26(suppl 1):S40–S51.
72. Hom AC, Buterbaugh GG. Estrogen alters the acquisition of seizures kindled by repeated amygdala stimulation or pentylenetetrazol administration in ovariectomized female rats. *Epilepsia* 1986;27:103–108.
73. Nicoletti F, Speciale C, Sortino MA, et al. Comparative effects of estradiol benzoate, the antiestrogen clomiphene citrate, and the progestin medroxyprogesterone acetate on kainic acid-induced seizures in male and female rats. *Epilepsia* 1985;26:252–257.
74. Spiegel E, Wycis H. Anticonvulsant effects of steroids. *J Lab Clin Med* 1945;30:947–953.
75. Woolley DE, Timiras PS. The gonad-brain relationship: effects of female sex hormones on electroshock convulsions in the rat. *Endocrinology* 1962;70:196–209.
76. Marcus EM, Watson CW, Goldman PL. Effects of steroids on cerebral electrical activity. *Arch Neurol* 1966;15:521–532.
77. Backstrom T, Zetterlund B, Blom S, Romano M. Effects of intravenous progesterone infusions on the epileptic discharge frequency in women with partial epilepsy. *Acta Neurol Scand* 1984;69:240–248.
78. Herzog AG. Intermittent progesterone therapy and frequency of complex partial seizures in women with menstrual disorders. *Neurology* 1986;36:1607–1610.
79. Landgren S, Backstrom T, Kalistratov G. The effect of progesterone on the spontaneous interictal spike evoked by the application of penicillin to the cat's cerebral cortex. *J Neurol Sci* 1978;36:119–133.
80. Logothetis J, Harner R, Morrell F, Torres F. The role of estrogens in catamenial exacerbation of epilepsy. *Neurology* 1958;9:352–360.
81. Herzog AG. Reproductive endocrine considerations and hormonal therapy for women with epilepsy. *Epilepsia* 1991;32(6):S27–S33.
82. Berman BM, Korenman SG. Measurement of serum LH, FSH, estradiol and progesterone in disorders of the human menstrual cycle: the inadequate luteal phase. *J Clin Endocrinol Metab* 1974;39:145–149.
83. Jones GS. The luteal phase defect. *Fertil Steril* 1976;27:351–356.
84. Strott CA, Cargille CM, Ross GT, Lipsett MB. The short luteal phase. *J Clin Endocrinol Metab* 1970;30:246–251.
85. Herzog AG. Progesterone therapy in women with complex partial and secondary generalized seizures. *Neurology* 1995;45:1660–1662.
86. Selye H. The antagonism between anesthetic steroid hormones and pentamethylenetetrazol (Metrazol). *J Lab Clin Med* 1941;27:1051–1053.
87. Kuhl DE, Engel J, Phelps M, Selin C. Epileptic pattern of local cerebral metabolism and perfusion in humans determined by emission computerized tomography of 18F-DG and 13NH3. *Ann Neurol* 1980;8:348–360.
88. Magistretti PL, Schomer DL, Blume HW, et al. Single photon tomography of regional cerebral blood flow in partial epilepsy. *Eur J Nucl Med* 1982;7:484–485.
89. Michaelis M, Quastel J. Site of action of narcotics in respiratory processes. *Biochem J* 1941;35:518–533.
90. Billiar RB, Little B, Kline I, Reier P, Takaoka Y, White PJ. The metabolic clearance rate, head and brain extractions and brain distribution and metabolism of progesterone in the anesthetized, female monkey *(Macaca mulatta)*. *Brain Res* 1975;94:99–113.
91. Gordon GS. Hormones and metabolism, influence of steroids on cerebral metabolism in man. *Recent Prog Horm Res* 1956;153–156.

92. Majewska MD, Harrison NL, Schwartz RD, Barker JL, Paul SM. Steroid hormone metabolites are barbiturate-like modulators of the GABA receptor. *Science* 1986;232:1004–1007.
93. Shavit G, Lerman P, Korczyn AD, Kivity S, Bechar M, Gitter S. Phenytoin pharmacokinetics in catamenial epilepsy. *Neurology* 1984;34:959–961.
94. Roscizewska D, Buntner B, Guz I, Zawisza L. Ovarian hormones anticonvulsant drugs and seizures during the menstrual cycle in women with epilepsy. *J Neurol Neurosurg Psychiatry* 1986;49:47–51.
95. Swanson TH, Phyllis JW. Progesterone in seizure therapy. *Neurology* 1987;37:1433.
96. Mattson RH, Cramer JA, Caldwell BV, Siconolfi BC. Treatment of seizures with medroxyprogesterone acetate: preliminary report. *Neurology* 1984;34:1255–1258.
97. Zimmerman AW, Holden KR, Reiter EO, Dekaban AS. Medroxyprogesterone acetate in the treatment of seizures associated with menstruation. *J Pediatr* 1973;83:959–963.
98. Dana Haeri J, Richens A. Effect of norethistrone on seizures associated with menstruation. *Epilepsia* 1983;24:377–381.
99. Livingston S. *Drug therapy for epilepsy.* Springfield, IL: CC Thomas, 1966;1–119.
100. Hall SM. Treatment of menstrual epilepsy with a progesterone-only oral contraceptive. *Epilepsia* 1977;18:235–236.
101. Cantor B. Induction of ovulation with clomiphene citrate. In: Sciarri JJ, ed. *Gynecology and obstetrics,* vol 5. Philadelphia: Harper & Row, 1984;1–7.
102. Herzog AG. Clomiphene therapy in epileptic women with menstrual disorders. *Neurology* 1988;38:432–434.
103. Login IS, Dreifuss FE. Anticonvulsant activity of clomiphene. *Arch Neurol* 1983;40:525.
104. Gloor P. Experiential phenomena of temporal lobe epilepsy: facts and hypothesis. *Brain* 1990;113:1673–1694.
105. Herzog AG. Perimenopausal depression: possible role of anomalous brain substrates. *Brain Dysfunct* 1989;2:146–154.
106. Post RM. Transduction of psychosocial stress into the neurobiology of recurrent affective disorder. *Am J Psychiatry* 1992;149:999–1010.
107. Nakajima T, Daval JL, Gleiter CH, et al. c-Fos mRNA expression following electrical-induced seizure and acute nociceptive stress in mouse brain. *Epilepsy Res* 1989;4:156–159.
108. Himmelhoch JM, Garfinkel ME. Sources of lithium resistance in mixed mania. *Psychopharmacol Bull* 1986;22:613–620.
109. Herzog AG. Neuroendocrine aspects of the emotional disorders associated with temporolimbic epilepsy. *Neuropsychiatry Neuropsychol Behav Neurol* 1996; (in press).
110. Geschwind N. Disconnexion syndromes in animals and man. I. *Brain* 1965;88:237–294.
111. Geschwind N. Disconnexion syndromes in animals and man. II. *Brain* 1965;88:585–644.
112. Geschwind N, Galaburda AM. Cerebral lateralization: biological mechanisms, associations, and pathology. I. A hypothesis and a program for research. *Arch Neurol* 1985;42:428–459.
113. Geschwind N, Galaburda AM. Cerebral lateralization: biological mechanisms, associations, and pathology: II. A hypothesis and a program for research. *Arch Neurol* 1985;42:521–552.
114. Geschwind N, Galaburda AM. Cerebral lateralization: biological mechanisms, associations, and pathology. III. A hypothesis and a program for research. *Arch Neurol* 1985;42:634–654.
115. Waxman SG, Geschwind NG. The interictal behavior syndrome of temporal lobe epilepsy. *Arch Gen Psychiatry* 1975;32:1580–1586.

Handedness, Cerebral Dominance, and Autoimmune Disease

28
Cerebral Asymmetries

Marjorie LeMay

Department of Radiology, Brigham and Women's Hospital, Boston, Massachusetts 02115.

Steven C. Schachter

Department of Neurology, Beth Israel Hospital, Boston, Massachusetts 02115.

Defining the range of human cerebral asymmetries, uncovering the factors that determine those asymmetries, and elucidating the behavioral associations of atypical asymmetries were major interests and lasting legacies of Norman Geschwind. He recognized that approximately 70% of the normal population share a particular pattern of cerebral asymmetries, which he designated as *standard structural dominance* (1). He called any deviation from standard structural dominance *anomalous structural dominance*. He argued that specific intrauterine factors such as testosterone and immune system elements could disrupt genetically programmed neuronal migration and maturation, thereby interfering with the development of standard structural dominance, resulting in anomalous standard and functional dominance. If this disruption occurred late in fetal life, when the left hemisphere grows more rapidly than the right, left hemisphere function would be predominantly affected; hence, language function might be adversely affected, resulting in a rightward shift of language dominance, language-based learning disabilities, or thought disorders.

This chapter will first present an overview of human brain development and the history of the field of cerebral asymmetry. Then, two aspects of Geschwind's hypothesis will be addressed: the evidence supporting the concept of standard structural dominance, and the behavioral associations of atypical cerebral asymmetry. Space does not allow for a discussion of nervous system asymmetries in animals (2) or the methodologic issues involved in procuring materials and measuring cerebral asymmetry (3–9). The relationship between handedness and cerebral asymmetry will be more fully discussed in Chapter 29.

THE DEVELOPMENT OF HUMAN CEREBRAL ASYMMETRY

The development of the human nervous system begins during the first few weeks of embryonic life. Primitive neural elements form, and then the neural plate becomes differentiated. The neural plate gives rise to the neural tube, which later develops into the central nervous system and the neural crest. The neural crest develops into the forebrain leptomeninges, portions of the peripheral nervous system, certain endocrine glands, epithelial components of the thymus gland, portions of the musculoskeletal system, and facial skin (including pigment cells) and bones.

The germinal zones form within the neural tube during the 6th week of gestation (10). Migration of neuronal and glial elements from the germinal zone to the growing cortical mantle then begins and continues until the 24th fetal week (11). As the cortical mantle thickens, newly migrating neurons move through the previously formed mature cortex and take their position on the surface. In this way, phylogenetically older cortical layers form earlier than the layers containing the newer granular neurons.

Cells destined to become part of different architectonic regions have separate origins within the germinal zone. As soon as neuroblasts arrive at their destination, they begin to differentiate and mature (10). Postmigration neurons establish dendritic and synaptic connections beginning during the 16th week in the deeper cortical layers, before migration of the less mature neurons to the superficial layers is complete. Myelinogenesis starts after neuronal connections are established and continues postnatally (12). A process of selected neuronal death and axonal attrition (13,14) occurs as neuronal connections are made, possibly under the control of the corpus callosum (15). The survival of presynaptic neurons may depend on the availability of postsynaptic sites.

Programmed asymmetries may begin with the formation of primitive neural elements, but they may not become evident until neuronal migration and maturation occur. Gross asymmetries in the shape of the sylvian fissures are apparent by the 16th fetal week, and in the shape of the frontal operculum and planum temporale by the 29th week (16). Geschwind suggested that intrauterine factors, probably chemical or hormonal, modified neuronal migration and maturation asymmetrically in the two hemispheres, which, in turn, would result in asymmetrical projections and asymmetrical preservation of neurons that had achieved synaptic relationships. Nonrandom asymmetries may also arise in the developing brain under the influence of the corpus callosum (15).

Lateralized differences in the rate of hemispheric development formed an integral part of Geschwind's theory. The right inferior frontal region develops before the left (17), and the sulcal pattern surrounding the right Heschl's gyrus is visible in the fetus 7 to 10 days earlier than the pattern surrounding the left (18). Further, the regions on the left that are destined to become larger than corresponding regions on the right initially may develop more slowly than their contralateral counterparts until late in gestation.

An alteration in or arrest of fetal cortical development may have clinical and/or behavioral consequences that range from subtle to devastating, depending on the timing and nature of the disruption. In general, the earlier the arrest in fetal development, the more profound the outcome (19).

STANDARD STRUCTURAL DOMINANCE

Historical Aspects

Paul Broca's well-publicized demonstration (20) of the lesioned brain from an aphasic patient challenged subsequent investigators to find the anatomic asymmetry that gave the left hemisphere dominance for language. Early work focused on the major fissures. Cunningham (21) and Eberstaller (22) showed that the posterior end of the right sylvian fissure curls up and terminates superior to the analogous region on the left. Eberstaller found that the ascending anterior sylvian limb, located in association with the frontal opercular region, is more often branched on the left (22).

In 1878, Heschl (23) noted differences in the surface of the right and left temporal lobes of human brains. He described transverse gyri and sulci on their superior anterior surfaces and noted they were different on the two sides. In addition, he observed that two transverse gyri were present more often on the right. In 1908, Flechsig (24) noted that the left temporal plane posterior to the transverse gyri described by Heschl was more often larger than the right. Pfeifer (25), a student of Flechsig, published a paper in 1936 that pointed out that the planum temporale, which was posterior to Heschl's gyri, was commonly larger on the left. In 1930, Von Economo and Horn (26) also reported that the planum temporale was larger on the left; in addition, they noted that Heschl's gyri was more often doubled on the right, observations that were confirmed by European and Japanese investigators (27,28) but unappreciated in the United States until the landmark paper of Geschwind and Levitsky in 1968 (29).

Asymmetries of the cerebral vascular sinuses were noted in fetal brains by Streeter in 1915 (30). He found that when the embryo was 22 cm in length, the superior sagittal sinus tended to drain to the right, as in adults.

The sylvian fissures can often be seen on endocranial casts of skulls. For example, the endocast of the skull of a La Chapelle-aux-Saints Neanderthal who lived over 40,000 years ago showed that the posterior end of the sylvian fissure was higher on the right than the left (31). Other asymmetries typically seen in *Homo sapiens* have been found in endocasts of Solo crania, which are anthropologically related to *Homo erectus* (32).

The behavioral significance of cerebral asymmetries has not always been acknowledged. Weil (33) compared endocranial casts of modern and ancient human beings and some anthropoid apes and concluded that the brain surfaces did not suggest there were significant asymmetries in the cerebral hemispheres of modern humans. Another persuasive opinion emerged from a symposium at Johns Hopkins University in 1961. At the end of that meeting, the speakers concluded that the evidence for cerebral asymmetries did not support a correlation between cerebral asymmetries and cerebral dominance (34).

In the early part of the 20th century, G. Elliot Smith, professor of anatomy at the University College in London and the Egyptian University in Cairo, studied a 2-million-year-old skull, which was discovered in Java in 1891. That skull showed reverse asymmetry, suggesting that Java man was left-handed (35,36).

In the modern area, cerebral asymmetries have been studied by gross dissection of postmortem specimens, histologic examination (cytoarchitectonics), and radiographic study of living subjects. *Cytoarchitectonics* refers to the structural features that microscopically distinguish one area of cortex from another. Cytoarchitectonic studies have described the microscopic counterparts to grossly visible cerebral asymmetries, especially regions closely associated with the lobar and regional asymmetries described below.

Temporal Lobe

Gross Anatomy

Temporal lobe asymmetries have received more attention than other lobar asymmetries. Geschwind and Levitsky, who were influenced by the findings of Pfeifer (25) and Von Economo and Horn (26) described previously, cut 100 adult brains postmortem in the planes of the sylvian fissures and compared the appearance of the left and right plana temporale using only a camera and a ruler. They found a larger left planum temporale in 65 of 100 brains, and a larger right planum in 11 (29). Juhn Wada (37) stated that his interest in morphologic asymmetries was greatly influenced by a lecture Geschwind gave in 1966, in which he described his study with Levitsky that reaffirmed the findings of Pfeifer and of von Economo and Horn. Shortly afterwards, Wada confirmed the findings of Geschwind and Levitsky (38). Subsequently, their findings have been repeatedly confirmed in adult, infant, and fetal brains (16,39–47). Men may be more likely to have reversed planum asymmetry than women (41), but not all the evidence supports this hypothesis (16).

Other modern studies have confirmed Heschl's observation that a second transverse temporal gyrus is more often found in the right temporal lobe than the left (18,41,48). One study found wider right superior temporal gyri in adult, but not infant, brains (49).

Cytoarchitectonics

Cytoarchitectonic area Tpt, located predominantly on the planum temporale and the posterior third of the superior temporal gyrus, is usually larger on the left (50). Further, the degree of asymmetry positively correlates with planum temporale asymmetries.

Radiologic Studies

Magnetic resonance imaging. Steinmetz et al. (51) evaluated left–right asymmetry of the planum temporale surface area using magnetic resonance imaging (MRI) and found larger left plana temporale in 22 out of 26 right-handed subjects.

Frontal Lobe

Gross Anatomy

Falzi et al. (39) measured the surface of the pars opercularis and pars triangularis, which are in Broca's area, and showed that the left frontal opercular region in the brains of right-handers contains an average of 22% more infolded cortex than the corresponding region on the right. Albanese et al. (52) measured the weight and surface area of the inferior frontal gyri and found that 63% of brains studied had leftward predominance of the anterior speech region (pars opercularis and caudal portion of the triangularis) and that 13% had rightward asymmetry, percentages that are intriguingly similar to those of the planum asymmetries found by Geschwind and Levitsky.

Cytoarchitectonics

Area 44 (of Brodmann), part of Broca's speech area, is located in the posterior portion of the third frontal gyrus within the frontal operculum and is identified by its unique pigmentation in lipofuscin stains. Area 44 was larger on the left in 8 of 10 brains studied by Galaburda (53).

Radiologic Studies

Computed tomography. LeMay and Kido (54) used computed tomography (CT) to measure frontal lobe widths. The frontal lobe was wider on the right than the left in 58% of right-handers, and the sides were equal in width in 30% and wider on the left in 12%. In an earlier study, LeMay (55) found forward protrusion of the right frontal bone in skulls and noted that this asymmetry correlated with CT-visualized lobar asymmetries. Chui and Damasio (56) found similar asymmetry of the frontal petalia (an extension of one hemisphere beyond the other as reflected in the inner table of the skull), as did Deuel and Moran (57) in a group of children. Finally, Bear et al. (58) measured the right–left differences of the frontal poles with CT scans and found larger right frontal poles. Further, men showed greater degrees of asymmetries than women, and reversal of the typical asymmetries was more common among women than men.

Occipital Lobe

Gross Anatomy

Murphy (59) measured the volume of striate cortex (area 17 of Brodmann; primary visual cortex) in 31 serially sectioned human brains from the Yakovlev collection at the Armed Forces Institute of Pathology in Washington, D.C. In 24 of 31 cases, the right striate cortex was larger, consistent with the known right hemisphere dominance for visual stimulus localization. Sex and age (from 33 weeks gestation to 94 years) were not associated with variations in striate cortical volume. Weinberger et al. (60) also utilized the Yakovlev collection and measured occipital lobe volume. In 32 of 40 brains, the left occipital lobe volume was larger than the right. The asymmetries in fetal and infant brains were similar to those in the adult brains; sex was not examined.

Radiologic Studies

Pneumoencephalography. McRae et al. (61) found that the left occipital horn of the lateral ventricle is usually longer than the right in right-handers. Strauss and Fitz (62) studied the pneumoencephalograms of 75 patients aged 5 months to 18 years. The occipital horn was longer on the left in 29 cases and longer on the right in 13 cases, consistent with a rightward asymmetry in mass of occipital brain tissue and the postmortem results of Murphy described earlier (59).
Computed tomography. LeMay and Kido (54) used CT to measure occipital lobe widths. Among right-handers, 75% had longer left occipital lobes and 9% had larger right occipital lobes. In an earlier study, LeMay (55) had found backward protrusion of the left occipital bone and had noted that this asymmetry correlated with CT-visualized lobar asymmetries. Bear et al. (58) measured the right-left differences of the occipital poles with CT scans and found larger left occipital poles. Further, as with frontal lobe asymmetries, men showed greater degrees of asymmetries than women, and reversal of the typical asymmetries was more common among women than men.
Magnetic resonance imaging. Kertesz et al. found that the left occipital lobe was wider than the right in 90% of right-handers (63).

Parietal Lobe

Cytoarchitectonics

Area PG, located on the angular gyrus and related to language function, is larger on the left in brains with a larger left planum temporale, whereas area PEG, possibly clinically relevant to disorders of attention and visuospatial functions and located on the dorsal lip of the inferior parietal lobule, is larger on the right (64).

Radiologic Studies

Cerebral arteriography. Stimulated by the findings of Geschwind and Levitsky (29), as well as by direct discussions with Geschwind, LeMay decided to look for cerebral asymmetries using angiography. Angiography was chosen because the branches of the carotid arteries lie within the temporal and parietal opercula and extend to the end of the sylvian fissures. LeMay and Culebras (65) found that coronal sections of carotid arteriograms through the posterior ends of the sylvian fissures showed that the left parietal operculum was larger, and it pressed the distal left middle cerebral artery downward as it exited the sylvian fissure. Further, the middle cerebral artery branches leaving the posterior end of the sylvian fissures were narrower on the left in 38 of 44 patients whose arteriograms were examined (90% were assumed to be right-handed). Bilateral arteriograms of 18 left-handed subjects showed that the angulation of the arteries leaving the sylvian fissures was equal in 15. Geschwind reviewed the paper and concluded that arteriography may play a role in localizing speech and other brain functions (66).

Hochberg and LeMay (67) extended these results by demonstrating that two thirds of right-handed patients who underwent cerebral angiograms had sylvian point angles that were over 10° larger on the right than the left. Further, the distal end of the venus sagittal sinus was commonly to the right of the midline, and the transverse sinus was higher on the right in 54% of right-handed subjects. These findings were subsequently confirmed by Ratcliff et al. (68) and Szikla et al. (69), who also reported the value of using stereotactic cerebral angiography in the evaluation of cerebral asymmetries in the posterior sylvian regions.

Magnetic resonance imaging. Habib et al. found leftward asymmetry of the parietal operculum with MRI, which, when present with convergent leftward planum asymmetry, strongly correlated with right-handedness (70). Kertesz et al. (63) found that the opercular parietal demarcation of sulci on MRI scan was sharper on the right side in 60% of right-handers.

Basal Ganglia

Gross Anatomy

Orthner and Sendler (71) measured the volumes of the lenticular nuclei (globus pallidus and putamen) and caudate nuclei of 58 normal brains and found that only the globus pallidus was consistently asymmetrical, being significantly larger on the left. Kooistra and Heilman (72) examined the size of the globus pallidus in postmortem specimens from the Yakovlev collection and found the left globus pallidus to be significantly larger than the right in 16 of 18, including 7 of 8 subjects below the age of 11 years; in two cases, the right globus pallidus was larger.

Radiologic Studies

Magnetic resonance imaging. Peterson et al. (73) measured basal ganglia volume with three-dimensional MRI reconstruction in 19 normal healthy adults. Fifteen right-handed subjects (12 men and three women) had a larger left lenticular nucleus and a larger right caudate nucleus. Asymmetry of the basal ganglia was not present in the four left-handed subjects.

Thalamus

Gross Anatomy

Eidelberg and Galaburda (74) examined the posterior thalami of nine normal brains in the Yakovlev collection for asymmetries and studied their cortical projections. The left lateral posterior nucleus, which connects with the left inferior parietal lobule, was larger than the right in the brains of right-handed subjects.

Summary

Standard structural dominance is characterized by the following interhemispheric asymmetries: the right frontal lobe is longer and wider, the left frontal opercular region contains more infolded cortex, area 44 (of Brodmann) is larger on the left, the left planum temporale is larger, areas Tpt and PG are larger on the left and parallel leftward planum temporale asymmetries, a second transverse temporal gyrus (of Heschl) occurs more often on the right, the right striate cortex is larger, the left occipital lobe is longer and wider, the left occipital horn of the lateral ventricle is longer, the parietal operculum is more developed on the left, area PEG is larger on the right, the globus pallidus and posterior nucleus of the thalamus are larger on the left, and the caudate nucleus is larger on the right.

LANGUAGE AND BRAIN ASYMMETRY

During the mid to late 19th century, Eberstaller (22) demonstrated the existence of cerebral asymmetries, and Paul Broca (20) established a correlation between language and the posterior portion of the left inferior frontal gyrus. Yet it remained for Geschwind and Levitsky (29), a century later, to combine these two observations by confirming the leftward hemispheric asymmetry of language-related cortex. Despite opinions in the literature doubting a structural–functional relationship (34), Geschwind and Levitsky specifically studied the left–right size asymmetry of the planum temporale, an area on the upper surface of the temporal lobe that contains auditory association cortex necessary for language (75). They concluded that the plana asymmetries were consistent with functional asymmetries in the two hemispheres. The impact of their study was quickly felt, as reflected in an article published that same year by Frank Benson and Geschwind (76) on cerebral dominance and asymmetrical function.

As noted earlier, Geschwind and Levitsky's results have been repeatedly confirmed with anatomic, radiographic, and cytoarchitectonic studies. In one study, Wada et al. (16) analyzed the brains of 100 adults and 162 infants who succumbed from nonneurological conditions. In the majority of these specimens, the left planum temporale was larger than the right and there was a greater degree of asymmetry in the adults. That is, although the planum asymmetries were present in the infant brains, the left planum appeared to have developed to an even larger size relative to the right in the adult brains.

The left frontal opercular region contains part of Broca's area, a region central to the expression of language. Studies quoted earlier have shown that the left frontal operculum is more infolded and contains more cortex than the right (39,52). Similar asymmetries have been found in a cytoarchitectonic area embedded within the operculum (53). One study, however, did not find significant left–right asymmetry or infant–adult differences in relative interhemispheric size of the frontal operculum (16).

Several studies have evaluated hemispheric dominance for language and cerebral asymmetries in living subjects. Ratcliff et al. (68) found that patients with right hemisphere language dominance have atypical asymmetries in the sylvian branches of the middle cerebral artery. In cerebral angiograms of patients with epilepsy, Strauss et al. (77) found a correlation between right-ear advantage on the dichotic listening test (suggestive of left hemisphere language dominance) and a wider left posterior sylvian region (width of the posterior temporal lobe at the level of the sylvian point). They also found a correlation between left-ear advantage and a wider right posterior sylvian region. These results were further developed by Foundas et al. (78) in a study of epileptic patients undergoing unilateral intracarotid amobarbital testing for determination of side of language dominance. MRI showed that all patients with left hemisphere language dominance on this test had leftward asymmetry of the planum temporale; the only patient with right hemisphere language dominance had a strong rightward asymmetry of the planum temporale. Both of these studies should be interpreted in light of evidence that speech lateralization in the epileptic population may not be representative of the normal population (79). Finally, Jancke and Steinmetz (80) did not find any correlation between degree of planum asymmetry and right- or left-ear advantage for dichotically presented verbal stimuli, suggesting that dichotic listening is unrelated to auditory functions subserved by the planum temporale.

As noted earlier, Eidelberg and Galaburda (74) found that the left lateral posterior nucleus of the thalamus is commonly larger than the right. This finding is interesting in light of reports of language deficits associated with lesions in the left, mainly posterior, thalamus (81–86).

Degree of language impairment and extent of resolution in patients with focal cortical lesions provide additional evidence that left-right asymmetries in language cortex have functional significance. Male patients with aphasia after stroke who have atypical posterior (occipital) asymmetries show better single-word recovery of comprehension, repetition, and naming than male patients with the usual asymmetries (87). Because aphasic patients who have right hemisphere or shared hemisphere dominance for language tend to have better prognoses after left hemisphere insults (88), these findings suggest that CT asymmetries correlate with localization of language function in males.

LEARNING AND COGNITIVE DISABILITIES AND BRAIN ASYMMETRY

The findings of Geschwind and Levitsky (29) have prompted research into the left–right asymmetries of language-related cortex in subjects with language-based disabilities such as dyslexia, and into the patterns of asymmetries in other behavioral disorders, including attention deficit–hyperactivity disorder (ADHD), Tourette's syndrome, and schizophrenia.

Dyslexia

Anomalous structural dominance was first associated with dyslexia by Drake (89). He examined the brain from an ambidextrous 12-year-old and found excessive numbers of neurons in the subcortical white matter, especially in the parietal region. Findings from another dyslexic's brain were reported by Galaburda and Kemper (90). Grossly, the left hemisphere was large because of an excessive volume of subcortical white matter. There were four distinct architectonic abnormalities: (a) micropolygyria where area Tpt is normally found; (b) clusters of neurons in layer one of cortex, especially in the left superior temporal and inferior frontal gyri; (c) clusters of neurons beneath the cortex, especially in left perisylvian areas; and (d) abnormally primitive layering and primitive neurons in many perisylvian and pericingulate areas on the left. The right hemisphere was virtually normal. Findings in three additional cases showed similar cortical dysplasias (91). In all of Galaburda's cases, the planum temporale was bilaterally symmetrical, indicative of anomalous structural dominance.

Radiologic studies of dyslexic subjects have assessed cerebral asymmetries *in vivo*. Examining CT scans of the head, Hier et al. (92) found that 10 (42%) of 24 selected dyslexics had reversal of the usual asymmetry, and that this finding correlated with low mean verbal IQ scores. Using MRI, Hynd et al. (93) noted smaller right anterior widths and left plana temporale in ten dyslexics than in age- and sex-matched controls. In contrast, Schultz et al. (94) used morphometric MRI to measure temporal lobe volume, overall brain volume, superior surface of the temporal lobe, and convolutional surface area of the planum temporale and found no differences between 17 dyslexic children and controls matched for age and brain size.

Attention Deficit–Hyperactivity Disorder

Hynd et al. (95) used MRI to evaluate the morphology of the head of the caudate nucleus in normal children and children with ADHD. Whereas nearly three quarters of the normal children had a leftward asymmetry, 64% of the children with ADHD had reversed asymmetry because of a significantly smaller left caudate nucleus. The findings were particularly striking in males.

Tourette's Syndrome

Peterson et al. (96) found that in patients with Tourette's syndrome, the usual leftward asymmetry of basal ganglia volume was lacking because the volume of the left lenticular region was reduced. The investigators also showed that certain subcortical nuclei (the caudate, lenticular, and globus pallidus) in patients with Tourette's syndrome had smaller mean volumes bilaterally than did controls. Similarly, Singer et al. (97) found a significant reduction in left–right asymmetry for putamenal and lenticular region volumes in children with Tourette's syndrome compared with controls. Further, the left globus pallidus was significantly smaller in children with both Tourette's syndrome and ADHD than in children with Tourette's syndrome only.

Schizophrenia

Gross Anatomy

Crow et al. (98) conducted a postmortem study of the brains of schizophrenic patients and found enlargement of the left temporal ventricular horn. In another postmortem study, Falkai et al. (99) found a 20% reduction in the volume of the left planum temporale and a 20% reduction in the anteroposterior diameter of the left planum temporale in the brains of 24 schizophrenic patients compared with age- and sex-matched controls.

Radiologic Studies

Luchins et al. (100) assessed cerebral asymmetries with CT in 57 right-handed schizophrenic patients without evidence of cerebral atrophy and found reversed frontal and occipital lobe asymmetries compared with controls. Similarly, Tsai et al. (101), in comparing CT scans of 36 schizophrenic patients with those of 18 right-handed male patients with mania, found a significant reversal of the usual occipital asymmetry in the schizophrenic patients. However, Andreasen et al. (102), in examining CT scans of right-handed schizophrenic patients and controls, found no differences in cerebral asymmetries when they compared the frontal and occipital petalia and frontal and occipital width. Similarly, in a study by Jernigan et al. (103), radiologists who were blinded to subject identity found no differences in the CT scans of schizophrenic patients and sex- and handedness-matched controls with respect to frontal and occipital width asymmetry.

Luchins et al. (104) studied 54 schizophrenic patients and evaluated the relationships between race, CT scan asymmetries, and HLA-A2. They found that in black patients with reversed cerebral asymmetry, the frequency of HLA-A2 was significantly higher than in black patients with normal asymmetries and in race-matched controls. In white patients, there was a similar trend that did not reach statistical significance.

In a volumetric study of brain and cerebrospinal fluid (CSF) using MRI, Gur et al. (105) found that schizophrenic patients had higher whole-brain CSF volume and higher ratios of ventricular and sulcal CSF to cranial volume than did normal controls. Stratta et al. (106) carried out a similar study and found significantly larger lateral ventricles and a smaller ratio of corpus callosum to brain in schizophrenic patients than in age- and sex-matched controls. Petty et al. (107) measured the surface area of the plana temporale in 14 right-handed schizophrenic patients using MRI reconstruction and found that the usual asymmetry, left side larger than right, was reversed in 13 of the patients; in contrast, the reversal was found in only 2 of 14 age-, sex-, handedness-, and race-matched controls. Further, there was an association between the severity of the thought disorder and planum asymmetry. In their study of MRI volume measurements, Shenton et al. (108) found that right-handed male schizophrenics had significant reductions in gray matter volume in the left anterior hippocampus-amygdala, the left parahippocampal gyrus, and the left superior temporal gyrus. As in the study by Petty et al. (107), the volume of the left posterior superior temporal gyrus correlated with the severity of the thought disorder.

Special Cognitive Abilities and Brain Asymmetry

Geschwind was fascinated by the concept of the pathology of superiority. He frequently noted clinical examples of special cognitive abilities in association with anomalous functional dominance, such as superior spatial skills in dyslexics (109). He explained this phenomenon by citing evidence that slowed or disrupted focal cortical development may foster additional growth or neural connectivity in other cortical or subcortical foci (110,111). One recent report in the literature that relates a special skill to structural dominance concerns perfect pitch. Schlaug et al. (112) used MRI morphometry to measure the plana temporale in professional musicians with and without perfect pitch. Musicians with perfect pitch had stronger leftward planum asymmetry than musicians without perfect pitch and age-, sex- and handedness-matched nonmusician controls. These results are consistent with observations made 20 years earlier that musically experienced listeners recognize simple melodies better when listening with the right ear than the left (113), and the results are particularly interesting in light of recent evidence from functional MRI imaging that the role of the superior temporal gyrus in language processing is the perception of acoustic–phonetic, rather than semantic, features of speech (114).

CONCLUSION

A major challenge for contemporary neuroscience is to explain the relationship between cerebral dominance and brain asymmetries. Mainly because of Geschwind's influence, patterns of brain asymmetries have been characterized by gross dissection, microscopic examination, and radiologic imaging, and they have then been correlated with lateralized dominance for handedness and language and with various cognitive disorders and learning disabilities.

Geschwind was motivated by intellectual curiosity and a deep-seated desire to help others. "The alleviation of suffering must be one of our major concerns. The continued elucidation of biological mechanisms of behavior will surely have its payoff in the treatment of patients" (115). The virtual explosion in cerebral asymmetry research that Norman Geschwind inspired has brought us closer to fulfilling his goal of expanding our knowledge of brain–behavior relationships (115). As neuroimaging techniques become more sophisticated in co-registering (superimposing) structural and functional measurements, additional gains will be made, especially when inconsistencies in study design are reduced and methods for defining, measuring, and analyzing cerebral asymmetries are established and widely applied.

REFERENCES

1. Schachter SC, Galaburda AM. Development and biological associations of cerebral dominance: review and possible mechanisms. *J Am Acad Child Psychiatry* 1986;25:741–750.
2. Bradshaw J, Rogers L. *The evolution of lateral asymmetries, language, tool use, and intellect.* San Diego, CA: Academic Press Inc, 1993.
3. Steinmetz H, Rademacher J, Huang Y, et al. Cerebral asymmetry: MR planimetry of the human planum temporale. *J Comput Assist Tomogr* 1989;13:996–1005.
4. Glicksohn J, Myslobodsky MS. The representation of patterns of structural brain asymmetry in normal individuals. *Neuropsychologia* 1993;31:145–159.
5. Bhatia S, Bookheimer SY, Gaillard WD, Theodore WH. Measurement of whole temporal lobe and hippocampus for MR volumetry: normative data. *Neurology* 1993;43:2006–2010.
6. Galaburda AM. The planum temporale. *Arch Neurol* 1993;50:457.
7. Witelson SF, McCulloch PB. Premortem and postmortem measurement to study structure with function: a human brain collection. *Schizophr Bull* 1991;17:583–591.
8. Habib M, Renucci RL, Vanier M, Corbaz JM, Salamon G. CT assessment of right-left asymmetries in the human cerebral cortex. *J Comput Assist Tomogr* 1984;8:922–927.
9. Witelson SF. Anatomic asymmetry in the temporal lobes: its documentation, phylogenesis, and relationship to functional asymmetry. *Ann NY Acad Sci* 1977;299:328–354.
10. Jacobson M. *Developmental neurobiology.* New York: Plenum Press, 1978;27–55, 115–217.
11. Marin-Padilla M. Prenatal and early postnatal ontogenesis of the human motor cortex: a Golgi study; I. The sequential development of the cortical layers. *Brain Res* 1970;23:167–183.
12. Flechsig P. *Anatomie des menschlichen Gehirns und Ruckenmarks auf myelogenetischen Grundlage.* Leipzig, Germany: George Thieme, 1920;9–37.
13. Cowan WM. Neuronal death as a regulative mechanism in the control of cell numbers in the nervous system. In: Rockstein M, ed. *Development and aging in the nervous system.* New York: Academic Press, 1973;19–41.
14. Hamburger V, Oppenheim RW. Naturally occurring neuronal death in vertebrates. *Neurosci Comment* 1982;1:39–55.
15. Lent R, Schmidt SL. The ontogenesis of the forebrain commissures and the determination of brain asymmetries. *Prog Neurobiol* 1993;40:249–276.

16. Wada JA, Clarke R, Hamm A. Cerebral hemispheric asymmetry in humans. Cortical speech zones in 100 adults and 100 infant brains. *Arch Neurol* 1975;32:239–246.
17. Herve G. *La circonvolution de Broca.* Paris, France: Delahage et Lecrosnier, 1888.
18. Chi JG, Dooling EC, Gilles FH. Gyral development of the human brain. *Ann Neurol* 1977;1:86–93.
19. Schachter SC. The neurobiology of epilepsy: developmental biology and clinical aspects. In: Hopkins A, Shorvon S, Cascino G, eds. *Epilepsy*, 2nd ed. London, England: Chapman & Hall, 1995;25–34.
20. Broca P. Nouvelle observation d'aphemie produite par une lesion de la moitie posterieure des deuxieme et troisieme circonvolutions frontal gauche. *Bull Soc Anthropol* 1861;35:398–407.
21. Cunningham DJ. *Contribution to the surface anatomy of the cerebral hemispheres.* Dublin, Ireland: Royal Irish Academy, 1892.
22. Eberstaller O. Zur oberflachen anatomie der grosshirn hemispharen. *Wien Med Blatter* 1884;7:479–482.
23. Heschl RL. *Die vordere quere Schlafenwindung des menschlichen Grosshirns.* Vienna, Austria: Braumuller, 1878.
24. Flechsig P. Bemerkungen uber die Horsphare des menschlichen Gehirns. *Neurol Zentralbl* 1908;27:2–7.
25. Pfeifer RA. Pathologie der Horstrahlung und der corticalen Horsphare. In: Bumke O, Foerster O, eds. *Handbuch der Neurologie.* Berlin, Germany: Springer, 1936;534–626.
26. Von Economo C, Horn L. Uber windungsrelief, masze und rindenarchitektonik der supratemporalflache. *Z Gesamte Neurol Psychiat* 1930;130:678–757.
27. Beck E. Typologie des Gehirns am Beispiel des dorsalen menschlichen Schlafenlappens nebst weiteren Beitragen zur Frage der Links-rechtshirnigkeit. *Dtsch Z Nervenheilkd* 1955;173:267–308.
28. Fukui T. Transverse gyri of temporal lobe in the Japanese brain. *Hokuetsu Igaku Zasshi* 1934;49:1025–1050.
29. Geschwind N, Levitsky W. Human brain: left-right asymmetries in temporal speech region. *Science* 1968;161:186–187.
30. Streeter GL. The development of the venous sinuses of the dura mater in the human embryo. *Am J Anat* 1915;18:145–178.
31. Boule M, Anthony R. L'encephale de l'homme fossile de la Chapelle-aux-Saints. *L'Anthropologie* 1911;22:129–196.
32. Holloway RL. Indonesian "Solo" (Ngandong) endocranial reconstructions: some preliminary observations and comparisons with Neandertal and *Homo erectus* groups. *Am J Phys Anthropol* 1980;53:285–295.
33. Weil A. Measurements of cerebral and cerebellar surfaces. *Am J Phys Anthropol* 1929;13:69–91.
34. Von Bonin G. Anatomical asymmetries of the cerebral hemispheres. In: Mountcastle WB, ed. *Interhemispheric relations and cerebral dominance.* Baltimore, MD: Johns Hopkins University Press, 1962.
35. Smith GE. On the asymmetry of the caudal poles of the cerebral hemispheres and its influence on the occipital bone. *Anat Anz* 1907;30:574–578.
36. Smith GE. Right- and left-handedness in primitive men. *Br Med J* 1925;1107–1110.
37. Wada JA. Pre-language and fundamental asymmetry of the infant brain. *Ann NY Acad Sci* 1977;299:370–379.
38. Wada JA. Interhemispheric sharing and shift of cerebral speech function. *Excerpta Med Int Congr Ser* 1969;193:296–297.
39. Falzi G, Perrone P, Vignolo LA. Right-left asymmetry in anterior speech region. *Arch Neurol* 1982;39:239–240.
40. Rubens AB, Mahowald MW, Hutton JT. Asymmetry of the lateral (sylvian) fissures in man. *Neurology* 1976;26:620–624.
41. Nikkuni S, Yashima Y, Ishige K, et al. Left-right hemispheric asymmetry of cortical speech zones in Japanese brains (author's transl). *No To Shinkei* 1981;33:77–84.
42. Foundas AL, Leonard CM, Heilman KM. Morphologic cerebral asymmetries and handedness. The pars triangularis and planum temporale. *Arch Neurol* 1995;52:501–508.
43. Kopp N, Michel F, Carrier H, Biron A, Duvillard P. Etude de certaines asymetries hemispheriques du cerveau humain. *J Neurol Sci* 1977;34:349–363.
44. Teszner D, Tzavaras A, Gruner J, Hecaen H. L'asymetrie droite-gauche du planum temporale; a propos de l'etude anatomique de 100 cerveaux. *Rev Neurol (Paris)* 1972;146:444–449.
45. Boss J, Godlewski G, Maurel JC. Study of right-left asymmetry of the temporal planum in the fetus. *Bull Assoc Anat* 1976;169:253–258.
46. Witelson SF, Pallie S. Left hemisphere specialization for language in the newborn. *Brain* 1973;96:641–646.
47. Pieniadz JM, Naeser MA. Computed tomographic scan cerebral asymmetries and morphologic brain asymmetries. Correlation in the same cases post mortem. *Arch Neurol* 1984;41:403–409.
48. Campain R, Minckler J. A note on the gross configurations of the human auditory cortex. *Brain Lang* 1976;3:318–323.
49. Hyde JB, Akesson EJ, Berinstein E. Asymmetrical growth of superior temporal gyri in man. *Experientia* 1973;29:1131.
50. Galaburda AM, Sanides F, Geschwind N. Human brain. Cytoarchitectonic left-right asymmetries in the temporal speech region. *Arch Neurol* 1978;35:812–817.
51. Steinmetz H, Volkmann J, Jancke L, Freund HJ. Anatomical left-right asymmetry of language-related temporal cortex is different in left- and right-handers. *Ann Neurol* 1991;29:315–319.
52. Albanese E, Merlo A, Albanese A, Gomez E. Anterior speech region. Asymmetry and weight–surface correlation. *Arch Neurol* 1989;46:307–310.
53. Galaburda AM. La region de Broca: observations anatommiques faites un siecle apres la mort de son decouvreur. *Rev Neurol (Paris)* 1980;136:609–616.

54. LeMay M, Kido DK. Asymmetries of the cerebral hemispheres on computed tomograms. *J Comput Assist Tomogr* 1978;2:471–476.
55. LeMay M. Asymmetries of the skull and handedness. Phrenology revisited. *J Neurol Sci* 1977;32:243–253.
56. Chui HC, Damasio AR. Human cerebral asymmetries evaluated by computed tomography. *J Neurol Neurosurg Psychiatry* 1980;43:873–878.
57. Deuel RK, Moran CC. Cerebral dominance and cerebral asymmetries on computed tomogram in childhood. *Neurology* 1980;30:934–938.
58. Bear D, Schiff D, Saver J, Greenberg M, Freeman R. Quantitative analysis of cerebral asymmetries. Fronto-occipital correlation, sexual dimorphism and association with handedness. *Arch Neurol* 1986;43:598–603.
59. Murphy GM. Volumetric asymmetry in the human striate cortex. *Exp Neurol* 1985;88:288–302.
60. Weinberger DR, Luchins DJ, Morihisa J, Wyatt RJ. Asymmetrical volumes of the right and left frontal and occipital regions of the human brain. *Ann Neurol* 1982;11:97–100.
61. McRae DL, Branch CL, Milner B. The occipital horns and cerebral dominance. *Neurology* 1968;18:95–98.
62. Strauss E, Fitz C. Occipital horn asymmetry in children. *Ann Neurol* 1980;8:437–439.
63. Kertesz A, Black SE, Polk M, Howell J. Cerebral asymmetries on magnetic resonance imaging. *Cortex* 1986;22:117–127.
64. Eidelberg D, Galaburda AM. Inferior parietal lobule. Divergent architectonic asymmetries in the human brain. *Arch Neurol* 1984;41:843–852.
65. LeMay M, Culebras A. Human brain—morphologic differences in the hemispheres demonstrable by carotid arteriography. *N Engl J Med* 1972;287:168–170.
66. Geschwind N. Cerebral dominance and anatomic asymmetry. *N Engl J Med* 1972;287:194–195.
67. Hochberg FH, LeMay M. Arteriographic correlates of handedness. *Neurology* 1975;25:218–222.
68. Ratcliff G, Dila C, Taylor L, Milner B. The morphological asymmetry of the hemispheres and cerebral dominance for speech: a possible relationship. *Brain Lang* 1980;11:87–98.
69. Szikla G, Hori T, Bouvier G. The third dimension in cerebral angiography; a stereotactic study on cortical localization and hemispheric asymmetry in living man. In: Solomon G, ed. *Advances in cerebral angiography*. Berlin, Germany: Springer-Verlag, 1975;236–250.
70. Habib M, Robichon F, Levrier O, Khalil R, Salamon G. Diverging asymmetries of temporo-parietal cortical areas: a reappraisal of Geschwind/Galaburda theory. *Brain Lang* 1995;48:238–258.
71. Orthner H, Sendler W. Planimetrische volumetrie an menschlechen gihirnen. *Fortschr Neurol Psychiat* 1975;43:191–209.
72. Kooistra CA, Heilman KM. Motor dominance and lateral asymmetry of the globus pallidus. *Neurology* 1988;38:388–390.
73. Peterson BS, Riddle MA, Cohen DJ, Katz LD, Smith JC, Leckman JF. Human basal ganglia volume asymmetries on magnetic resonance images. *Magn Reson Imaging* 1993;11:493–498.
74. Eidelberg D, Galaburda AM. Symmetry and asymmetry in the human posterior thalamus. I. Cytoarchitectonic analysis in normal persons. *Arch Neurol* 1982;39:325–332.
75. Meyer A. *The collected papers of Adolf Meyer*. Baltimore, MD: The Johns Hopkins University Press, 1950.
76. Benson DF, Geschwind N. Cerebral dominance and its disturbances. *Pediatr Clin North Am* 1968;15:759–769.
77. Strauss E, Lapointe JS, Wada JA, Gaddes W, Kosaka B. Language dominance: correlation of radiological and functional data. *Neuropsychologia* 1985;23:415–420.
78. Foundas AL, Leonard CM, Gilmore R, Fennell E, Heilman KM. Planum temporale asymmetry and language dominance. *Neuropsychologia* 1994;32:1225–1231.
79. Woods RP, Dodrill CB, Ojemann GA. Brain injury, handedness, and speech lateralization in a series of amobarbital studies. *Ann Neurol* 1988;23:510–518.
80. Jancke L, Steinmetz H. Auditory lateralization and planum temporale asymmetry. *Neuroreport* 1993;5:169–172.
81. Fisher CM. The pathologic and clinical aspects of thalamic hemorrhage. *Trans Am Neurol Assoc* 1959;84:56–59.
82. Penfield W, Roberts L. *Speech and brain mechanisms*. Princeton, NJ: Princeton University Press, 1959.
83. Mohr JP, Watters WC, Duncan GW. Thalamic aphasia. *Brain Lang* 1975;2:3–7.
84. Samarel A, Wright TL, Sergay F, Tyler HR. Thalamic hemorrhage with speech disorder. *Trans Am Neurol Assoc* 1976;101:283–305.
85. Bell DS. Speech functions of the thalamus inferred from the effects of thalomotomy. *Brain* 1968;91:619–638.
86. Ojemann GA. Asymmetric function of the thalamus in man. *Ann NY Acad Sci* 1977;299:380–395.
87. Pieniadz JM, Naeser MA, Koff E, Levine HL. CT scan cerebral hemispheric asymmetry measurements in stroke cases with global aphasia: atypical asymmetries associated with improved recovery. *Cortex* 1983;19:371–391.
88. Luria AR. *Traumatic aphasia*. The Hague, the Netherlands: Mouton, 1970.
89. Drake WE. Clinical and pathological findings in a child with a developmental learning disability. *J Learn Disabil* 1968;1:486–502.
90. Galaburda AM, Kemper TL. Cytoarchitectonic abnormalities in developmental dyslexia: a case study. *Ann Neurol* 1979;6:94–100.
91. Galaburda AM, Sherman GF, Rosen GD, Aboitiz F, Geschwind N. Developmental dyslexia: four consecutive patients with cortical anomalies. *Ann Neurol* 1985;18:222–233.
92. Hier DB, LeMay M, Rosenberger PB, Perlo VP. Developmental dyslexia. Evidence for a subgroup with a reversal of cerebral asymmetry. *Arch Neurol* 1978;35:90–92.

93. Hynd GW, Semrud-Clikeman M, Lorys AR, Novey ES, Eliopulos D. Brain morphology in developmental dyslexia and attention deficit disorder/hyperactivity. *Arch Neurol* 1990;47:919–926.
94. Schultz RT, Cho NK, Staib LH, et al. Brain morphology in normal and dyslexic children: the influence of sex and age. *Ann Neurol* 1994;35:732–742.
95. Hynd GW, Hern KL, Novey ES, et al. Attention deficit-hyperactivity disorder and asymmetry of the caudate nucleus. *J Child Neurol* 1993;8:339–347.
96. Peterson B, Riddle MA, Cohen DJ, et al. Reduced basal ganglia volumes in Tourette's syndrome using three-dimensional reconstruction techniques from magnetic resonance images. *Neurology* 1993;43:941–949.
97. Singer HS, Reiss AL, Brown JE, et al. Volumetric MRI changes in basal ganglia of children with Tourette's syndrome. *Neurology* 1993;43:950–956.
98. Crow TJ, Ball J, Bloom SR, et al. Schizophrenia as an anomaly of development of cerebral asymmetry. A post-mortem study and a proposal concerning the genetic basis of the disease. *Arch Gen Psychiatry* 1989;46:1145–1150.
99. Falkai P, Bogerts B, Schneider T, et al. Disturbed planum temporale asymmetry in schizophrenia. A quantitative post-mortem study. *Schizophr Res* 1995;14:161–176.
100. Luchins DJ, Weinberger DR, Wyatt RJ. Schizophrenia: evidence of a subgroup with reversed cerebral asymmetry. *Arch Gen Psychiatry* 1979;36:1309–1311.
101. Tsai LY, Nasrallah HA, Jacoby CG. Hemispheric asymmetries on computed tomographic scans in schizophrenia and mania. A controlled study and a critical review. *Arch Gen Psychiatry* 1983;40:1286–1289.
102. Andreasen NC, Dennert JW, Olsen SA, Damasio AR. Hemispheric asymmetries and schizophrenia. *Am J Psychiatry* 1982;139:427–430.
103. Jernigan TL, Zatz LM, Moses JA, Cardellino JP. Computed tomography in schizophrenics and normal volunteers. II. Cranial asymmetry. *Arch Gen Psychiatry* 1982;39:771–773.
104. Luchins DJ, Weinberger DR, Torrey EF, Johnson A, Rogentine N, Wyatt RJ. HLA-A2 antigen in schizophrenic patients with reversed cerebral asymmetry. *Br J Psychiatry* 1981;138:240–243.
105. Gur RE, Mozley PD, Resnick SM, et al. Magnetic resonance imaging in schizophrenia. I. Volumetric analysis of brain and cerebrospinal fluid. *Arch Gen Psychiatry* 1991;48:407–412.
106. Stratta P, Rossi A, Gallucci M, Amicarelli I, Passariello R, Casacchia M. Hemispheric asymmetries and schizophrenia: a preliminary magnetic resonance imaging study. *Biol Psychiatry* 1989;25:275–284.
107. Petty RG, Barta PE, Pearlson GD, et al. Reversal of asymmetry of the planum temporale in schizophrenia. *Am J Psychiatry* 1995;152:715–721.
108. Shenton ME, Kikinis R, Jolesz FA, et al. Abnormalities of the left temporal lobe and thought disorder in schizophrenia. A quantitative magnetic resonance imaging study. *N Engl J Med* 1992;327:604–612.
109. Geschwind N, Galaburda AM. Cerebral lateralization. Biological mechanisms, associations, and pathology: I. A hypothesis and a program for research. *Arch Neurol* 1985;42:428–459.
110. Goldman PS, Galkin TW. Prenatal removal of frontal association cortex in the fetal rhesus monkey: anatomical and functional consequences in postnatal life. *Brain Res* 1978;152:451–485.
111. Schneider GE. Early lesions and abnormal neuronal connections. *TINS* 1981;4:187–192.
112. Schlaug G, Jancke L, Huang Y, Steinmetz H. In vivo evidence of structural brain asymmetry in musicians. *Science* 1995;267:699–701.
113. Bever TG, Chiarello RJ. Cerebral dominance in musicians and nonmusicians. *Science* 1974;185:537–539.
114. Binder JR, Rao SM, Hammeke TA, et al. Functional magnetic resonance imaging of human auditory cortex. *Ann Neurol* 1994;35:662–672.
115. Geschwind N. Anatomical asymmetry as the basis for cerebral dominance. *Fed Proc* 1978;37:2263–2266.

29

Handedness Measurement and Correlation with Brain Structure

Steven C. Schachter

Department of Neurology, Beth Israel Hospital, Boston, Massachusetts 02215.

In 1981, I began my residency in the Longwood Neurology Training Program in Boston along with eight other neurology residents. Tragically, we would be the last residents to fully train under Dr. Geschwind. We had come to Boston to learn about higher cortical functions, such as aphasia, from Dr. Norman Geschwind. Yes, we were taught about aphasia. But when Dr. Geschwind examined a patient, he was captivated by seemingly trivial details such as hair color or family history of autoimmune disease, and he would then explain how these characteristics were anything but coincidental in the patient's case. Little did we know that he was beginning to articulate a set of ideas that would later become known as the Geschwind-Behan-Galaburda (GBG) hypothesis, as published in the *Archives of Neurology* with Albert Galaburda (1–3).

There was no apparent limit to the breadth of Dr. Geschwind's ideas, and his enthusiasm was infectious to the open-minded listener. I became fascinated by his assertions that brain structure was in part dependent on the fetal environment and that handedness and gender were associated with distinct patterns of cerebral asymmetries.

One day he mentioned that architects were more likely to be left-handed (LH) than the general population and predicted that librarians would be more strongly right-handed (RH) than the general population. Finding this hard to believe, I proposed a study to evaluate the handedness of various professionals. Dr. Geschwind welcomed the idea, suggested possible professional groups to look at, and recommended that the Edinburgh Handedness Inventory (EHI) be used as the tool to measure handedness (4). In addition, he encouraged me to ask about hair color and history of learning disabilities. I did not know why he wanted me to obtain this information but did as he asked.

I found any excuse I could to visit with him in his office as the project proceeded. His office reminded me of Freud's last office in suburban London—cluttered with interesting artifacts, gifts, and books, many of them personally inscribed. These visits were surprisingly easy to carry out. His door was always open. Asking him a simple question would lead to a long, fascinating discussion. Often these discussions would leave me breathless and often they continued as he left his office to go somewhere. I can still picture him talking to me outdoors about handedness on one occasion, seemingly oblivious to the fact we were in a driving rainstorm.

Over 1,100 questionnaires out of the 2,700 that I sent were returned, and I spent many exciting nights entering the data into a computer. I presented the initial results to him with great anticipation. After spending about 10 minutes in silence (which was distinctly unusual for him) looking over the data, he began scribbling furiously and then he frowned. He asked me how I had arrived at the handedness scores, called laterality quotients (LQs), and I showed him. He told me that I had not calculated the LQs correctly and I left somewhat dejected, sure that I had no future in academia. I went back and read Oldfield's instructions for scoring the EHI and saw my error (4). However, the more I thought about my method (which I had intuitively arrived at), the more I thought that it made more sense than the LQ method (see later). So I went back and explained the differences to Dr. Geschwind, who was soon convinced that my method was better. He called it the laterality score (LS) to distinguish it from the LQ. From that point forward, he recommended the LS method as the scoring method of choice for handedness studies based on the EHI.

We then began to look at the results of the study. I can still remember watching Geschwind do his own chi square calculations by hand and gleaming with the results. We found that subjects with blond hair were more likely to be non-right-handed (NRH) than nonblonds (which fit perfectly with his predictions—see Chapter 30 for a fuller exposition). Architects were the most LH, as were subjects with a history of learning disabilities, and librarians were the most RH (also as he predicted). The correlations between hair color, learning disabilities, and handedness were published (5), but the professional group correlations were published only just recently (6) because at that time he "wasn't quite sure what to make of it." He was particularly intrigued by subjects with intermediate handedness, an interest that I have since pursued further.

During those precious months, I made myself a ready and willing listener whenever Dr. Geschwind reviewed or developed his ideas out loud. He asked me to comment on the rough draft of the GBG hypothesis manuscript. This request greatly impressed me because I was barely out of my internship. After working through this manuscript and engaging in many far-ranging and often one-way discussions with Dr. Geschwind, I developed an overall perspective of his theory and saw how the pieces were beginning to fit together into a breathtaking whole.

Dr. Geschwind turned over several handedness studies to me that he had conceived, such as measuring handedness in women exposed to diethylstilbestrol (DES), and he included me as a consultant for other ongoing handedness studies. This was my first introduction to many of his colleagues outside of the Beth Israel area, several of whom have written for this book. When I expressed doubt as to the value of my research and fear that my papers would be rejected, he quickly dispelled my insecurity by saying that some of the most important papers in the literature were initially rejected, such as the Krebs cycle paper. He had a disarming way of boosting everyone's sense of importance, no matter what their relationship to him.

Geschwind was a pioneer in defining the anatomic bases and biological associations of cerebral dominance in groups of normals and subjects with anomalous dominance and then deducing possible mechanisms governing the development of lateralized dominance (7). Since his death, I have continued to pursue (and defend) his interests in handedness studies, and, in particular, the usefulness of handedness studies in supporting his theories of cerebral dominance (8). However, the full contribution of handedness studies in clarifying the developmental origins of cerebral dominance has yet to be realized because of a lack of standardization in handedness measurement and *in vivo* measurements of brain structure.

The following sections will address these issues in greater detail. First, the GBG hypothesis on the development of lateralized dominance will be outlined. Then the measurement, definition, and analysis of handedness will be discussed. Finally, studies that correlate handedness with brain structure will be reviewed. Ironically, a guiding principle of this work was published the year Dr. Geschwind died: "No index of group difference, no matter how reliable, is a useful laterality measure unless it can be shown that the task is related to underlying brain asymmetry" (9).

THE GBG HYPOTHESIS AND ASSOCIATED PREDICTIONS

The GBG hypothesis is based on two general sets of observations. First, specific interhemispheric asymmetries in brain structure are found in approximately 70% of normal subjects, who are defined as possessing standard structural dominance (7,10). Anomalous structural dominance is defined as any deviation from standard structural dominance. Second, there are quantifiable biological attributes that correlate with anomalous structural dominance, including non-right-handedness, right- or mixed-hemisphere language dominance, and certain learning disabilities. Those attributes and others are therefore defined as examples of anomalous functional dominance.

Besides these two observations, there are three assumptions central to the GBG hypothesis. First, intrauterine factors operating at critical times in fetal cortical development influence genetically programmed neuronal migration and maturation. Because of lateralized differences in the rate that the cerebral hemispheres form, intrauterine factors affect brain development asymmetrically, especially late in fetal life, when left hemisphere growth accelerates. Factors that affect brain development at these critical times (the GBG hypothesis proposed testosterone and immune system factors) may therefore be associated with anomalous structural and functional dominance—for example, as measured by neuroimaging studies or handedness.

Second, intrauterine factors, especially testosterone, affect the developing fetal immune system, perhaps via the thymus (10,11) or hypothalamus (12), resulting in elevated frequencies of immune-mediated diseases in subjects with anomalous structural and functional dominance.

Third, intrauterine factors that slow or disrupt focal development may foster additional growth or neural connectivity in other cortical or subcortical foci (13,14), which may lead to unusual cognitive abilities in association with anomalous structural and functional dominance (2,15). Corollaries to these assumptions would anticipate interrelationships between these effects, such as elevated frequencies of allergies in dyslexics (16), increased immune disorders in dyslexics (17,18), and unusual cognitive abilities in people with allergies (19).

The remainder of this chapter will focus primarily on the relationships between handedness and anomalous structural dominance as reflected in correlations between non-right-handedness and atypical cerebral/lobar asymmetries. Relationships between handedness and the anatomy of the corpus callosum will not be presented here but are discussed elsewhere (20–24).

HANDEDNESS

Measurement

Two methods are generally used to measure handedness: (a) determining hand preference for everyday tasks, and (b) measuring manual performance in a defined task such as moving pegs. The cross-correlations of these two forms of measurement, preference and performance, are reviewed elsewhere (25–28). Most studies in the adult literature use preference measures, in particular, handedness batteries or questionnaires, and therefore measures of manual skills and performance will not be discussed.

Handedness batteries measure hand usage for commonly performed tasks through subject report or interview, or by direct observation of the subject. Several questionnaires have been developed and adapted to a variety of cultural groups and age ranges.

Geschwind, along with many others, used the EHI because of its ease of administration and its brevity (4). The EHI originated when Oldfield submitted a questionnaire with 20 handedness preference items to 1,100 undergraduate psychology students in England and Scotland. After performing a statistical analysis, he selected 10 items for the final questionnaire. Some items were left off because they were culturally specific, such as using a cricket bat. There are two columns next to the ten handedness items. The subject places a plus sign (+) in the left or right column for each item according to which hand is usually preferred. When one hand is always used for an item or "where the preference is so strong that you [the subject] would never try to use the other hand unless absolutely forced to," then the subject puts two pluses (++) in the appropriate column. If there is no preference, a + is put in both columns. The extensive use of this questionnaire in the literature has substantiated Oldfield's call for "a measure of hand laterality . . . simply applied and widely used." Another popular questionnaire, derived and published by Annett (29), contains 12 tasks. The subject indicates hand usage for each item without regard to degree of preference.

Another way to measure handedness is simply to ask the subject, "Are you RH, LH, or ambidextrous?" Some studies leave out "ambidextrous" as a choice. This method is usually called self-described handedness (SDH).

Scoring Methods

The scoring method recommended by Oldfield for the EHI was based on an accepted index of handedness, (R–L)/(R+L), and results in the laterality quotient (LQ, range –100 to +100) (4). In Oldfield's words, " . . . to calculate the L.Q., all that has to be done is to add all the +'s for each hand, subtract the sum for the left from that for the right, divide by the sum of both and multiply by 100." This scoring method has also been used with Annett's questionnaire (30).

An alternative method for scoring the EHI was first described in the literature by White and Ashton (31) and has been used since in several other studies (5,32,33). In one method, which I inadvertently devised and which was adopted by Geschwind as described earlier, each of the five possible responses to an item was given an associated score: "always left" (–10), "usually left" (–5), "no preference" (0), "usually right" (+5), or "always right" (+10) (5). Scores for the ten items are summed and the total is the laterality score (LS); the range varies from –100 to +100 by integral units of 5. The results are quickly and easily tabulated. Both the LQ and LS methods agree in the separation of subjects above and below 0. Tan (34) referred to the LS as the Geschwind score. A similar scoring modification for Annett's questionnaire (29) was described by Briggs and Nebes (35). We emphasized the advantages of this scoring method, as illustrated by the following examples (5):

	Left	Right
1 Writing		++
2 Drawing		++
3 Throwing		++
4 Scissors		++
5 Toothbrush		++
6 Knife		++
7 Spoon		++
8 Broom (upper hand)		++
9 Striking match		++
10 Opening box		++

Laterality quotient = $(20 - 0)/20 \times 100 = +100$
Laterality score = $(10 \times 10) = +100$

In the preceding example, the subject always uses the right hand for all ten items. Both the LQ and the LS are the same, +100.

However, in the next example, the subject usually uses the right hand for all items. Although the LQ is still +100, the LS is +50, thereby reflecting the difference in degree of preference.

	Left	Right
1 Writing		+
2 Drawing		+
3 Throwing		+
4 Scissors		+
5 Toothbrush		+
6 Knife		+
7 Spoon		+
8 Broom (upper hand)		+
9 Striking match		+
10 Opening box		+

Laterality quotient = $(10 - 0)/10 \times 100 = +100$
Laterality score = $(10 \times 5) = +50$

These two examples show that the LQ score of +100, often called "complete right-handedness," combines subjects with an LS of +50 together with those with an LS of +100. In effect, as pointed out by McMeekan and Lishman (36), if the subject uses the same hand for all ten items (whether + or ++), the LQ is always −100 or +100 (for left- or right-hand usage); for those subjects, LQ scores do not reflect degrees of preference: that is, whether one hand is usually or always used for an item. Use of LQ in studies of the biological correlations of handedness assumes that subjects with equivalent scores also share other similar biological attributes. However, evidence to the contrary will be presented later. To confuse the issue further, in one study the LS method was used except for those subjects who checked "usually right" for all ten items—they were given a score of +100 (33).

The following example further points out the counter-intuitiveness of the Oldfield scoring method. A subject who always (++) uses the right hand for nine items and usually the left hand for the tenth item has a lower LQ (+89) than a subject who usually (+) uses the right hand for every item (LQ = +100). The respective LS scores are +85 and +50, which again more accurately reflects the degree of preference. This example is particularly noteworthy because the item "top hand on a broom" weakly correlates with the other items, as described later (4,37).

	Left	Right
1 Writing		++
2 Drawing		++
3 Throwing		++
4 Scissors		++
5 Toothbrush		++
6 Knife		++
7 Spoon		++
8 Broom (upper hand)	+	
9 Striking match		++
10 Opening box		++

Laterality quotient = (18 − 1)/19 × 100 = +89
Laterality score = (9 × 10) + (−5) = +85

Compared with quantitative measures such as the LS or LQ, SDH may be less informative, perhaps because of an overlap of self-described right-handedness in the strong and weak RH ranges of quantified handedness distributions. For example, the distribution of subjects in our study was divided into 86% self-described RH ($N = 958$), 4% ambidextrous ($N = 46$), and 10% LH ($N = 113$) (5). Among all subjects with weak RH scores (LS 0 to +70; $N = 152$), most were self-described right-handers (85%) and yet blond hair and learning disabilities were significantly more common in the subjects with an LS of 0 to +70 than in the LS > +70 group (which was 99% self-described RH). These results suggest that the self-description of RH may not reflect biological associations as sensitively as the LS. In addition, SDH may not correlate with actual performance on manual dexterity tasks (38,39). Utilizing "hand used for writing" as a handedness measure may also obscure potential associations of handedness, especially in populations with widely varying ages (see later), although perhaps not in narrow age ranges (40,41). Similarly, although the family history of handedness is often obtained by inquiring about hand used for writing (42), the usefulness of quantifying family handedness has been demonstrated (18,19).

Several studies have evaluated the test/retest reliability of handedness preference measurements. Raczkowski et al. (28) asked approximately 650 undergraduates to fill out a 23-item questionnaire and selected 47 for further study in order to include a large percentage of apparent LH subjects. Subjects were given three possible responses for each item: right, left, or both. Degree of preference was not studied. One month later, 27 of the 47 subjects filled out the same questionnaire a second time and the investigators evaluated how often the responses to a given item were the same, although data were not included for subjects who answered "both" for a particular item on one questionnaire and "right" or "left" on the other questionnaire for that same item. For 17 of 23 items, there was agreement in the responses for at least 90% of subjects. The other six items showed less than 90% agreement, and one of these—"Which hand is on top of the handle when you sweep the floor with a straight broom?"—showed agreement in only 74%

of subjects. That is, one in four subjects who answered this item "right" or "left" the first time gave the opposite response the second time. A very similar item appears on the EHI. Chapman and Chapman (26) performed a similar study using 14 items found by Raczkowski et al. (28) to have the highest test/retest agreement, and this showed a 97% correlation in responses to items for men ($N = 79$) and 96% correlation for women ($N = 187$) when these subjects answered two identical questionnaires 6 weeks apart. Six of these 14 items appear in similar form on the EHI.

The EHI was subjected to reliability analysis by McMeekan and Lishman (36) in 73 LH and ambidextrous volunteers. Sixty-two subjects changed the strength of hand preference without changing the laterality of hand preference on at least one item at retest, and 47 changed the laterality of hand preference (i.e., "right"/"left"/"either") on at least one item. We also evaluated the test/retest reliability of the EHI by sending this questionnaire to the 1,117 subjects who participated in our first study, 18 months after each subject returned the EHI the first time (43). A total of 735 subjects sent the questionnaire back. A comparison of the subjects' scores on the test and on the retest showed a high degree of reliability.

Methods of Analysis

In addition to selecting appropriate methods for measuring and scoring handedness, handedness researchers must control for many variables, including age, and use suitable statistical methods for describing handedness distributions and differences between groups.

Advancing age correlates with increasing right-handedness (5,44–46). Plato et al. (46) noted that 11.8% of white men under age 40 taken from a study on aging wrote with the left hand, compared with 3.5% of men over age 60. Similarly, we found that 40% of subjects under age 30 had an NRH LS ($N = 58$) compared with 25% of subjects over age 30 ($N = 1,059$) (5). Further, the younger group used the left hand for writing more than twice as often as the older group; both age-related differences were statistically significant. One possible explanation is a decrease in cultural pressures to use the right hand for writing, so that more naturally LH subjects in the younger age groups may be allowed to write with the left hand. However, there has not been a longitudinal study of handedness to exclude other factors beyond the early elementary years, and at least one study found an opposite relationship between age and handedness (11). Age is therefore an important variable to control, particularly if handedness is assessed by the hand used to write.

The distribution of handedness is strikingly asymmetric when measured by batteries. Annett (29) and others (28,47) have pointed out the continuum of discrete measurement intervals in the distribution of handedness between complete left- and right-handedness. Many investigators have found bimodal distributions, called J-shaped (4,5,27,35,48). Because handedness distributions are bimodal, parametric statistical methods may not be applicable for their analysis. That is, measures of central tendency, such as mean, do not accurately describe typical handedness distributions. Despite this fact, many studies analyze preference score means and most do not show the handedness distributions for the study and control populations (16,31,48–53).

Other studies often rely on chi square statistics, yet many have insufficient numbers of subjects or controls to show significant differences between the study and control groups. For example, if the frequency of left-handedness (irrespective of definition) in a control group is 10% and a study group has a threefold increase (30%), then there must be a minimum of 71 subjects and 71 controls to demonstrate statistical significance at the 0.05

level with a power of 0.80 (20% chance of missing the effect) (54). If the actual elevation in the study group is less than 3 times the control group, or the frequency of left-handedness in controls is greater than 10%, even larger numbers are necessary. Yet some studies conclude that the frequency of left-handedness is not increased when as few as 14 study subjects and equal numbers of controls are used, in which case left-handedness would have to be 6 times more frequent in the study population (with a power of 0.80) to show statistical significance at the 0.05 level (assuming 10% frequency of left-handedness in controls) (55). Therefore, studies should include sufficient numbers of subjects and controls based on the anticipated difference in handedness frequencies, and nonparametric statistics should be used, because handedness is not generally normally distributed.

Additional methodologic problems in laterality research are created when investigators adopt different definitions for RH and LH. One investigator used the EHI but ignored the scores and labeled anyone as LH who expressed a preference for using any item with the left hand (56). Geschwind and Behan (10,57) used LQ = +100 and -100 as the criteria for RH and LH, respectively. Others define left-handedness as an LQ <0, after Oldfield (4,19,33,48,51,53,57–62). As noted earlier, separating right-handedness from left-handedness using a score of 0 has the advantage of identifying the same groups regardless of the scoring method (LS or LQ) used and, to some extent, regardless of the questionnaire used; as a result, this approach simplifies cross-study comparison (48). In addition, it readily distinguishes laterality of hand preference (LH versus RH) and agrees well with SDH. For example, we noted that 97% of self-described LH subjects scored ≤0 (on LS) and that 99% of self-described RH subjects scored >0 (5). When LH is defined as a score <0, there is no advantage to using the LS method over the LQ, although this point is not generally stated (61).

The term *NRH* designates all subjects other than strong RH subjects and has been defined as an LS or LQ ≤+60 to +70 (5,18,48,63,64). Geschwind picked LS +70 as a cutoff point based on the cross-correlation of LS and SDH in our study (5). He noted that among self-described RH (N = 958), the distribution of LS was 86% >+70, 13% 0 to +70, and 1% <0. Further, among those with LS >+70 (N = 826), 99% were self-described right-handers. Therefore, he defined subjects with an LS >+70 as RH and subjects with an LS ≤+70 as NRH. This method of defining handedness emphasizes *degree* of hand preference rather than direction and was an important feature of Geschwind's approach to handedness measurement after his initial studies.

In some studies, the definitions used for RH and LH exclude some of the subjects from entering into the analysis because only a limited portion of the entire handedness range is evaluated. Such methods typically emphasize direction, but not degree, of hand preference. For instance, if an investigator defines RH and LH as LQ = +100 and LQ = –100, respectively, and then compares the frequencies of these two scores in subjects and controls, those with LQs between these extremes will not be included. Similarly, if the same battery and scoring methods are used, and subjects with LQ ≤0 are defined as LH and compared with controls, then those with an LQ of >0 will be excluded. Potentially useful information may be lost in this manner if a biological trait is overrepresented in the segment of the handedness range excluded from analysis, or if there are insufficient numbers of subjects (e.g., LQ = –100). In support of this observation, several studies suggest that *degree* of hand preference may be more important than *direction* of hand preference with respect to anomalous functional dominance. In our study of handedness and hair color using the EHI and LS, there was no significant correlation of blond hair with an LS <0 (5). However, the percentage of blonds among those with an LS 0 to +70 was almost 2½ times greater than the percentage of nonblonds. As a result, blond hair color correlated with LS ≤70 because the LS 0 to +70 range strongly contributed to the statistical association. Further, the frequency of learning disability was higher in those with LS 0 to +70 (11%) than in those with LS <0 (8%).

Other studies further illustrate the usefulness of considering the full handedness range. Dellatolas et al. (48) found that stuttering was more than doubled in those with handedness scores equivalent to LS ≤+70 compared with LS >+70, and Lahita (11) established that the percentage of patients with systemic lupus erythematosus who had an LQ between 0 and +50 was significantly increased compared with controls. Another study compared the LS distributions among women exposed to DES *in utero* to those of controls (65). There was a shift from strong RH (LS +70 to +100) to weak RH (LS 0 to +70) among the DES-exposed women compared with controls. Finally, Bakan et al. (66) showed that ambidextrous subjects were twice as likely as RH subjects to report pregnancy and birth complications.

Other scoring methods may present additional problems in defining handedness. For instance, Pennington et al. (16) measured LQ on the EHI and defined handedness in a way that classified a subject with an LS +80 as mixed-handed and a subject with an LS +45 as RH. As mentioned earlier, the usual LQ scoring method combines LS +50 (usually the right hand for all 10 items) with LS +100 (both have an LQ of +100). Yet the preceding examples suggest that the lower LS (LS +50) is associated with different frequencies of certain biological traits than the higher LS. Therefore, use of the LQ scoring method or analysis of restricted segments of the handedness range (such as less than 0) could potentially obscure biological correlations through exclusion of data from pertinent domains of the laterality range.

The methodologic issues raised in the previous sections illustrate the problems found in the handedness literature. Whenever possible, handedness studies should include an appropriate number of study and control subjects to demonstrate statistical significance and must control for age and gender as well as other factors not discussed, including educational background and familial handedness (56). A sensitive, validated measuring instrument (e.g., the EHI rather than SDH) should be given in the same manner to subjects and controls and scored quantitatively with a method such as LS, which assigns a score parallel with the degree and direction of handedness. The distribution of the entire range of scores should be tested for normality, and segments of the handedness range should be selected and assessed for differences between study and control groups using the appropriate statistics based on the distribution of scores. Finally, the selection of segments along the handedness spectrum that include as many subjects as possible will enable investigators to explore further which segments are most informative for particular biological variables.

HANDEDNESS STUDIES AND BRAIN STRUCTURE

Although the existence of cerebral asymmetries has been known for over 100 years, gross anatomic cerebral asymmetries have not been clearly correlated with handedness (67). Geschwind's interest in cerebral asymmetries grew out of a desire to "explore the possibility that the human brain was endowed with anatomical asymmetries that could account for the various aspects of cerebral dominance" (68). In 1968, Geschwind and Levitsky (69) reported a larger left planum temporale in 65 of 100 brains studied. However, they were unable to obtain handedness information. Rubens et al. (70) evaluated cerebral asymmetries only in RH subjects. Other studies that documented cerebral (usually temporal lobe) asymmetries in adults and infants did not evaluate handedness

(71–78). McRae et al. (79) evaluated the dominant hand used for a variety of tasks in 100 consecutive patients undergoing pneumoencephalography and ventriculography but had too few LH and ambidextrous subjects to test whether these groups showed different patterns of ventricular asymmetry from RH subjects.

LeMay and Culebras (80) retrospectively compared the cerebral arteriograms of 18 patients stated in their hospital records to be LH with 44 other consecutive arteriograms from other patients. The investigators assumed that 90% of these control angiograms belonged to RH patients and found a more highly developed parietal operculum on the left in 38 of 44 controls, whereas 15 of 18 LH patients had bilaterally equal parietal opercularization. Hochberg and LeMay (81) defined handedness using self-report or the hand used for writing and analyzed bilateral cerebral angiograms in 123 RH and 38 LH subjects. In 67% of the RH subjects, sylvian point angles were over 10° greater on the right than the left; the same finding occurred in only 21% of the LH subjects.

Several studies have evaluated handedness and cerebral asymmetries noted on computed tomography (CT) scans. LeMay and Kido (82) correlated frontal and occipital lobe widths with SDH in 165 patients. Among the 80 RH, 75% had longer left occipital lobes and only 9% had larger right occipital lobes. The frontal lobe was wider on the right than the left in 58% of RH and equal in 30%, whereas only 12% of RH had wider left frontal lobes. The LH group ($N = 85$) showed an almost equal distribution of subjects with wider right occipital lobes (32%), wider left occipital lobes (34%), and occipital lobes of equal size (34%). Similarly, there were nearly equal numbers of LH subjects with wider right frontal lobes (35%), wider left frontal lobes (31%), or symmetrical frontal lobes (34%). Although the pattern of cerebral asymmetries seemed to differ between the two handedness groups, there was no statistical analysis given. In another study, LeMay (83) found similar trends in lobar asymmetries on CT related to handedness as well as skull asymmetries in RH analogous to the CT findings, but again no statistical analysis was done.

Koff et al. (60) measured handedness with a questionnaire in 146 dextral and 26 sinistral patients aged 16 to 80. Although the method used to define handedness was quantitative, the scores lumped together strong RH with subjects in the upper middle range. No correlation was found between handedness and lobar asymmetries (frontal and occipital), nor between degree of handedness and degree of asymmetry. Similarly, Chui and Damasio (84) found no relation between handedness and frontal and occipital asymmetries except for left occipital width predominance in NRH compared with RH. Deuel and Moran (85) studied 94 children and could not correlate parent-reported hand preference with CT asymmetries.

Bear et al. (63) used the EHI and the LQ scoring method in 66 patients. Non-right-handers ($N = 16$; LQ $\leq +70$) had a reduction or reversal of left occipital predominance, especially for width, compared with RH ($N = 50$; LQ $> +70$) but no difference in frontal asymmetries. Kertesz et al. (86) used preference and performance measures to classify 20 subjects as either RH or LH, although the scoring method, statistical findings, and classification criteria were not detailed. Magnetic resonance imaging (MRI) showed the opercular parietal demarcation of sulci to be sharper on the right side in 60% of RH and 10% of LH subjects. Occipital width was larger on the left in 90% of RH and 30% of LH subjects. The anterior frontal width, parietal width, and sulcal demarcations taken together predicted handedness in 19 of 20 subjects.

CONCLUSION

The GBG hypothesis asserts that intrauterine factors influence fetal brain development. Geschwind's insight into these processes represented a brilliant advance in the nature–nurture concept of behavior, suggesting that nurturing actually begins before birth. The studies done over the past 10 years have kept the debate limited to the two putative influences suggested by Geschwind, Behan, and Galaburda (but not critical to the argument): testosterone and the immune system. Further, most studies of the GBG hypothesis have used indirect measures of cortical organization (namely, studies of handedness, dichotic listening, and visual field presentation), with relatively little correlation to actual brain structure. Consequently, the results of this initial approach to validating the GBG hypothesis have been disappointing (87). Pursuing the GBG hypothesis with handedness studies will continue to be difficult until they are done in a more uniform manner. Further gains will depend on reducing inconsistencies in study design and establishing accepted and widely applied methods for defining, measuring, and analyzing handedness.

The GBG hypothesis gives special importance to handedness correlation studies by seeking to increase our understanding of the interrelationships between structural and functional cerebral dominance. Some of the preceding evidence lends support to an association between handedness and cerebral asymmetries—in general, LH people have less interhemispheric structural differences than RH people, and among RH people, the right frontal and left occipital lobes tend to be larger than the corresponding lobes of the other hemisphere. However, some of the studies find no statistical association, and therefore the goal of correlating right-handedness with standard structural dominance and left-handedness or non-right-handedness with anomalous structural dominance has not been completely achieved. Importantly, more studies of handedness and cerebral asymmetries are needed (88), especially as new *in vivo* methods for quantifying cerebral anatomy and function are developed (89,90) and methodologic issues in quantifying cerebral morphology are resolved (91). Then, the handedness measures that correlate best with specific lobar or even gyral asymmetries may be identified.

Once handedness measures are identified in this manner, further studies of these handedness measures and biological variables that reflect the fetal environment may be performed. However, even if well-designed handedness studies fail to support a role for either testosterone or immune factors in fetal brain development, the core assumption of the GBG hypothesis will not be denied. There may yet be new associations of handedness or anomalous structural dominance identified and hence other potential intrauterine influences on brain development will emerge, continuing the search for the solution to the puzzle of cerebral dominance and perpetuating the influence of Norman Geschwind on our age-old struggle to understand ourselves.

REFERENCES

1. Geschwind N, Galaburda AM. Cerebral lateralization. Biological mechanisms, associations, and pathology: I. A hypothesis and a program for research. *Arch Neurol* 1985;42:428–459.
2. Geschwind N, Galaburda AM. Cerebral lateralization. Biological mechanisms, associations, and pathology: II. A hypothesis and a program for research. *Arch Neurol* 1985;42:521–552.
3. Geschwind N, Galaburda AM. Cerebral lateralization. Biological mechanisms, associations, and pathology: III. A hypothesis and a program for research. *Arch Neurol* 1985;42:634–654.
4. Oldfield RC. The assessment and analysis of handedness: the Edinburgh inventory. *Neuropsychologia* 1971;9:97–113.
5. Schachter SC, Ransil BJ, Geschwind N. Associations of handedness with hair color and learning disabilities. *Neuropsychologia* 1987;25:269–276.
6. Schachter SC. Ambilaterality: definition from handedness preference questionnaires and potential significance. *Int J Neurosci* 1994;77:47–51.
7. Schachter SC, Galaburda AM. Development and biological associations of cerebral dominance: review and possible mechanisms. *J Am Acad Child Psychiatry* 1986;25:741–750.

8. Schachter SC. Evaluating the Bryden-McManus-Bulman-Fleming critique of the Geschwind-Behan-Galaburda model of cerebral lateralization. *Brain Cogn* 1994;26:199–205.
9. Schwartz S, Kirsner K. Can group differences in hemispheric asymmetry be inferred from behavioral laterality indices? *Brain Cogn* 1984;3:57–70.
10. Geschwind N, Behan PO. Laterality, hormones, and immunity. In: Geschwind N, Galaburda AM, eds. *Cerebral dominance: the biological foundations.* Cambridge, MA: Harvard University Press, 1984;211–224.
11. Lahita RG. Systemic lupus erythematosus: learning disability in the male offspring of female patients and relationship to laterality. *Psychoneuroendocrinology* 1988;13:385–396.
12. Wofsy D. Hormones, handedness, and autoimmunity. *Immunol Today* 1984;5:169–170.
13. Goldman PS, Galkin TW. Prenatal removal of frontal association cortex in the fetal rhesus monkey: anatomical and functional consequences in postnatal life. *Brain Res* 1978;152:451–485.
14. Schneider GE. Early lesions and abnormal neuronal connections. *Trends Neurosci* 1981;4:187–192.
15. Marx JL. Autoimmunity in left-handers: left-handedness may be associated with an increased risk of autoimmune disease. Is testosterone the link between the two? *Science* 1982;217:141–144.
16. Pennington BF, Smith SD, Kimberling WJ, Green PA, Haith MM. Left-handedness and immune disorders in familial dyslexics. *Arch Neurol* 1987;44:634–639.
17. Hugdahl K. Functional brain asymmetry, dyslexia, and immune disorders. In: Galaburda AM, ed. *Dyslexia and development: neurobiological aspects of extra-ordinary brains.* Cambridge, MA: Harvard University Press, 1990;133–154.
18. Urion DK. Nondextrality and autoimmune disorders among relatives of language-disabled boys. *Ann Neurol* 1988;24:267–269.
19. Benbow CP. Physiological correlates of extreme intellectual precocity. *Neuropsychologia* 1986;24:719–725.
20. Witelson SF, Goldsmith CH. The relationship of hand preference to anatomy of the corpus callosum in men. *Brain Res* 1991;545:175–182.
21. Witelson SF. Hand and sex differences in the isthmus and genu of the human corpus callosum: a postmortem morphological study. *Brain* 1989;112:799–835.
22. Steinmetz H, Jancke L, Kleinschmidt A, Schlaug G, Volkmann J, Huang Y. Sex but no hand difference in the isthmus of the corpus callosum. *Neurology* 1992;42:749–752.
23. Kertesz A, Polk M, Howell J, Black SE. Cerebral dominance, sex, and callosal size in MRI. *Neurology* 1987;37:1385–1388.
24. Habib M, Gayraud D, Oliva A, Regis J, Salamon G, Khalil R. Effects of handedness and sex on the morphology of the corpus callosum: a study with brain magnetic resonance imaging. *Brain Cogn* 1991;16:41–61.
25. Bishop DVM. Does hand proficiency determine hand preference? *Br J Psychol* 1989;80:191–199.
26. Chapman LJ, Chapman JP. The measurement of handedness. *Brain Cogn* 1987;6:175–183.
27. Johnstone J, Galin D, Herron J. Choice of handedness measures in studies of hemispheric specialization. *Int J Neurosci* 1979;9:71–80.
28. Raczkowski D, Kalat JW, Nebes R. Reliability and validity of some handedness questionnaire items. *Neuropsychologia* 1974;12:43–47.
29. Annett M. A classification of hand preference by association analysis. *Br J Psychol* 1970;61:303–321.
30. Lindesay J. Laterality shift in homosexual men. *Neuropsychologia* 1987;25:965–969.
31. White K, Ashton R. Handedness assessment inventory. *Neuropsychologia* 1976;14:261–264.
32. Bryden MP. Measuring handedness with questionnaires. *Neuropsychologia* 1977;15:617–624.
33. Messinger HB, Messinger MI, Graham JR. Migraine and left-handedness: is there a connection? *Cephalalgia* 1988;8:237–244.
34. Tan U. The distribution of hand preference in normal men and women. *Int J Neurosci* 1988;41:35–55.
35. Briggs GG, Nebes RD. Patterns of hand preference in a student population. *Cortex* 1975;11:230–238.
36. McMeekan ERL, Lishman WA. Retest reliabilities and interrelationship of the Annett hand preference questionnaire and the Edinburgh handedness inventory. *Br J Psychol* 1975;66:53–59.
37. Williams SM. Factor analysis of the Edinburgh Handedness Inventory. *Cortex* 1986;22:325–326.
38. Benton AL, Meyers R, Polder GJ. Some aspects of handedness. *Psychiatr Neurol* 1962;144:321–337.
39. Satz P, Achenbach K, Fennell E. Correlations between assessed manual laterality and predicted speech laterality in a normal population. *Neuropsychologia* 1967;5:295–310.
40. Hugdahl K, Ellertsen B, Waaler PE, Klove H. Left and right-handed dyslexic boys: an empirical test of some assumptions of the Geschwind-Behan hypothesis. *Neuropsychologia* 1989;27:223–231.
41. Van Strien JW, Bouma A, Bakker DJ. Birth stress, autoimmune diseases, and handedness. *J Clin Exp Neuropsychol* 1987;9:775–780.
42. Bishop DVM. Measuring familial sinistrality. *Cortex* 1980;16:311–313.
43. Ransil BJ, Schachter SC. Test-retest reliability of the Edinburgh handedness inventory and global handedness preference measurements, and their correlation. *Percept Motor Skills* 1994;79:1355–1372.
44. Fleminger JJ, Dalton R, Standage KJ. Age as a factor in the handedness of adults. *Neuropsychologia* 1977;15:471–473.
45. Lansky LM, Feinstein H, Peterson JM. Demography of handedness in two samples of randomly selected adults (N = 2083). *Neuropsychologia* 1988;26:465–477.
46. Plato CC, Fox KM, Garruto RM. Measures of lateral functional dominance: hand dominance. *Hum Biol* 1984;56:259–275.

47. Cernacek J. Handedness as a quantitative estimation. *J Neurol Sci* 1964;1:152–159.
48. Dellatolas G, Annesi I, Jallon P, Chavance M, Lellouch J. An epidemiological reconsideration of the Geschwind-Galaburda theory of cerebral lateralization. *Arch Neurol* 1990;47:778–782.
49. Nass R, Baker S, Speiser P, et al. Hormones and handedness: left-hand bias in female congenital adrenal hyperplasia patients. *Neurology* 1987;37:711–715.
50. Neils JR, Aram DM. Handedness and sex of children with developmental language disorders. *Brain Lang* 1986;28:53–65.
51. Schur PH. Handedness in systemic lupus erythematosus. *Arthritis Rheum* 1986;29:419–420.
52. Searleman A, Fugagli AK. Suspected autoimmune disorders and left-handedness: evidence from individuals with diabetes, Crohn's disease and ulcerative colitis. *Neuropsychologia* 1987;25:367–374.
53. Weinstein RE, Pieper DR. Altered cerebral dominance in an atopic population. *Brain Behav Immunol* 1988;2:235–241.
54. Fleiss JL. *Statistical methods for rates and proportions*. New York: Wiley, 1981;262.
55. Bender BG, Puck MH, Salbenblatt JA, Robinson A. Hemispheric organization in 47 XXY boys. *Lancet* 1983;1:132.
56. McGee MG, Cozad T. Population genetic analysis of human hand preference: evidence for generation differences, familial resemblance, and maternal effects. *Behav Genet* 1980;10:263–275.
57. Geschwind N, Behan P. Left-handedness: association with immune disease, migraine, and developmental learning disorder. *Proc Natl Acad Sci USA* 1982;79:5097–5100.
58. Behan P, Geschwind N. Dyslexia, congenital anomalies, and immune disorders: the role of the fetal environment. *Ann NY Acad Sci* 1985;457:13–18.
59. Cosi V, Citterio A, Pasquino C. A study of hand preference in myasthenia gravis. *Cortex* 1988;24:573–577.
60. Koff E, Naeser MA, Pieniadz JM, Foundas AL, Levine HL. Computed tomographic scan hemispheric asymmetries in right- and left-handed male and female subjects. *Arch Neurol* 1986;43:487–491.
61. Meyers S, Janowitz HD. Left-handedness and inflammatory bowel disease. *J Clin Gastroenterol* 1985;7:33–35.
62. Smith J. Left-handedness: its association with allergic disease. *Neuropsychologia* 1987;25:665–674.
63. Bear D, Schiff D, Saver J, Greenberg M, Freeman R. Quantitative analysis of cerebral asymmetries: fronto-occipital correlation, sexual dimorphism and association with handedness. *Arch Neurol* 1986;43:598–603.
64. Betancur C, Velez A, Cabanieu G, Le Moal M, Neveu PJ. Association between left-handedness and allergy: a reappraisal. *Neuropsychologia* 1990;28:223–227.
65. Schachter SC. Handedness in women with intrauterine exposure to diethylstilbestrol. *Neuropsychologia* 1994;32:619–623.
66. Bakan P, Dibb G, Reed P. Handedness and birth stress. *Neuropsychologia* 1973;11:363–366.
67. Eberstaller O. Zur Oberflachen-Anatomie der Grosshirn-Hemispharen. *Wien Med Blatter* 1884;7:644.
68. Geschwind N. Anatomical asymmetry as the basis for cerebral dominance. *Fed Proc* 1978;37:2263–2266.
69. Geschwind N, Levitsky W. Human brain: left-right asymmetries in temporal speech region. *Science* 1968;161:186–187.
70. Rubens AB, Mahowald MW, Hutton JT. Asymmetry of the lateral (sylvian) fissures in man. *Neurology* 1976;26:620–624.
71. Beck E. Typologie des Gehirns am Beispiel des dorsalen menschlichen Schlafenlappens nebst weiteren Beitragen zur Frage der Links-Rechtshirnigkeit. *Dtsch Z Nervenheilk* 1955;173:267–308.
72. Campain R, Minckler J. A note on the gross configurations of the human auditory cortex. *Brain Lang* 1976;3:318–323.
73. Chi JG, Dooling EC, Gilles FH. Gyral development of the human brain. *Ann Neurol* 1977;1:86–93.
74. Falzi G, Perrone P, Vignolo LA. Right-left asymmetry in anterior speech regions. *Arch Neurol* 1982;39:239–240.
75. Teszner D, Tzavaras A, Gruner J, Hecaen. H. L'asymetrie droite-gauche du planum temporale: a propos de l'etude anatomique de 100 cerveaux. *Rev Neurol (Paris)* 1972;146:444–449.
76. Wada JA, Clarke R, Hamm A. Cerebral hemispheric asymmetry in humans: cortical speech zones in 100 adults and 100 infant brains. *Arch Neurol* 1975;32:239–246.
77. Weinberger DR, Luchins DJ, Morihisa J, Wyatt RJ. Asymmetrical volumes of the right and left frontal and occipital regions of the human brain. *Ann Neurol* 1982;11:97–100.
78. Witelson SF, Pallie W. Left hemisphere specialization for language in the newborn: neuroanatomical evidence of asymmetry. *Brain* 1973;96:641–646.
79. McRae DL, Branch CL, Milner B. The occipital horns and cerebral dominance. *Neurology* 1968;18:95–98.
80. LeMay M, Culebras A. Human brain—morphologic differences in the hemispheres demonstrable by carotid arteriography. *N Engl J Med* 1972;287:168–170.
81. Hochberg FH, LeMay M. Arteriographic correlates of handedness. *Neurology* 1975;25:218–222.
82. LeMay M, Kido DK. Asymmetries of the cerebral hemispheres on computed tomograms. *J Comput Assist Tomogr* 1978;2:471–476.
83. LeMay M. Asymmetries of the skull and handedness. Phrenology revisited. *J Neurol Sci* 1977;32:243–253.
84. Chui HC, Damasio AR. Human cerebral asymmetries evaluated by computed tomography. *J Neurol Neurosurg Psychiatry* 1980;43:873–878.
85. Deuel RK, Moran CC. Cerebral dominance and cerebral asymmetries on computed tomogram in childhood. *Neurology* 1980;30:934–938.

86. Kertesz A, Black SE, Polk M, Howell J. Cerebral asymmetries on magnetic resonance imaging. *Cortex* 1986;22:117–127.
87. Bryden MP, McManus IC, Bulman-Fleming MB. Evaluating the empirical support for the Geschwind-Behan-Galaburda model of cerebral lateralization. *Brain Cogn* 1994;26:103–167.
88. Schachter SC. Studies of handedness and anomalous dominance: problems and progress. In: Galaburda AM, ed. *Dyslexia and development: neurobiological aspects of extra-ordinary brains.* Cambridge, MA: Harvard University Press, 1993;269–296, 358–365.
89. Jouandet ML, Tramo MJ, Herron DM, et al. Brainprints: computer-generated two-dimensional maps of the human cerebral cortex in vivo. *J Cogn Neurosci* 1990;1:88–117.
90. Binder JR, Rao SM, Hammeke TA, et al. Lateralized human brain language systems demonstrated by task subtraction functional magnetic resonance imaging. *Arch Neurol* 1995;52:593–601.
91. Weis S, Haug H, Holoubek B, Orun H. The cerebral dominances: quantitative morphology of the human cerebral cortex. *Int J Neurosci* 1989;47:165–168.

30

Left-handed Blonds and Other Odd Correlations

Stanley Coren

Department of Psychology, University of British Columbia, Vancouver, British Columbia, Canada V6T 1Z4.

I can't recall whether it was at the Orton Society meetings or the American Academy of Neurology meetings, but I found myself standing in a line where coffee was being poured into styrofoam cups. A man built a bit shorter than average was standing in front of me. He turned and glanced back at my conference badge. "Coren, huh? You did a bit on handedness and birth stress, didn't you?" he asked. For a number of years my laboratory had been looking at birth stressors and a number of other factors (genetic and pathological) that seemed to be correlated with left-handedness, so I nodded. "Look, if you have a little free time I would like to talk to you about handedness. Do you have some time now?"

Because my cup of coffee was already in my hand, I allowed myself to be steered to an empty padded bench nearby and listened as the man continued talking. He spoke at a rapid pace, spinning out a continuous train of ideas and opinions. He was totally intent on the scientific subject matter and had not even stopped to introduce himself, but I noted that his badge read "Norman Geschwind, Harvard University." At the outset, he indicated that he knew of several of my publications, and he made it clear that although he felt that my research was "interesting," I should understand that "birth stress is only a small part of the story" and "simple genetics only explains a minor portion of the problem." I suppose that I should have been put off by this apparent dismissal of my work, but there appeared to be no malice intended and some of the ideas that he was outlining were really interesting and exciting and I wanted to hear more.

At one point during our conversation I was reminded of a story told to me about a well-known physicist who had a "creativity machine." It consisted of a large container filled with a number of slips of paper. Each slip had on it a brief description of a fact, research finding, concept, or situation. Each morning he would stir the papers around, grab two of them, and then try to form some association between them or develop some idea that connected them. At first, Geschwind's suggestions seemed just as random, yet when one listened carefully, it became clear that he had firmly grasped the "handedness slip" and was systematically working through a number of possible correlates. Each of the "second slips" was a research finding, an observation, or something from case histories. There was no randomness, however, involved. Each idea came out with "hooks" firmly grounded in current neurological data or theory.

A WEB OF ASSOCIATIONS

Our discussion ranged quite far afield. We both agreed that handedness had many correlates, and there were data indicating that left-handedness was associated with a number of problems. As of today, for instance, we know that left-handedness has shown significant correlations with:

age
aggression
alcoholism
attempted suicide
autism
birth complications requiring the use of forceps
brain damage
breathing difficulties at birth
breech delivery
chromosomal damage
clinical depression
criminality
deafness
drug abuse
emotionality
epilepsy
excessive smoking
high and low extremes in numerical ability
high and low extremes in spatial ability
homosexuality
low birth weight
manic–depressive psychosis
mental retardation
neuroticism
older mothers at parturition
poor verbal ability
premature birth
prolonged labor during delivery
reduced adult height
reduced adult weight
Rh incompatibility with mother
schizophrenia or schizotypal thinking
school failure
sex
shortened life span
sleep difficulty
slow maturation
strabismus
stuttering
sudden heart attack death
transsexuality
twinning
variations in fingerprint patterns
vegetarianism

Geschwind and his collaborators had already confirmed, or would soon confirm, many of these associations. Furthermore, they would eventually expand this list significantly so that it would include correlations of handedness with:

allergies
anatomic asymmetries in the brain
asthma
celiac disease
Crohn's disease
dyslexia
epilepsy
Hashimoto's thyroiditis
hay fever
hypopigmentation
infection susceptibility
juvenile onset diabetes
language problems
learning disabilities
migraine headaches
myasthenia gravis
neural tube defects
regional ileitis
testosterone exposure during gestation
ulcerative colitis
urticaria

To the casual observer, these lists probably seem to be overinclusive. In much the same way that the popular press seems to claim that there is no human activity that does not ultimately lead to heart failure, it would almost seem that neuropsychologists are claiming that there is no negative aspect of human health or behavior that is not associated with left-handedness. Does that make sense?

HANDEDNESS AS A PATHOLOGICAL MARKER

We must understand that left-handedness has to be viewed as a "soft sign" for possible pathology. The linkage between handedness and these various pathological conditions comes about because of both neurological and statistical considerations. The statistical component has been mathematically explored in the form of the rare trait marker model, which notes that a number of statistically rare traits are associated with a range of pathological conditions (1). Examples include rare-colored animals; "blue-marl" collies, white dogs, and albino human beings, for instance, often have major sensory deficits that affect their vision or hearing. Rare palm crease patterns, rare distributions of toe lengths, and even rare ear shapes are often associated with cognitive or physical deficits. Left-handedness, which affects only about 10% of the population, qualifies as a rare trait.

Given a trait such as handedness, which has both common and rare forms, we need only add the possibility that the appearance of the rare form, as opposed to the common form, can be influenced by pathological factors. If both of these conditions are met, then, because of statistical considerations, we have all that is needed to create a clinical soft sign for pathology. As a simple illustration, suppose that we started with a population in which, if development proceeded naturally, 90% would become right-handers and 10%, left-handers. Suppose that there was some disturbance in development, some aberrant condition or some birth risk factor that caused 10% of each group to deviate from their targeted handedness. The result would be 9% (10% of the 90% who would be right-handed) "pathologically" shifting from right-handedness to left-handedness, in contrast to only 1% (10% of the 10% targeted to be sinistral) shifting from left-handedness to right-handedness. The final result is that 50% of the phenotypical left-handers (9% out of the total of 18% sinistrals) are pathological, whereas only 1.2% of the right-handers are. Thus, the relative risk of a left-hander being pathological is around 41% greater than that of a right-hander. How well a trait predicts pathology depends upon its distribution in the population and the likelihood of pathological change. Just by chance, the roughly 10% incidence of left-handedness falls into the optimal predictive range of values (1).

The neurological reason why left-handedness is a useful soft sign for pathology is related to the *diffuse control system* of handedness. This term refers to the fact that the control of handedness is neurologically complex, involving various brain sites and neural pathways. A study of a number of reviews of upper limb coordination (e.g., 2–5), leads to the conclusion that a variety of different neurological systems are involved in hand control. Specifically implicated are three motor systems that originate in the cerebral cortex, several subcortical sites, a sensory system, and several commissural systems. In the cortex, Brodmann's areas 1, 2, 3, 4, 5, and 6 have all been shown to play a role in upper limb control. The corticospinal or pyramidal tract, the ventromedial brain stem system (including the reticulospinal tract), and the lateral brainstem system (including the rubrospinal pathway) all perform significant functions in manual activities. Among the subcortical sites mentioned as important to the regulation of hand use are the basal ganglia structures. The corpus callosum, which transfers information between the two cerebral hemispheres, also seems to be a factor in hand control. Sensory systems include, at the minimum, proprioceptive and kinesthetic systems in the postcentral cortex. In all, at least 23 neural centers or systems have been mentioned as important to manual control.

The extended and complex nature of hand control was recognized by Geschwind. Implicit in some of his theorizing is the notion that anything that disturbs or disrupts the normal functioning of any of the many sites or systems that control hand use, or any variable that might alter the expected pattern of cerebral dominance might also alter the natural development of handedness. In general, Geschwind seemed to hold the idea that the natural state of affairs is right-handedness and that, therefore, any shifts caused by random or pathological events are apt to be toward non-right-handedness. Geschwind believed that the period of vulnerability to such pathological influences occurs quite early in development. In his view, the most important events are likely to be those that might alter the natural course of development, including the conditions surrounding the maturing fetus.

Although Geschwind was a bit dismissive, in our conversation, of the importance of birth stressors in the development of left-handedness, it was clear from his case work and research that he accepted them as possible contributors to or, at least, correlates of sinistrality. An example appears in a letter that he wrote to Dr. Harrison Pope on May 14, 1981: "It is certainly clear that among those people who have difficult deliveries there is an increased incidence of left-handedness and of brain damage...."

Later, however, Geschwind modified his stance somewhat to suggest that visible lesions or alterations of brain structure are more likely to have been the result of processes influencing development during the intrauterine period, not merely at the time surrounding delivery. He summarized this view by saying that "it seems to us that difficult birth is much more likely to be a parallel manifestation rather than the cause of these disorders; in other words, the same influences that alter brain development also lead to disturbance of the birth process" (6).

Geschwind strongly favored the idea that hormonal imbalances or other physical factors that can cause defects in neuronal migration and assembly may result in alterations of cortical organization, motor system control, or pathway mapping. Regardless of the causal agent, however, he was certainly comfortable with the prediction that many forms of abnormal development may manifest themselves in association with an increased probability of left-handedness. Under this hypothesis, left-handedness becomes a sensitive marker of pathology because the genesis of abnormal shifts in hand dominance may be a number of different types of insults or disturbances that could have had an impact on any one of the numerous neural centers and systems involved in handedness. Handedness is a useful indicator of other pathology because of the likelihood that the same patterns of disturbed development that affect the control of handedness also affect other control centers and pathways involved with other functions. Thus the pattern of disturbed development that causes left-handedness might also interfere with normal learning or language processes; produce emotional, neurotic, or psychotic symptoms; affect the immune system; or even reduce adaptive and survival ability in various ways.

Although the preceding discussion suggests that left-handedness might be a sensitive marker for a number of pathological conditions, left-handedness lacks specificity as a marker. Left-handedness might be seen as a soft sign indicating increased risk of many problems. However, which specific problems a person might have and which neural loci might be involved are not determinable. Thus, if all that is known about a person is that he or she is left-handed, one can list the many problems that the person is at increased risk for but one cannot tell which of them that particular left-hander is most likely to have, which part of the nervous system is most apt to be damaged, or the probable source of the pathology. One can say with some certainty that the more diffuse the pathological events, the higher the likelihood of non-right-handedness and also the higher the probability that functions other than handedness will also be disturbed.

AN ODD ASSOCIATION

I recall several highlights of my conversation with Geschwind. The first one was the suggested link between testosterone and sinistrality. Put simply, the notion was that testosterone results in a delay in the growth of the left hemisphere, which in turn reduces the probability of right-handedness. That idea was really exciting because it promised to explain the often-observed fact that males are about one-third more likely to be left-handed than females. Geschwind's hypothesis seemed a lot cleaner and less convoluted than the best one that I had come up with at that time (mine started off with the relative vulnerability of male fetuses to birth stress). I remember mentioning to Geschwind that his hypothesis seemed to deal with this issue considerably more convincingly. He looked at me as one might look at a particularly dense student and said, "Of course!" Then, as if the interruption had never occurred, he moved the discussion forward, extrapolating the initial idea into the prediction that testosterone also slows the growth of the thymus, which should produce an association between handedness and immune system function. Specifically, he predicted more problems, such as allergies, migraine headaches, and asthma, in left-handers. I was considerably less comfortable with that extrapolation, although a number of years later my own laboratory was destined to produce data that supported those very predictions (7).

Perhaps the oddest association that Geschwind offered, and certainly the one of which I was most skeptical, was that blonds should have a higher incidence of left-handedness. The story unfolded as a pattern of "noticed" associations but ended, as usual, with a solid scientific explanation that made this correlation seem more sensible. According to

Geschwind, the lay literature on dyslexia suggested that light hair and early graying of the hair are more common among dyslexics than nondyslexics. Furthermore, there was some evidence that Nordic peoples, the majority of whom are blond, are more likely to have autoimmune system disorders than non-Nordic peoples. These observations started Geschwind thinking about hypopigmentation as a marker for the same types of neural disorganization associated with left-handedness and led directly to the suggestion that the incidence of left-handedness is increased in blonds.

As he spelled out the argument, Geschwind explained that he had just recently read a book by Nichole Le Douarin (8) on the neural crest and was excited about several aspects of it. The neural crest appears early in embryonic development. The sequence starts with the development of two longitudinal ridges, or neural folds, on the dorsal surface of an embryo. These ridges then unite to form the neural tube, the structure from which the brain and spinal cord will eventually develop. The neural crest is a band of pigmented cells extending down the length of the neural tube. These cells will eventually form the autonomic and spinal ganglia, glia and neurons in the peripheral nervous system and visual system, the adrenal medulla, and several other important structures, some of which are associated with the immune system. They also provide the pigment cells that color hair, eyes, and skin. Le Douarin believed that the vast majority of pigmented cells in the body were of neural crest origin. The importance of these pigmented cells in the neural crest is that they serve as neuronal cell guides, directing the migration of neural tube cells to the sites where they will form various central nervous system centers. This concept was later presented formally (6,9). At the time that Geschwind was thinking about the pigmented cells of the neural crest, there was some evidence from albino cats and human beings that these melanin-bearing cells play a vital role in the development of the optic pathways (10,11). It was also suggested that a number of problems related to neural tube defects, such as spina bifida, are more common among white infants than black ones (the former have fewer pigment cells) (6) and more common in the British Isles than in the Orient (12), again suggesting that reduced numbers of pigment-bearing cells were associated with developmental disorders. More recent studies have used genetically manipulated mice to show that embryonic neural growth is disrupted when there is an insufficiency of pigment (melanin) cells (13,14), and *in vitro* studies have shown that the presence of pigment cells makes it more likely that neurons will form the cellular clusters during development that would be precursors to formation of neural ganglia (15).

Once this groundwork has been prepared, the prediction becomes quite simple. Lightly pigmented persons have fewer or less effective neuronal guide cells. The absence of an adequate set of guide cells will interfere with normal cell migration, perhaps altering final site locations and connections. This disrupted neural migration and development will cause broadly dispersed effects and will probably affect many brain sites and centers. Because the resulting pathology, although mild, is also widely distributed, the likelihood is high that one or more of the resultant problems will affect one or more of the brain sites or pathways involved in establishing manual dominance. The outcome should then be an increase in left-handedness.

I admit that while I understood the argument and appreciated its cleverness, I remained a bit skeptical. I was about to pursue the issue further when I felt a hand on my shoulder. It was a Canadian colleague, who asked, "Isn't your paper supposed to be given in about 15 minutes?" I looked at my watch and gasped. We had been talking for nearly 2 hours. My coffee, virtually untouched, was resting beside me, now stone cold. I had been totally caught up in the conversation and my head was now filled with a series of possible hypotheses about conditions associated with handedness. I checked to make sure that I had the slides for my talk and stood up to go. Geschwind also stood and said, "I plan on being at your talk. If I leave the session a little early, don't be upset. It's just that I made arrangements to talk about handedness with someone else this morning."

LEFT-HANDED BLONDS

The conversation with Geschwind was important to me because it alerted me to his handedness research, little of which had been published at that time. As the testosterone link with handedness became better known and the handedness and immune system link began to be explored, some of my own research began to include measures of variables related to these hypotheses as well. When I heard of Geschwind's untimely death, I was much saddened. I wondered how many of those "wild" or "odd" associations were still untested and how many might now never be tested. I found myself particularly wondering about Geschwind's hypothesis about left-handed blonds.

Some time later, I encountered the paper by Schachter, Ransil, and Geschwind (16). I smiled when I read that they had found the frequency of non-right-handers among blonds to be nearly twice that among nonblonds. "He was right, I guess," I thought to myself.

A few years ago, it dawned on me that one could push the hypopigmentation hypothesis a bit further. The trigger for this idea was an almost accidental observation I made during some research that our laboratory was doing on individual differences in perception. This research, which had nothing to do with issues of laterality, produced some data that seemed to indicate that blue-eyed persons have poorer hearing than brown-eyed ones, at least for higher tonal frequencies (17). The only reason that I had bothered to look for this difference is that I had stumbled across a report that people with blue eyes suffer more from noise-induced threshold elevation than do people with brown eyes (18). When I looked for an explanation, I found that there was evidence suggesting that a lack of melanin around the strial capillaries in the cochlear region is often found to be associated with reduced auditory function (e.g., 19). These cochlear melanin cells, like the pigment cells in the iris of the eye, are of neural crest origin. Once these facts were in hand, I found myself, much like the physicist mentioned earlier who randomly pulled slips of paper out of a box, thinking of a report by Bonvillian et al. (20). The mental association that triggered this thought was probably the fact that these researchers were working with hearing; however, their predictor variable was not pigmentation but handedness. In their sample of 226 deaf persons, they reported 28% left-handedness as opposed to only 11% in 210 normally hearing subjects. As I mused about this finding, my mind contained thoughts about hearing, eye color, and now handedness. Eye color, like hair color, is a simple sign of pigmentation levels in human beings. Blue or gray eyes represent virtually unpigmented irises. Suddenly the random associations linked and I found myself thinking about pigmentation and handedness again, that odd hypothesis that Geschwind had come up with several years before.

Because we were engaged in a large data acquisition project, I had an opportunity to test and extend Geschwind's notions without adding much expense to the research. Thus, we added questions about hair color and eye color to a larger survey on issues of laterality and health status in young adults. Participants in the survey were mostly university students, but this group was supplemented with some persons recruited from church and social groups in Vancouver, Canada. The final sample consisted of 3,495 subjects (2,136 women and 1,359) men, whose mean age was 20.1 years.

Hair color data were obtained by simply asking each subject whether his or her natural hair color (before any graying or coloring) was black, brown, red, or blond. Eye color data were obtained by asking whether the person's eyes were gray, blue, green, hazel, brown, or black.

MEASURING HANDEDNESS

Geschwind was quite interested in the issue of assessing handedness, which is more difficult to assess than eye or hair color. He recognized that one could not necessarily base handedness classification upon the response obtained from asking a person, "Are you left- or right-handed?" In our laboratory, we have encountered numerous instances of people not accurately reporting their own handedness. For example, in one case a person confidently told us that he was a right-hander. We were surprised to find that when we tested him to see which hand he used to throw a ball, aim a dart, use scissors, and so forth, he performed every single action with his left hand. His only right-handed activity seemed to be writing. Given the glaring inconsistency between his self-classification and his actual behaviors, at the end of the session we asked him, "Since you seem to have done every test here with your left hand, we were wondering why you describe yourself as being right-handed?" He replied, "I *am* right-handed. It's just that I do *some things* with my left hand." "Some things" in this case translated to everything except writing. Global self-classification is a poor predictor of specific hand use. Thus, when Satz et al. (21) compared such self-classification with hand use in a number of everyday activities, their results indicated that 7% of the group actually did more things with their supposedly nondominant hand than with their supposedly dominant hand.

The obvious solution to determining handedness from self-report is to use specific behavioral items. Thus one might ask, "Which hand would you use to hold a knife while cutting?" Presumably, people ought to be able to recall which hand they use for a common behavior such as this. Unfortunately, not all specific questions are equally successful in determining handedness. Questions like "Which hand do you use to hold a pitcher when pouring?" or "Which hand is nearest the top of the handle when you sweep the floor with a straight broom?" get answers that are wrong from too many people. When given a chance to actually *demonstrate* how they pour a pitcher or use a broom, more than 1 out of every 5 people will *not* use the hand they had said they used (22). However, it is possible to select sets of items for which people are not only accurate but consistent in describing their behaviors. By selecting self-report items of this latter sort, one can obtain both a valid and reliable estimate of a person's handedness (22,23).

The fact that people seem to be able to describe their own hand-use patterns accurately for some types of activities but not for others suggests that there may be several types of handedness. Different patterns of handedness may manifest themselves in different situations. Some of these varieties of handedness appear to be quite stable and consistent, but others, weak or unstable. Peters (24) explained this state of affairs by suggesting that there is a distinct set of handedness patterns for behaviors and activities that "matter" as opposed to activities that "don't matter." What he apparently meant is that, in certain instances, the extra skill that is attained by using the dominant hand is needed but that, in other instances, that skill is irrelevant.

Geschwind contributed to the debate about the complexity of handedness in the paper by Healey et al. (25). In this analysis, he suggested that specific types of handedness might be defined by characteristic muscle and movement patterns. Steenhuis and Bryden (26) generally confirmed that there might be up to four distinct handedness patterns similar to those suggested by Geschwind. They labeled these patterns according to the types of actions involved. The first type of handedness involves actions that require some skill (these are the situations where handedness matters, according to Peters' classification). Such *skilled actions* include using a hammer, swinging a tennis racquet, throwing a dart, striking a match, and similar activities. If one uses a needle to sew on a button, one is bound to hold it in the dominant hand. If one uses the other hand, the job will take much longer, be done less precisely, and be more difficult to accomplish without harming oneself. The same goes for writing. For such actions people know their handedness well and they show strong, consistent handedness patterns.

The three other dimensions or types of handedness appear to be less behaviorally salient. That is, they all involve activities in which handedness, in terms of the relative skill of the two hands, is not a significant factor. The second type of handedness involves *reaching actions*. When one reaches for a book or an apple on a table, it really doesn't matter which hand does the reaching. Either hand can manage the task equally well. There is no particular cost to using the nonpreferred hand and no real advantage to using the preferred hand. A third form of handedness involves *power actions*. An example is carrying a heavy suitcase. Although one might choose the strongest hand to begin with, the choice is not very stable because of the inclination to switch hands a lot when one is carrying a heavy load, so that ultimately both hands will be used. A final form of handedness involves *bimanual actions,* or actions that require two hands. For these last three classes of actions, people are less consistent in their hand use patterns and much more likely to use their hands interchangeably than they are for skilled actions.

Usually when we consider handedness, we are speaking only about the hand used for skilled activities. When Geschwind originally began to study handedness, he started out by using Oldfield's Edinburgh Handedness Battery (27). This battery, however, is not a pure measure of skilled activities because it contains a bimanual item, a reaching item, and two items not directly addressing handedness at all. For this reason Geschwind soon began to "tinker" with the questions. He altered the wording of some items and modified the scoring procedures as well, finally settling on a 10-item battery.

My own solution to measuring handedness follows Geschwind's in emphasizing the skilled movement dimension. However, I use a considerably shorter scale that my laboratory developed and validated over several years. My measure is the handedness subscale of the Lateral Preference Inventory (LPI), which also assesses other aspects of lateral preference (28). The four-item handedness scale determines the hand used to draw, throw a ball, remove the top card when dealing cards, and erase something on paper. The behavioral validity of these items has been determined by testing them against actual laboratory performance of these actions, and there is 97% concordance between the actual behaviors and the self-reports for these actions (23). We also measured test/retest reliabilities over a period of a full year and found an average concordance of 98% (29). One of the more interesting aspects of the LPI is that it has been empirically shown that this scale is highly correlated ($r = 0.95$) with an extended (12-item) scale (which contains all the skilled hand use items contained in Geschwind's version of the Edinburgh Inventory, plus several others). Furthermore, when used to classify subjects dichotomously into left- versus right-handed, there is a 98.9% concordance between the LPI brief scale and the extended handedness battery. The final point in favor of using the LPI handedness measure is that extensive normative data are available on this scale (28,30).

OTHER ASPECTS OF LATERALITY

When Geschwind first considered the hypopigmentation hypothesis, he was concerned solely with handedness. Handedness, however, is only one of several forms of lateral preference. Lateral preferences manifest themselves both in the motoric and sensory realms, in which one member of a bilateral pair of limbs or sense organs is habitually used in a variety of behavioral coordinations. We have already discussed handedness, which might be demonstrated when one hand is preferentially used for writing. Similarly, footedness is demonstrated when one foot is regularly used to kick a ball, eyedness when one eye is habitually used for sighting down a telescope, and earedness when one ear is regularly used to listen to the faint ticking of a watch. Whenever measures of these lateral preferences are taken, results indicate that human populations are biased toward right-sidedness on all four indexes. However, the degree of dextral bias varies among the various preference indexes, being strongest for handedness (88% right-handed) and weaker for the other indexes, with 81% right-footed, 71% right-eyed, and 60% right-eared (30). The specific proportions may vary somewhat from one study to another, depending on the stringency of the operational definition used. The same statistical and neurological arguments used for handedness as a marker or soft sign for pathology can be made for any of the other indexes of laterality. However, it is important to remember that, according to the way the model works, the more extreme the distributional split between the proportion of left- and right-dominant persons, the more strongly the index will be associated with pathology. Accordingly, we might expect hand preference to be a good indicator of risk, foot preference to be less good, and eye and ear preference to be the weakest predictors, based on the relative rarity of sinistrality in the four indexes. In my research, I often lean toward inclusion of all four indexes of lateral preference, partly for the sake of completeness but also to provide an indication of the strength of the effects that are obtained. Weaker effects may significantly involve handedness only, whereas stronger effects may produce significant shifts in all four indexes. Operating on this usual bias, I decided to include foot, eye, and ear preference as well as handedness in this look at hypopigmentation and laterality.

Although there are several self-report inventories for the measurement of handedness (see refs. 30,31 for reviews), very few questionnaires have been developed that can provide a quick, valid measure of all four indexes of lateral preference. The LPI provides not only a valid and reliable measure of handedness but also measures of foot, eye, and ear preferences (28). The LPI contains only 16 items (four items per subscale) and takes only 2 or 3 minutes to complete. Despite its brevity, experiments have demonstrated a 92% average concordance between self-reports for the LPI items and performance testing (23,30). As in the case of handedness, these measures showed high reliabilities over a period of a full year (29), and large-sample normative data are available for the foot, eye, and ear preference subscales in this inventory (28,30).

DEFINING RIGHT-HANDERS

Before the actual data can be discussed, one more measurement issue must be dealt with, the criterion to be used to define left- versus right-handedness (or sidedness). Various investigators use different criteria to distinguish dextrals from sinistrals. Traditionally, the data are dichotomized for any given scale. When the majority rule is used in scoring handedness, people who claimed that they performed more actions with the left hand are classified as left-handed, whereas people who claimed that they performed more actions with the right hand are classified as right-handed. Balanced mixed-handers, or ambidexters, who either claimed that they did everything with either hand or checked an equal number of items for left and right, are rare (usually 1% or less) and are traditionally lumped together with the left-handers (30).

When Geschwind became seriously involved in the collection of handedness data, he soon abandoned the simple majority rule classification procedure and adopted a considerably more stringent criterion. In his scoring of the ten-item Edinburgh Inventory, subjects could indicate for each item a degree of handedness by responding "always left," "usually left," "no preference," "usually right," or "always right." The laterality scores assigned to these responses by his resident, Steve Schachter, were –10, –5, 0, 5, and 10, respectively, and the person's handedness was simply the algebraic total, giving scores that run from –100 (strongly left-handed for everything) to +100 (strongly right-handed for everything). According to several letters that he wrote in 1982 and 1983, Geschwind was impressed by the fact that virtually no one who globally classified himself or herself as either a left-hander or an ambidexter ever had a score above 70 when this measuring scheme was used. Furthermore, around 75% of the population, all self-classified right-handers, had scores higher than 70. Thus the data seemed to suggest a natural, yet stringent, cutoff point, defining those with scores above 70 as right-handers and those with scores of 70 or below as non-right-handers. This dichotomy contrasts strong or consistent right-handers with all other handedness groups. Geschwind thought that inspection of the distribution of scores obtained would suggest how subjects and scores should be grouped for classification purposes.

This same theme appears in several other places in Geschwind's work. Although he first derived the stringent criterion for handedness based on the concordance between global handedness self-classifications and various Edinburgh Inventory scores, Geschwind soon came to believe that his strong criterion for right-handedness represented a measure of the degree of right hand dominance needed to accurately classify a person as belonging to a nonimpaired group. For example, in a letter to Peter Behan dated October 14, 1983, after a discussion with Robert Lahita, a clinician who worked with lupus erythematosus patients, he wrote:

> Lahita thought that left-handedness would not be elevated in lupus. But I have been over every questionnaire (about 150 so far). I did the laterality scores by the new method I wrote you. . . . [Here he describes the method again.] Now in the lupus cases there were almost no scores above +70 [underlined in the original]. On the other hand scores less than zero were not particularly frequent. Thus it appears that the curve is shifted to the left quite significantly. The big shift is therefore to the 0 to +70 range, but a cut-off of zero fails to pick up this very big shift.

Using dyslexia rather than lupus as his marker, Geschwind noted, in a letter to Camilla P. Benbow dated March 16, 1984, a replication of the case for the strong criterion for handedness:

> We then inspected the data carefully and found the following. The rate of dyslexia ran at 9% to 10% through all of the ranges from –100 to +70. Above +70 the rate fell abruptly to about 3%. . . . As you note in our series in which we studied dyslexia we let the data show us where the cut-off point was rather than choosing a cut-off point in advance which is after all not necessary.

With the shorter LPI handedness scale, one can produce the traditional dichotomy or a more stringent Geschwind-type dichotomy for classifying handedness. This is done by assigning a +1 for each response of "right," –1 for each response of "left," and 0 for each response of "either" or "both." An algebraic total is then computed (28). The score for handedness thus goes from 4 for consistent right-handedness (all activities done with the right hand, equivalent to Geschwind's +100) to –4 for consistent left-handedness (all activities done with the left hand, equivalent to Geschwind's –100). A score of 0 represents ambilaterality and is the same as Geschwind's score of 0. The traditional criterion defines right-handers as any subjects with scores greater than 0, and left-handers as subjects with scores less than or equal to 0. This is simply the majority rule definition of handedness (28,30,31). According to this criterion, about 87% of the population is right-handed. The stricter, Geschwind-type criterion dichotomizes the sample into a consistent right-handed group (with an LPI-based handedness index of 4) versus a non-right-handed group (with any scores less than 4). Thus the only people who are classified as right-handed are those who perform all of the four tested activities with their right hand. Although this may seem to be a more extreme cutoff than that used by Geschwind, when this criterion was used, the proportion of right-handers in the sample was 77%, which is similar to the approximately 75% noted by Geschwind using his +70 score cutoff on the Edinburgh Inventory.

The importance of where one sets the classification criterion for handedness has gradually forced itself into my consciousness during various research endeavors. In one case, I was specifically interested in Geschwind's suggestion that there is a relationship between handedness and allergic response (this issue is discussed in detail in Behan's chapter in this book). In my study (7), subjects were classified as allergic if they reported hypersensitivity to any one (or more) of a list of items, including several ingested substances (cow's milk, chocolate, eggs, wheat, oranges, apples, beef, fish, and bubble gum), inhaled and contact allergens (cats, dogs, dust, feathers, sun exposure, bee stings, and other insect bites), and a few common drugs (e.g., quinine, penicillin, sulfonamides). Using the traditional majority rule criterion for handedness, I found a small increased incidence of left-handedness in the allergic group (15.4% compared with 12.8%). However, because this difference was not statistically significant [$\chi^2(1) = 0.61$], the data failed to support the expected autoimmune relationship with handedness. The picture was quite different when I used the stricter, Geschwind-type definition of handedness. With this latter classification scheme I found 26.9% non-right-handers in the allergic group compared with only 18.4% in the nonallergic group, and this difference was statistically significant [$\chi^2(1) = 4.41; p < 0.05$]. This latter analysis clearly provides support for the handedness–autoimmune system link suggested by Geschwind. It also points out the increased sensitivity apparently obtained by using a more stringent cutoff for classifying right-handers.

To be consistent with Geschwind's scoring procedures in testing the relationship between laterality and hypopigmentation, I have used the more stringent criterion. This criterion is used not only for handedness but also for footedness, eyedness, and earedness. Specifically, then, for each laterality dimension we will contrast consistent right-siders (all four measured actions showing a right-hand preference) with those who are left-sided or ambidextral on any action, who would be classified as "non-right-siders" (a better label might be "adextrals"). When this scoring procedure is used to determine foot, eye, and ear preference, consistent right-sidedness is much rarer than right-handedness.

HYPOPIGMENTATION AND HANDEDNESS REVISITED

Let us now turn to the issue of hypopigmentation and sidedness, based on our 3,495 subjects. First, let us consider the effects of blond hair alone as a marker for increased likelihood of non-right-sidedness. Table 1 presents these data. Each value represents the number of adextrals, or non-right-siders, for each index. The table shows that there was a significantly higher percentage of non-right-handers in the group with the lightly pigmented, blond hair, confirming the findings of Schachter et al. (16). In addition, blonds were more likely to be non-right-footed. However, there were no significant differences for eye or ear preference.

Geschwind's laboratory looked only at hair color; however, as noted earlier, eye color is also a marker of reduced pigmentation, with blue-eyed persons generally being con-

Table 1. *An index of laterality: the percentage of non-right-siders for hand, foot, eye, and ear preference, as a function of hair color and eye color considered separately and conjointly*

	Hair color		Eye color		Hair and eye color combined	
	Blond	Not blond	Blue-eyed	Not blue-eyed	Both light	Not both light
Hand	22.0[a]	17.5*	21.8	17.3**	25.6	17.6**
Foot	61.1	54.1*	62.0	53.2***	62.2	54.4*
Eye	38.7	40.2	37.0	40.4	38.2	39.9
Ear	59.7	62.6	61.1	62.8	60.0	62.9

Statistical significance: *$p < 0.05$; **$p < 0.01$; ***$p < 0.001$.
[a]Entries are percentages of subjects who are not consistently right-sided.

siderably fairer and having fewer melanin-bearing cells than persons with darker eyes. Table 1 also presents the results comparing blue-eyed people with those with darker eye pigmentation. The pattern of results is quite similar to that observed for hair color. People with lighter eyes were more likely to be non-right-handed and non-right-footed, although there were no sinistral shifts found for eye or ear preference. These data help to generalize the Geschwind contention, extending the results to include eye color as a marker for hypopigmentation.

If blond hair and blue eyes are both adequate markers for reduced pigmentation, the effect should be accentuated if both markers are present. The final pair of columns in Table 1 report the results of comparing persons who are both blond and blue-eyed (lightly pigmented) with those who are not. Again, significant leftward shifts are found for lightly pigmented people when both handedness and footedness are considered, but not when eye or ear preference is indexed.

One way to estimate the size of the effects in Table 1 is to use a measure of relative risk (RR). For any given outcome, the relative risk would be defined as the ratio of the incidence of a condition in the group having what we hypothesize to be a pathological marker, to the incidence in the group without the marker. If the marker makes no difference, RR = 1.00. The relative risk of being non-right-handed if one is blond is 1.25. This means that if one is blond, the chance of being non-right-handed increases by 25%. Being blue-eyed produces virtually the same results (RR = 1.24). Combining the two markers raises the risk of adextral handedness in an almost simple additive manner, so that it is now 46% (RR = 1.46).

If the appearance of non-right-sidedness follows the rare trait marker model, then we should expect weaker effects on the other indexes of lateral preference, because their population splits are not as extreme, with footedness representing the best chance for additional significant effect. This is quite clearly the case, as shown in Table 1. The only significant impact that hypopigmentation has in the form of a shift away from right-sidedness in the other indexes of laterality is for footedness. Here, the effect of being blond raises the risk of adextrality to RR = 1.12, and the effect of being blue-eyed raises the risk to RR = 1.16. With both markers, there is no additivity (RR = 1.14). Eye and ear preference do not indicate any significant risk of reduced right-sidedness.

Now, more than a decade after Geschwind first suggested it, I find myself looking at a data set that confirms the "odd" prediction that light hair is associated with some developmental neural deficits expressed more in non-right-handed blonds. The fact that this phenomenon is actually due to a hypopigmentation factor, perhaps reducing the effectiveness of neural guides during development, is also supported here. The idea that hypopigmentation is causal comes from the fact that another marker of reduced pigmentation (namely, iris pigmentation) can also predict the same effects, at least for handedness. Persons with both markers for hypopigmentation have a higher risk of being non-right-handed than persons with only one of the markers. Finally, these results show that the underlying process produces effects that are strong enough to manifest themselves in measures of footedness. These findings would surely have made Geschwind quite happy, because footedness, like handedness, has often been explained with reference to dominance of the contralateral hemisphere of the brain.

I have dwelt on Geschwind's hypopigmentation and handedness hypothesis not because it is regarded as among his most important contributions, but because it reveals how his mind worked and perhaps something about his courage (or feistiness), which manifested itself in his willingness to express ideas that might elicit skepticism or outright disbelief at first hearing. His ideas always had certain characteristics that distinguished them from the combination of random associations of a "creativity machine." They were always about interesting topics, and they brought together interesting associations. Perhaps more important, his ideas did not exist as self-contained entities. They were all hooked together by an overriding theoretical framework that contained both implicit and explicit components. Thus, the hypopigmentation and handedness link was, when I first heard it, quite a bizarre notion. Yet, over time, I came to see it as just another outcropping of the larger theoretical structure from which Geschwind worked. This outcropping contained elements that reflected on the "grand questions" of neural development, and it influences every aspect of our behavior and our being.

I am reminded of something that the French mathematician Henri Poincaré wrote in 1902 (32): "Science is built of facts the way a house is built of bricks: but the accumulation of facts is no more science than a pile of bricks is a house." In my eyes, Geschwind first seemed to be a man with a great pile of brick-like associations. Yet as I got to know his work, it soon became easy to see that he had shaped from those "bricks" a sound scientific "house." It is the architectural vision that produced that theoretical structure, not the results of individual experiments or associative bricks, that is his legacy.

ACKNOWLEDGMENTS

This research was supported in part by grants from the Natural Sciences and Engineering Research Council of Canada, the British Columbia Health Care Research Fund, and the Medical Research Council of Canada. I would like to gratefully acknowledge the assistance of David Wong, Wayne Wong, Joan Coren, Marion Buday, Susan Dixon, Kevin Donelly, Geof Donelly, and Tanya Jackson, and all the other members of the research staff of the Human Neuropsychology and Perception Laboratory of the University of British Columbia who helped with various aspects of the data collection.

REFERENCES

1. Coren S, Searleman A. Birth stress and left-handedness: the rare trait marker model. In: Coren S, ed. *Left-handedness: behavioral implications and anomalies. Advances in psychology,* no. 67. Amsterdam, the Netherlands: North-Holland, 1990;3–32.
2. Brodal A. *The central nervous system: structure and function.* New York: Oxford University Press, 1992.
3. Goodwin AW, Darian-Smith I. *Hand function and the neocortex.* New York: Springer-Verlag, 1985.
4. Lewis OJ. *Functional morphology of the evolving hand and foot.* New York: Oxford University Press, 1989.
5. Kuypers HGJM. The anatomical and functional organization of the motor system. In: Swash M, Kennard C, eds. *Scientific basis of clinical neurology.* Edinburgh, Scotland: Churchill Livingstone, 1985;3–18.

6. Geschwind N, Galaburda AM. *Cerebral lateralization: biological mechanisms, associations, and pathology.* Cambridge, MA: MIT Press, 1985.
7. Coren S. Handedness and allergic response. *Int J Neurosci* 1994;76:231–236.
8. Le Douarin N. *The neural crest.* Cambridge, England: Cambridge University Press, 1982.
9. Geschwind N, Galaburda AM. Cerebral lateralization: biological mechanisms, associations, and pathology. III. A hypothesis and a program for research. *Arch Neurol* 1985;42:521–552.
10. Creel D, O'Donnell FE, Witkop CJ Jr. Visual system anomalies in human ocular albinos. *Science* 1978;201: 931–933.
11. Guillery RW, Okoro AN, Witkop CJ Jr. Abnormal visual pathways in the brain of a human albino. *Brain Res* 1975;96:373–377.
12. Ghosh A, Woo JSK, Poon IML, Ma HK. Neural-tube defects in Hong Kong Chinese. *Lancet* 1981;2:468–469.
13. Huszar D, Sharpe A, Jaenisch R. Migration and proliferation of cultured neural crest cells in W mutant neural crest chimeras. *Development* 1991;112:131–141.
14. Perris R, Lofberg J, Fallstrom C, von Boxberg Y, Olsson L, Newgreen DF. Structural and compositional divergencies in the extracellular matrix encountered by neural crest cells in the white mutant axolotl embryo. *Development* 1990;109:533–551.
15. MacDonald JF, Brandes L, Deverill M, Mody I, Salter MW, Theriault E. Mammalian neurons in dissociated cultures form clusters in the presence of retinal pigment epithelium. *Exp Brain Res* 1991;83:643–655.
16. Schachter SC, Ransil BJ, Geschwind N. Associations of handedness with hair color and learning disabilities. *Neuropsychologia* 1987;25:269–276.
17. Coren S. Eye color and pure-tone hearing thresholds. *Percept Motor Skills* 1994;79:1373–1374.
18. Barrenas ML, Lindgren F. The influence of eye colour on susceptibility to TTS in humans. *Br J Audiol* 1991;25: 303–307.
19. Cable J, Huszar D, Jaenisch R, Steel KP. The effects of mutations at the W locus (c-*kit*) on inner ear pigmentation and function in the mouse. *Pigment Cell Res* 1994;7:17–32.
20. Bonvillian JD, Orlansky MD, Garland JB. Handedness patterns in deaf persons. *Brain Cogn* 1982;1:141–157.
21. Satz P, Achenbach K, Fennel E. Correlations between assessed manual laterality and predicted speech laterality in a normal population. *Neuropsychologia* 1967;5:295–310.
22. Raczkowski D, Kalat JW, Nebes R. Reliability and validity of some handedness questionnaire items. *Neuropsychologia* 1974;12:43–47.
23. Coren S, Porac C, Duncan P. A behaviorally validated self-report inventory to assess four types of lateral preference. *J Clin Neuropsychol* 1979;1:55–64.
24. Peters M. Phenotype in normal left-handers: an understanding of phenotype is the base for understanding mechanism and inheritance of handedness. In: Coren S, ed. *Left-handedness: behavioral implications and anomalies. Advances in psychology,* no. 67. Amsterdam, the Netherlands: North-Holland, 1990;167–194.
25. Healey JM, Liederman J, Geschwind N. Handedness is not a unidimensional trait. *Cortex* 1986;22:33–53.
26. Steenhuis RE, Bryden MP. Different dimensions of hand preference that relate to skilled and unskilled activities. *Cortex* 1989;25:289–304.
27. Oldfield RC. The assessment and analysis of handedness: the Edinburgh Inventory. *Neuropsychologia* 1971;9: 97–113.
28. Coren S. The Lateral Preference Inventory for measurement of handedness, footedness, eyedness and earedness: norms for young adults. *Bull Psychonomic Soc* 1993;31:1–3.
29. Coren S, Porac C. The validity and reliability of self-report items for the measurement of lateral preference. *Br J Psychol* 1978;69:207–211.
30. Porac C, Coren S. *Lateral preferences and human behavior.* New York: Springer-Verlag, 1981.
31. Coren S. *The left-hander syndrome: the causes and consequences of left-handedness.* New York: Free Press, 1992.
32. Poincaré H. *La science et l'hypothese.* Paris, France: Fammariaon, 1902/1968.

31

Handedness and Autoimmune Disease

Peter O. Behan

Department of Neurology, Institute of Neurological Sciences, Southern General Hospital, Glasgow G514TF.

EARLY EXPERIENCES

I went to Boston City Hospital to complete a year as a research fellow in psychiatry before beginning my residency in neurology. While there, I attended Dr. Geschwind's lectures and immediately fell under his spell. I decided then that I wished to be trained by Dr. Geschwind. I realized soon after I joined his service that he had a rigorous but somewhat unusual method of working. In the morning he would stay in his room, reading voraciously from a wide range of material. Once he had finished reading, he felt compelled to discuss whatever he had found interesting with virtually anyone who would listen. I remember many occasions when I was ready to leave work at 6:00 PM but was still listening well past 8:00 PM to Dr. Geschwind's discussion of some particular item.

During my early years with Norman, two interesting patients were admitted to the hospital in close succession. One was a man in whom acute hemorrhagic leukoencephalitis was diagnosed after he had undergone a cerebral biopsy; the other was a man in whom a strange neurological disorder with coma developed after he was stung on the testicle by a bee. The latter patient turned out to have atypical multiple sclerosis in association with hypertrophic polyneuritis. Both these patients were found to have atypical lymphocytes in their peripheral blood, lymphoblastoid cells that were actively synthesizing DNA (1). These cells immediately became the focus of Norman's attention. I was dispatched to Boston with slides of the cells to show to leading authorities on hematology and immunology. This is an illustration of another of Norman's working principles: If he did not understand something, he readily asked for advice, without feeling humiliated, from someone who did.

I dutifully showed the cells to a variety of professors and was informed that they were immunoblasts from patients who were actively undergoing an allergic reaction. Norman's mind was at once turned on to what it could be that these patients were allergic to, and after much discussion, the culprit antigens were posited to be neural in type, possibly myelin basic proteins. I was then sent to the laboratory of Dr. John David to learn *in vitro* techniques of macrophage inhibition, and to other laboratories to master lymphocyte culture and transformation. Both these techniques were soon standardized in a small room in the Veterans' Administration Hospital that became devoted to neuroimmunologic research. The results of these experiments showed that in patients with postinfectious encephalomyelitis, and in others with idiopathic polyneuropathy, the pathogenesis was mediated by immunologic processes (2–4). Indeed, this was the first demonstration that postinfectious encephalomyelitis is an autoimmune disorder and that delayed-type hypersensitivity to encephalitogenic myelin basic protein develops secondary to a viral infection. This finding is now well established (5).

Based on our early findings, we began to investigate experimental allergic encephalomyelitis. Nonhuman primates rather than small animals were used for the research because Norman believed that the results would be more akin to what occurred in human beings. We soon found that baboons and monkeys immunized to develop experimental allergic encephalomyelitis had cells similar to those immunoblasts that we had found in humans with demyelinating diseases in their peripheral blood. We also found that, using the same *in vitro* techniques mentioned previously, we could demonstrate delayed-type hypersensitivity to encephalitogenic myelin basic proteins in these animals (4). Indeed, by varying the immunizing dose we were able to reproduce an exact animal model for both postinfectious encephalomyelitis and acute hemorrhagic leukoencephalitis (4). Further studies ensued, including detailed immunopathological and pathological analyses of acute hemorrhagic leukoencephalitis in human beings, so that a precise comparison with the animal models was made at all levels (6). The encephalitogenic myelin basic proteins were supplied by the late Dr. Marian Kies from the National Institutes of Health, and fruitful collaborative research was established with her laboratory. Many papers were published during this time, and all our experiments were the result of long, protracted discussions with Norman, who would advocate the principle that a pencil and a piece of paper, with the topic discussed ad nauseam, was by far the best preparation for any experiment (i.e., prolonged discussions are necessary for any good experimental design). Because of Norman's interest, patients with rare cases were often obtained for testing, and in some of these patients we were able to demonstrate that a variant of the Miller-Fisher syndrome had the same pathogenesis and similar immunologic mechanisms as those found in Guillain-Barré polyneuritis (7).

One of the original patients whom we had tested using *in vitro* techniques became afflicted with a bizarre neurological condition after he received a bee sting, as mentioned previously. He was later shown to have multiple sclerosis with peripheral nerve involvement. Norman followed the man's case very carefully, always giving the patient attentive personal care. Until the patient's death, I was sent on many occasions to collect blood samples and repeat experiments on his blood. The patient's postmortem examination showed that he had multiple sclerosis with hypertrophic polyneuropathy. We repeatedly discussed among ourselves and with a variety of experts why both entities had occurred in the same patient; these discussions resulted in a major paper being published in *Brain* by Dr. Schoene from the Peter Bent Brigham Hospital in Boston. Additional cases were contributed to this study by Dr. Stirling Carpenter from McGill (8). One other fascinating feature about this patient was that he had a brother with multiple sclerosis, a fact that immediately caused Norman to become acutely interested in the role of genetics in multiple sclerosis and genetics in general.

Geschwind's understanding of genetics was evident in his subsequent papers and in his many discussions of cerebral lateralization and the biological associations with anomalous dominance. Some years later, we published a paper in *Immunology Today* on hormones, handedness, and immunity, which was commented on by a physician who disagreed with some of our conclusions. It can be seen from Norman's reply (resulting from letters and telephone calls between Glasgow and Boston) that he had a very deep and critical knowledge of genetics, particularly the role of the major histocompatibility antigens and immune response genes (9). Around this time he discussed with me, when I was compiling a book on the genetics of muscle diseases, some very important observations on how the major histocompatibility complex loci control immune responses.

THE DEVELOPMENT OF HIS EARLY OBSERVATIONS ON DOMINANCE

On my return to Great Britain, I was appointed lecturer at the University of Glasgow. My interest in neuroimmunology continued, focusing on muscle diseases because my chief was Professor John A. Simpson, who was the first to suggest that myasthenia gravis is an autoimmune disease. From time to time, Norman would visit Glasgow and give lectures, and we would discuss our various lines of research. He had been at the National Hospital, Queen Square, with both John Walton and Ian Simpson, and his visits to Glasgow were always a delight. A dinner party was invariably arranged, at which Norman would entertain us with monologues on such diverse topics as the selection of roots for different good vines and why diabetes mellitus is more common in broad-shouldered women. He had an enormous range of interests, and his discussions were those of a very cultured man. At these university dinners he often demonstrated his marvelous skill as a raconteur, regaling us with jokes and stories, often bursting into peals of laughter before he came to the point of his story. So well liked and popular was he in Scotland that it was very easy to get him elected Honorary Fellow of the Royal College of Physicians and Surgeons of Glasgow upon my initial proposal.

My wife and I spent some time in late 1980 working at Massachusetts General Hospital with Dr. E. P. Richardson. At that time, Norman had already begun his major work on cerebral dominance. While we were having dinner at his home one evening, the question arose whether any of us had observed an association between any diseases and left-handedness. Curiously, I had just treated two cases of progressive dementia in patients who had premature white hair and who were strongly left-handed. These patients were also interesting for another reason: they each had thyroiditis and had responded to thyroid replacement therapy. Norman stated that he had seen a patient with a similar history that week. He also immediately recalled a professor and his daughter whom he knew intimately and both of whom were left-handed and had premature gray hair and possible early dementia.

These associations intrigued Norman greatly, and we decided to conduct a formal study, which we carried out in Glasgow. The results were published in the *Proceedings of the National Academy of Sciences* in 1982 and received great attention (10). In 1984, the first World Congress of Neuroimmunology was held at Stresa, Italy, where Sir John Walton, now Lord Walton, gave the initial address entitled "Neuroimmunology Comes of Age" (11). In this talk, he referred to Panum's observation in 1846 that a single attack of measles confers lifelong immunity. This clinical observation, which demonstrated two of the most important features of immunology—its specificity and its memory—may not have received, at the time, the attention it merited, but like Norman's observation, it had enormous implications.

The hypothesis put forward by Norman likewise has had wide-ranging effects, and his major paper in the *Archives of Neurology* will continue to generate research ideas for some time to come. At the 1984 World Congress of Neuroimmunology, Norman was asked to deliver a talk on the immunologic associations of cerebral dominance. Even at this stage, his contributions were recognized as seminal. Now with the explosion that has occurred in neuroimmunology and molecular biology, the mechanisms exist to develop and explore his theories. At the congress he stood among the world's leading neuroimmunologists and gave a splendid account of what he saw as the biological foundations of cerebral dominance, particularly as it involved immune factors. With his extraordinary depth of knowledge, he reviewed the history of learning disabilities and left-handedness and showed that the incidence of certain immune disorders is increased among persons with learning disabilities. He highlighted the increased incidence of atopic disorders in patients who stutter and showed that there is an increased incidence of certain autoimmune diseases, particularly celiac disease, among children with autism. He further illustrated the role of genetics by showing that the incidence of autoimmune thyroid diseases is elevated in the parents of children with celiac disease and that the incidence of Down syndrome is often increased in the relatives of children with autism (12).

We now know a great deal about the effects of testosterone on the immune system, and research continues in this very important area. In 1981, while Norman and I were on a train from Dublin to Cork, where Norman was to address the Irish Neurological Association, he told me that his readings had left him without any doubt that it was the effects of testosterone combined with genetic influences that lay behind the curious biological associations of left-handedness. At that time, some data existed, but now we know much more about the effects of androgens on the immune response, particularly because of the work of Stimson and his colleagues in Glasgow (13) and other researchers worldwide. Immunoglobulin levels are higher in females (14), females mount greater primary and secondary responses to a number of pathogens, including viruses (15), and cellular-mediated immunity is also greater in females. These facts may very well explain the increased incidence of autoimmunity in females and the protective effect of testosterone. Some enteroviral infections in infancy attack only male children. Norman was forever pointing out that atopic illnesses were more common in boys before puberty, but they decreased with the production of testosterone and increased again as testosterone waned (12). That testosterone can increase a person's susceptibility to infection and interfere with experimentally induced autoimmune diseases is now recognized. Testosterone can have similar effects on the immune system and the nervous system; the latter can be beautifully demonstrated by a morphologic analysis of Onuf's nucleus in murine models, in which testosterone increases the proliferation of cells in this nucleus (16).

VERIFICATION OF A HYPOTHESIS

Castration and restoration experiments in animals have demonstrated that testosterone affects both helper and suppressor cells (17). In experiments on the New Zealand F_1 mouse, testosterone has been shown to affect immunity *in vivo* (18). Testosterone has been demonstrated to cause thymic atrophy in animals, and a number of investigators have demonstrated the presence of specific androgen receptors on the thymic epithelium. The fact that these receptors have been demonstrated on the thymic epithelium but not on lymphocytes suggests that one method of producing their immunomodulatory effects is through inducing changes in thymic processing of lymphocytes via the thymic epithelium (13). Likewise, as experiments with birds have shown, testosterone has an effect on the bursa of Fabricius and, presumably, a similar effect on the mammalian equivalent in bone marrow. Indeed, Sullivan and Wira (19) have demonstrated a bursal testosterone receptor. McCruden and Stimson (13) recently reviewed the effects of sex hormones on the immune system, and it is clear from a wide variety of experiments that the sex steroids play a major role in the differentiation of not only sexual and central nervous tissue but also lymphoid tissue and its function.

A vast amount of clinical observation and experimentation have now shown a clear-cut relationship between the immune and nervous systems. Indeed, modulation by the central nervous system of immunologic reactions may be lateralized (20). The association between left-handedness and autoimmune disease has now been confirmed by other investigators, particularly for Crohn's disease, ulcerative colitis, and diabetes type I (21), whereas other researchers have shown that there is an association between left-handedness and atopic disorders, including urticaria, asthma, and eczema (22). Children who are allergic to mites have an increased incidence of left-handedness (23), and young children, particularly boys who are mathematically gifted, have an increased incidence of allergy and left-handedness (24). There is a significant increase in both autoimmune and allergic disorders in dyslexic patients (25). A number of other studies, including detailed family histories of Nobel laureates whose grandparents were also Nobel laureates, have demonstrated the same association. Animal studies have also shown an association between handedness and immune disorders (26). Some studies have not confirmed this association (27), but there are valid reasons why they did not reach such a conclusion. For instance, in one study of handedness and allergy in children, the age range of the children went up to 16 years (27). Including older children in that study may well have masked the relationship between left-handedness and allergies that exists only in early life, as Norman pointed out on many occasions.

I am continually being reminded about Norman's observations when I am in the clinic and in discussions with colleagues who are studying sex hormones, and I have confirmed many of his predictions.

In other studies, we had found that some patients with dyslexia had a high titer of anti-Ro antibodies (28). In evaluating anti-Ro antibody, we confirmed that it was present in women who had given birth to children with congenital heart disease and also in women who had recurrent abortions. This finding of course brought us back to lupus erythematosus, and the question of hormones was raised again in the study of these patients. One other discovery was the finding of anti-Ro antibodies in patients with depressed levels of complement, who turned out to have connective tissue disorders, particularly lupus and polymyositis, and who themselves often had conductive tissue anomalies of their hearts (29).

Great scientists are said to fall into two categories, those who are intuitive and those who are cartesian. Norman Geschwind was certainly of the intuitive variety: he possessed unique powers not only of observation but also of understanding and manufacturing. He had, as the late Patrick Surander from Gothenburg often stated, enormous fantasy and vision. I will continue to mourn his loss.

REFERENCES

1. Behan PO, Lamarche JB. A new cell in demyelinating disease? *Lancet* 1968;2:52–53.
2. Behan PO, Geschwind N, Lamarche JB, Lisak RP, Kies M. Delayed hypersensitivity to encephalitogenic protein in disseminated encephalomyelitis. *Lancet* 1968;2:1009–1012.
3. Behan PO, Lamarche JB, Behan WMH, Feldman RG, Kies M. Immunopathological mechanisms of allergic neuritis in animals, primates and man. *Trans Am Neurol Assoc* 1969;94:219–222.
4. Behan PO, Behan WMH, Kies MW, Feldman RG. Cell-mediated hypersensitivity to neural antigens: occurrence in human patients and nonhuman primates with neurological diseases. *Arch Neurol* 1972;27:145–152.
5. Johnson RT, Griffen DE, Hirsch RL, Wolinsky JS, Roedenbeck S, De Soriano IL, Vaisberg A. Measles encephalomyelitis: clinical and immunologic studies. *N Engl J Med* 1984;310:137–141.
6. Lamarche JB, Behan PO, Segarra JM, Feldman RG. Recurrent acute necrotizing haemorrhagic encephalopathy. *Acta Neuropathol (Berl)* 1972;22:79–87.
7. Behan PO, Geschwind N. The ophthalmoplegic form of the Guillain-Barré syndrome: an immunologic study. *Acta Ophthalmol* 1973;51:529–542.
8. Schoene WC, Carpenter S, Behan PO, Geschwind N. The simultaneous occurrence of multiple sclerosis and hypertrophic neuropathy. (A study zof four autopsied cases and review of the literature.) *Brain* 1977;100:755–773.
9. Geschwind N, Behan PO. Hormones, handedness and immunity. *Immunol Today* 1984;5:190–191.
10. Geschwind N, Behan PO. Left-handedness: association with immune disease, migraine and developmental learning disorder. *Proc Natl Acad Sci* 1982;79:5097–5100.

11. Walton J. Neuroimmunology comes of age. In: Behan P, Spreafico F, eds. *Neuroimmunology*. New York: Raven Press, 1984;1–9.
12. Geschwind N. Immunological associations of cerebral dominance. In: Behan P, Spreafico F, eds. *Neuroimmunology*. New York: Raven Press, 1984;451–461.
13. McCruden AB, Stimson WH. Effects of estrogens/androgens on the immune response. In: Grossman CJ, ed. *Bilateral communication between the endocrine and immune systems*. New York: Springer-Verlag, 1994;36–50.
14. Rowley MJ, MacKay IR. Measurement of antibody-producing capacity in man. *Clin Exp Immunol* 1969;5:407–418.
15. London WI, Drew JR. Sex differences in the response to hepatitus B infection among patients receiving chronic dialysis treatment. *Proc Natl Acad Sci USA* 1977;74:2561–2563.
16. Keir SD. *The role of testosterone in the development of neuroanatomical lesions associated with specific learning disorders* [thesis]. Glasgow, Scotland: University of Glasgow, 1993.
17. Aboudkhil S, Bureau JP, Garrelly L, Vago P. Effects of castration, depotestosterone and cyproterone acetate on T-lymphocyte subsets in mouse thymus and spleen. *Scand J Immunol* 1991;34(5):647–653.
18. Burnet FM, Hornes MC. The natural history of the NZB/NZW F_1 mouse: a laboratory model of systemic lupus erythematosis. *Australas Ann Med* 1965;14:185–191.
19. Sullivan DA, Wira CR. Sex hormone and glucocorticoid receptors in the bursa of Fabricius of immature chicks. *J Immunol* 1979;122:2617–2623.
20. Biziere K, Guillaumin JM, Deguenne D, Renoux M, Renoux G. Lateralized neocortical modulation of the T-cell lineage. In: Guillemin R, Cohn M, Melnechuk T, eds. *Neural modulation of immunity*. New York: Raven Press, 1985;81–94.
21. Searleman A, Fugagli AK. Suspected autoimmune disorders and left-handedness: evidence from individuals with diabetes, Crohn's disease and ulcerative colitis. *Neuropsychologia* 1987;25:367–374.
22. Smith J. Left-handedness: its associations with allergic disease. *Neuropsychologia* 1987;25:665–674.
23. Lelong M, Thelliez F, Thelliez P. Les gauchers sont-ils plus souvent des allergiques? *Allerg Immunol* 1986;18:10–13.
24. Benbow CP, Benbow RM. Biological correlates of high mathematical reasoning ability. *Prog Brain Res* 1984;61:469–490.
25. Pennington BF, Smith SD, Kimberling WJ, Green PA, Haith MM. Handedness and immune disorders in familial dyslexics. *Arch Neurol* 1987;44:634–639.
26. Denenberg VH. Behavioral asymmetry. In: Geschwind N, Galaburda AM, eds. *Cerebral dominance: the biological foundations*. Cambridge, MA: Harvard University Press, 1984;114–133.
27. Bishop DVM. Is there a link between handedness and hypersensitivity? *Cortex* 1986;22:289–296.
28. Behan WMG, Behan PO, Geschwind N. Anti-Ro antibody in mothers of dyslexic children. *Dev Med Child Neurol* 1985;27:538–542.
29. Behan WMH, Behan PO, Gairns J. Cardiac damage in polymyositis associated with antibodies to tissue ribonucleoproteins. *Br Heart J* 1987;57:176–180.

Epilogue

32

Norman Geschwind (1926–1984)*

Albert M. Galaburda

Department of Neurology, Beth Israel Hospital, Boston, Massachusetts 02215.

On November 4, Norman Geschwind died suddenly at his home in Brookline, Massachusetts. With his passing, the broad community of neuroscience has suffered a heavy and premature loss. Dr. Geschwind played a unique role in neurology and neuropsychology, the effects of which will be felt for years to come.

Norman Geschwind was born in New York City on January 8, 1926. Near the turn of the century, his parents had come to the United States from the region of Tarnow and Mielec in Polish Galicia, then a part of Austro-Hungary. When Norman was only 4 years old, his father died of pneumonia, and the family, which consisted of his mother and his older brother Irving, moved to the Brooklyn section of New York. There, the young Geschwind attended first the Hebrew Institute of Boro Park and subsequently the prominent Boys High School. In his high school years he was keenly interested in Latin, French, English literature and mathematics, and he received several honors in these subjects.

Beginning in 1942, Geschwind, on a Pulitzer Scholarship, attended Harvard College, where he concentrated in mathematics. However, his studies were interrupted by the war; he joined the United Stares Army and was shipped to Europe in 1944 and to Japan in 1945. After the war ended, he returned to Harvard, where he finished his studies leading to the Bachelor of Arts degree (magna cum laude).

Geschwind attended Harvard Medical School from 1947 to 1951 and carried out a medical internship at the Beth Israel Hospital from 1951 to 1952. Subsequently, he traveled to London on a Moseley Scholarship, where he spent 3 years at the National Hospital (Queen Square) working with Ian Simpson. During that time, he studied the problem of myotonia and its treatment with procaine amide.

In 1955, Geschwind returned to Boston as chief Neurology resident in the service of Derek Denny-Brown at the Boston City Hospital. Following that tenure, he joined the staff of Francis O. Schmitt, at the Massachusetts Institute of Technology, to work on axonal physiology.

By 1958, Geschwind's interests had turned from neurophysiology to psychology, and he joined Fred Quadfasel at Boston's Veterans Administration Hospital, where his work on the higher functions began. Quadfasel retired and Geschwind replaced him as chief of the service in 1963. The Boston University Aphasia Center was established by 1966, and Geschwind became its director and professor and chairman of the Department of Neurology.

In 1969, Geschwind returned to Harvard as the James Jackson Putnam Professor and Director of the Harvard Neurological Unit of the Boston City Hospital. In 1975, the Har-

---

*Reprinted with permission of *Neuropsychologia* 1985;23:297-304 and the author.

vard unit moved to the Beth Israel Hospital, where Geschwind remained as chief until the time of his death.

Although Geschwind made several important contributions to general neurology, his influence was felt most strongly in the neurology of behavior and neuropsychology. During the early years of his involvement in psychology, Geschwind, as almost everyone else at that time, had been greatly influenced by the holistic views of Hughlings Jackson, Kurt Goldstein, and Henry Head. However, an important change took place soon after he had arrived at the Veteran's Hospital and was exposed to large numbers of patients with cognitive disorders. The rationale for this change is best expressed by his own words, written in 1964 in his critique of the role of Kurt Goldstein in the history of aphasia:

> Somewhere about 1960, I awoke, perhaps belatedly, to my own profound confusion. . . . I was persistently troubled by the fact that people who had left their mark so indelibly in many areas of neurology, such as Wernicke, Bastian, Déjérine, Charcot, and many others, could apparently have shown what was asserted to be the sheerest naivete and incompetence in the area of the higher functions. . . . Rather than accept the authority of even so distinguished a group as Marie, von Monakow, Head, and Goldstein, [I decided to] go back to the original literature and see for [myself] whether indeed the evidence was so poor as had been suggested. . . . The picture that emerged from this study was not the classic one of the chaotic confabulations of a group of tedious imperceptive German scholars, but rather that of the healthy active disagreements of a lively science. (1, p. 215)

With this introduction, Geschwind launched a revival of this lively science, and by this action, he became known around the world as its clearest and most incisive champion.

At around that time, Geschwind was introduced by Edith Kaplan to a patient known as Mr. K. The patient had had surgery for a left frontal glioblastoma, and he showed a strong grasping reflex in his right hand—a perfect opportunity for Dr. Kaplan to test the Bouman and Grunbaum hypothesis that pure agraphia was caused by a grasping reflex. As it turned out, the patient showed aphasia in writing only with his left hand. Geschwind carried out a detailed neurological examination and reasoned that, during surgery, the anterior cerebral artery had been ligated, which resulted in infarction of the anterior portion of the corpus callosum, thus disconnecting the left-hemisphere language zones from the right-hemisphere areas controlling the left hand. A case report was prepared for Neurology, and, while the paper was still in press, Mr. K. died. His brain was examined at postmortem, and the lesion predicted by Geschwind was found; these new findings were added in footnote to the article (2).

The syndrome of the corpus callosum had been described recently by Sperry in cats, but the work of Akelaitis had suggested that it did not exist in humans. The findings in Mr. K., however, reinforced in Geschwind the notion that the old observations needed to be taken seriously, and this led to the massive literature search and intellectual effort that culminated in the publication of the paper "Disconnexion syndromes in animals and man" (3). Furthermore, the rebirth of the connexional approach led to modern descriptions of conduction aphasia and pure alexia, and uncovered the previously unknown isolation of the speech area.

The second major chapter in Geschwind's contribution to neuropsychology was inaugurated with his study (with Walter Levitsky) of anatomic asymmetries in the language areas (4). He had come across a statement by Gerhard von Bonin, in which the anatomist had written that there were no anatomic asymmetries in the human brain to account for the striking functional lateralization it exhibits. Geschwind again delved into the classic literature and discovered a cornucopia of findings of anatomic asymmetry in the brains of animals and men. He then repeated and expanded the study of Richard Pfeifer, a student of Paul Flechsig, and demonstrated the striking asymmetry of the planum temporale.

Several workers confirmed these findings, and still others found additional asymmetries in autopsy brains, in radiologic studies and in endocasts of primitive man. Subsequently Geschwind stimulated the study of brain asymmetries at the microscopic level, asymmetries during brain development, and the asymmetries in animals.

In addition to his work on aphasia and its related disorders, and on cerebral dominance and its anatomic substrates, Geschwind made important inroads to the understanding of the behavioral effects of limbic epilepsy and of traumatic amnesia. However, his last major contribution is apt to become the most original and most significant of his career. During the last few years, Geschwind became interested in the developmental learning disabilities, and he set out to uncover its neurological substrates. His keen clinical acumen led to his noticing that mothers of dyslexic children often reported left-handedness, atopic illnesses, and thyroid disease. With Peter Behan, in Glasgow, he then designed a study of over 1,000 left-handed individuals coming to a shop for left-handed utensils in London, and showed that there was a significant increase in the incidence of stuttering, dyslexia, colitis, thyroid disease, and myasthenia gravis in the population of strongly left-handed individuals (5). Follow-up studies expanded these findings to include other illnesses as well, and found associations between laterality scores, learning disabilities, blond hair, and occupation. Furthermore this work led to the finding in immune defective mice of developmental brain changes and learning disorder.

Geschwind's work evolved from the reestablishment of classic thinking to the forging of new frontiers, thus reinforcing the idea that in order to make progress, it is necessary to know the useful past. Geschwind's last work, like his early writings, remains an invitation to the world community of neuroscience to test his hypotheses for right or wrong, always in the spirit of lively science he so much believed in.

REFERENCES

1. Geschwind N. The paradoxical position of Kurt Goldstein in the history of aphasia. *Cortex* 1964;1:214–224.
2. Geschwind N, Kaplan E. A human deconnection syndrome: a preliminary report. *Neurology* 1962;12:675–685.
3. Geschwind N. Disconnexion syndromes in animals and man. (2 parts). *Brain* 1965;88:237–294, 585–644.
4. Geschwind N, Levitsky W. Human brain: left-right asymmetries in temporal speech region. *Science* 1968;161:186–187.
5. Geschwind N, Behan P. Left-handedness: association with immune disease, migraine, and developmental learning disorder. *Proc Natl Acad Sci USA* 1983;79:5097–5100.

Subject Index

A

Abstract behavior, 80
Academy of Aphasia, founding, 18
Achromatopsia, 121
Acoustical study, affective prosody, 185–187
Acute confusional state
 agraphia, 134
 descriptions, 133
 etiology, 136–137
 lesions associated, 133–138
 right middle cerebral artery territory infarction, 136–137
 systemic metabolic disturbance, 133
 unilateral neglect, 135
Acute dementia, stroke, 136
Acute hemorrhagic leukoencephalitis, 287
Adenosine, progesterone, 232
Affective gesture
 right hemisphere, 184
 right hemisphere infarction, 185
Affective prosody
 acoustical study, 185–187
 aphasia, 186
 hemispheric lateralization, 185–187
 right hemisphere, 184
 right hemisphere infarction, 185
 Wada test, 187–188
Age, handedness, 263
Aggressive character disorder, 218
Aggressiveness
 complex partial seizure, 213
 temporal lobe epilepsy, 215, 218
Agraphia, 116
 acute confusional state, 134
 alexia, 74
Akinetopsia, 121
Alexia, 74, 116
 agraphia, 74
 color, 83
Allergy, handedness, 282
Alzheimer's disease, 165
 conceptual apraxia, 180
 olfaction, 167
American Academy of Neurology, 18
 behavioral neurology section, 76
American Neurological Association, 3–4, 15

Amnestic aphasia, 80
Amorphosynthesis, 10
Amygdala, 214
 ventromedial hypothalamus, 224
 visual pathway, 221f
Androgen, epilepsy, 224
Androgen deficiency
 antiseizure medication, 225–227
 enhancement of testosterone conversion to estradiol, 225–227
 gonadal steroid synthesis suppression, 225
 sex-hormone-binding globulin synthesis induction, 225
 causes, 224–227
 epilepsy, 224–225
Angular gyrus of left temporoparietal region, anomia, 83
Anomalous functional dominance, 259
Anomia, 79–87
 anatomic basis, 83
 angular gyrus of left temporoparietal region, 83
 contemporary approaches, 84–87
 historical aspects, 79–81
 1950s concepts, 79–81
 varieties, 82–84
Anomic aphasia, 79
Anosognosia, 129
Anterior temporal cortex, 221, 221f
Anti-Ro antibody, dyslexia, 291
Antiseizure medication, androgen deficiency, 225–227
 enhancement of testosterone conversion to estradiol, 225–227
 gonadal steroid synthesis suppression, 225
 sex-hormone-binding globulin synthesis induction, 225
Anxiety, reproductive endocrine disorder, 234, 235f
Aphasia, 8–9, 41, 71–77, 89, 117, 171, 296
 affective prosody, 186
 classification, 75
 historical aspects, 71–72
 information-processing system, 171

left hemisphere lesion, 172
repetition of spoken language, 73–74
representation, 171
typology, 80
Apraxia, 122–123, 171–181. *See also* Specific type
 asymbolia, 172
 callosal disconnection, 173, 174
 characterization, 122–123
 defined, 171
 handedness, 173
 historical aspects, 171
 left hemisphere lesion, 172, 173
 left supramarginal gyrus, 174–175
 principal deficits, 123
 representational hypothesis, 176
 terminology, 118
Aprosodia, 185
Aprosodia battery, 186
Archives of Neurology, 4
Arcuate fasciculus, 175f
Aromatase inhibitor, seizure, 227
Arteriovenous malformation, seizure, 196
Asperger syndrome, 144, 150–151
 pregnancy, 150, 151
Association area, 120–122
Association bundle, 117
Association cortex, stuttering, 103
Asymbolia, 171
 apraxia, 172
Attention, 127–139
 coherence, 134, 135, 138
 components of normal, 134
 distractibility, 134, 138
 organization, 138
 overview, 127, 139
 selectivity, 134, 138
 sensitivity, 134, 138
 universality, 134, 138
Attention deficit-hyperactivity disorder, cerebral asymmetry, 251
Attention disorder, 127–139
 global deficits of attention, 127
 unilateral disorders of attention, 127
Attentional matrix, mental state examination, 45
Atypical multiple sclerosis, 287

SUBJECT INDEX

Auditory affective agnosia, right posterior sylvian infarction, 184
Auditory masking device, stuttering, 103
Auditory neglect, 128
Autism, 143–154
  autopsy studies, 153
  bilateral temporal horn enlargement, 144
  characterized, 143
  clinical cases, 148–151
  complex partial seizure, 149
  executive function, 152
  Geschwind's influence on recent advances, 151–154
  historical aspects, 144–146
  Korsakoff's amnestic syndrome, 143
  language disorder, 144
  magnetic resonance imaging, 153, 154
  National Institutes of Health 1995 conference on autism, 154
  neurologic model, 145
  prefrontal cortex, 152
  pregnancy, 150, 151
  seizure, 144
  serotonin, 144
  sexuality, 148–149
  social cognition, 152
  theory of mind, 152
Autistic spectrum, 144
Autoimmune disorder, 203
  handedness, 287–291
  testosterone, 290
Autoimmune thyroid disorder, 146
Autonomic dysfunction, temporal lobe epilepsy, 198–199

B

Basal ganglia, cerebral asymmetry, 248
  gross anatomy, 248
  radiologic studies, 248
Behavioral analysis, anatomic and mechanistic model, 115
Behavioral neurology, 102
  revival, 18
  using historical studies, 63–65
Benton, Arthur, 53
Bilateral temporal horn enlargement, autism, 144
Birth stress, handedness, 271, 274
Blond hair, handedness, 275–276, 277, 282, 283t
"The Borderland of Neurology and Psychiatry: Some Common Misconceptions," 44
Boston Neuroscience Association, 17
Brain
  connection to behavior, 124
  cytoarchitectural, 120–121
  function, 7
  functional divisions, 120–121
  handedness
    development, 274
    structure, 265–266
Brain plasticity, 199
Brain substrate
  anomalous, 234
  hormone, 234
Broca's area, 249
Brodmann's area 7, 10
Buccofacial apraxia, 17

C

Callosal disconnection, 18–19, 174–175
  apraxia, 173, 174
Callosal syndrome, 116
Capgras syndrome, 134
Case report, 42
Catamenial epilepsy
  menstrual cycle, 230, 231f
  progesterone, 231–232
Cerebral abscess, epilepsy, 211–212
Cerebral asymmetry, 243–253, 296–297
  anomalous structural dominance, 243, 259
  attention deficit-hyperactivity disorder, 251
  basal ganglia, 248
    gross anatomy, 248
    radiologic studies, 248
  cognitive disability, 250–253
  development, 243–244
  dyslexia, 250–251
  frontal lobe, 246–247
    cytoarchitectonics, 246
    gross anatomy, 246
    radiologic studies, 246–247
  handedness, 265–266
  learning, 250–253
  occipital lobe, 247
    gross anatomy, 247
    radiologic studies, 247
  parietal lobe, 247–248
    cytoarchitectonics, 247
    radiologic studies, 248
  schizophrenia, 251–252
    gross anatomy, 251
    radiologic studies, 252
  special cognitive abilities, 252–253
  standard structural dominance, 243, 244–249, 259
    historical aspects, 244–245
  temporal lobe, 245–246
    cytoarchitectonics, 246
    frontal lobe, 246–247
    gross anatomy, 245–246, 246
    radiologic studies, 246
  thalamus, 249
    gross anatomy, 249
    language, 249–250
  Tourette's syndrome, 251
Cerebral cortex, hierarchical organization, 128
Cerebral dominance, 19
  anatomic substrates, 296–297
  handedness, 258
  immunologic associations, 289–290
Cerebral lateralization, 4
Cerebral white matter, 117
Cerebrovascular disease, management, 37
Chronic brain syndrome, 164
Classical anomia, 83
  mechanisms, 83–84
Clinical association, 35–36
Clomiphene, seizure, 227, 233
Cochlear melanin cell, 277
Cognition, as multidisciplinary endeavor, 43
Cognitive disability, cerebral asymmetry, 250–253
Cognitive testing, 196
Coherence, attention, 134, 135, 138
Color, alexia, 83
Color vision, 121
Communicating hydrocephalus, 17
Complex partial seizure, 198, 214
  aggression, 213
  autism, 149
  depomedroxyprogesterone, 233
Conceptual apraxia, 180
  Alzheimer's disease, 180
Conduction aphasia, 117, 118, 171
Conduction apraxia, 177–179
Confusional state, 36, 134–135
  clinical characteristics, 134–135
  focal right hemisphere lesion, 135–137
  stroke, 136
  types, 134–135
Congenital hemihypoplasia, 197
Contralateral limb, neglect, 130–131
Controversy, 43–44
Corpus callosum, ideomotor apraxia, 172–173
Cortical connectivity, 121
Corticocortical connectivity, hierarchical nature, 127
Craniologic method, 65–66
Creativity, 47–51
  defined, 48
  dimensions, 47–48
  field, 50
  intellectual power, 48
  and learning, 48
  personality traits, 49
  synthesis, 48
  types, 47–48
  variables, 48–50
Cybernetics, stuttering, 106

D

Deafness, handedness, 277
Deja vu, 123

Delayed auditory feedback, stuttering, 104
Dementia
 diagnosis, 165
 differential diagnosis, 159
 Geschwind's case notes, 164–166
 Geschwind's publications on, 163–164
 handedness, 289
 olfaction, 167–168
 recent advances, 166
 stroke, 130
 treatment, 165
Dementing disorder, 163–168
Denny-Brown, D., 6, 10, 17
Depomedroxyprogesterone
 complex partial seizure, 233
 epilepsy, 233
Depression
 neurology, 185
 temporal lobe epilepsy, 201
DeRenzi, Ennio, 54–55
Development disorder, 143–154
Developmental dyslexia, 143
Developmental learning disability, neurological substrates, 297
Diethylstilbestrol, handedness, 258
Disassociation apraxia, 179
Disconnection anomia, 83
 mechanisms, 83–84
Disconnection syndrome, 3–4, 19, 115–124, 129
 historical aspects, 115–118
 localization, 118
Disconnection theory, 74–75
"Disconnexion Syndromes in Animals and Man," 19, 115, 118–120, 123–124
 outline, 119–120
 style, 119
Disorder of motor movement, stuttering, 107–108
Display behavior, differential hemispheric processing, 187–188, 189t
Distal sensory loss, 32–33
Distractibility, attention, 134, 138
Dysexecutive syndrome, 160
Dyslexia, 146
 abnormal phonologic processing, 95–96
 abnormalities of brain development, 19
 as acquired disorders, 90
 anatomy, 89–97
 anti-Ro antibody, 291
 cerebral asymmetry, 250–251
 disturbed perception of rapidly changing sounds, 95–96
 etiology, 92
 Geschwind-Behan-Galaburda model, 92–93
 handedness, 281
 hypothesis, 90
 propagation of changes, 95–97
 spatial skills, 252

E
Ectopia, 91, 94–95
 state of the field, 93–94
Edinburgh Handedness Inventory, 257, 258, 260, 262–263
Embolic infarction
 left primary auditory area, 6–7
 subcortical matter, 6–7
Emotion
 differential hemispheric processing, 187–188, 189t
 estrogen, 234
 hormone, 233–234
 neurology
  right hemisphere hypothesis, 188
  valence hypothesis, 188
 progesterone, 234
 right hemisphere syndrome, 183–189
Emotional disorder
 hormone, 234, 235f
 temporal lobe epilepsy, 234, 235f
Epilepsy. *See also* Seizure
 androgen, 224
 androgen deficiency, 224–225
 behavioral characteristics, 198
 cerebral abscess, 211–212
 depomedroxyprogesterone, 233
 hormone
  in men, 224–227
  reproductive dysfunction, 224
  reproductive endocrine disorder, 228, 229
  sexual dysfunction, 224
  therapy, 227
  in women, 228–233
 language, 208–209
 mechanisms of behavioral change, 218–220
 memory, 197
 neuroendocrinology, 223–237
  overview, 223–224, 236–237
 progestin, 233
 schizophrenia-like psychosis, 214–215
 temporal lobe hamartoma, 197–198
 testosterone, 224
Estrogen, emotion, 234
Executive function, autism, 152
Experimental allergic encephalomyelitis, 288
Expressive aphasia, 35
Eye color, 277
 handedness, 282–283, 283t

F
Facial expression, multiple motor pathways, 123
Familial disease, 35–36
Fetus
 immune system factor, 259
 testosterone, 259
Flechsig's rule, 118, 127
Focal right hemisphere lesion
 confusional state, 135–137
 right hemisphere dominance for attention, 136
Focused attention, 134
Frontal arcuate sulcus, unilateral lesions, 128
Frontal lobe, cerebral asymmetry, 246–247
 cytoarchitectonics, 246
 gross anatomy, 246
 radiologic studies, 246–247
Frontal lobe epilepsy, 220
Frontal lobe syndrome, 157–160
 characteristics, 158–159
 current trends, 160
 Geschwind's formal teachings on, 159
 Geschwind's writings on, 158–159
 historical aspects, 157–158
 utilization behavior, 159
Functional disease, 37
Functional symmetry, anatomic substrates, 15–16

G
Geschwind, Norman, 16f
 as advisor, 27–29
 anatomy of naming, 81–82
 aphasia contributions, 73–75
 autism
  clinical issues, 146–147
  research, 146–147
 background, 18
 bedside evaluations, 23
 Beth Israel Hospital, 35
  Professor's Rounds, 35–37
  weekly rounds, 37–38
 Boston City Hospital
  Harvard Neurological Unit, 128
  infrastructure, 10–11
  Professor's Rounds, 31
 Boston Veterans Administration Hospital, 17
 career, 115, 295–297
 case reports, 22, 42
 Child Neurology Service, 24–25
 clinical associations, 35–36
 clinical teaching, 129, 135
 as colleague, 21–26
 as creative genius, 47–51
 creativity, 271, 284
 cultural cluster, 50
 development of philosophical outlook, 40
 developmental dyslexia anatomy, 89–97
 early life, 295
 education, 295
 as educator, 5–13
 familial disease, 35–36
 fostering students, 8, 24
 historical antecedents to, 63–69
 on history and scientific progress, 40–41

influence on colleagues, 75–76
intellectual strengths of, 72–73
as international figure, 53–55, 56
late work, 49–50
learning from mistakes, 9–10
lengthy discourses, 23–24
as linguist, 55
    patient treatment, 57
    as physician, 57–59
medical students, 8, 24
as mensch, 15–19
as mentor, 12–13, 31–33, 39–45
monologues, 8–9
papers, 19, 22, 115, 118–120, 123–124
pathology of superiority, 252–253
persistence, 8–9
personal qualities, 3, 124
and phrenology, 89
residents, 24, 28–29
    academic careers of, 28–29
    respect for patients, 27–28
as role model, 31–33
on role of specialist, 26
Royal Society of London address, 134
as scientist and human being, 51
seminal papers, 18–19
standard setting, 11–12
on stupid questions, 12
style, 123
as synthesizer, 3, 203, 271
as teacher, 35–38
as theorist, 3–4
tutorials, 123
understanding of genetics, 288
University Hospital, Boston University, 17
using historical studies, 63–65
on value of controversy, 43–44
varieties of anomia, 82–84
Wednesday "brain-cutting" session, 25–26
wrong diagnosis, 10, 25
Geschwind-Waxman syndrome, 32
Global attentional disturbance, 133–135
Gonadal steroid, seizure, 228–230
Goodglass, Harold, 17
Grasp reflex, 115

H

Handedness, 257–267, 297
age, 263
allergy, 282
analysis methods, 263–265
anatomic substrates, 15–16
apraxia, 173
autoimmune disease, 287–291
birth stress, 271, 274
blond hair, 275–276, 277, 282, 283t
brain development, 274
brain structure, 265–266
cerebral asymmetry, 265–266
cerebral dominance, 258
correlations with, 272–273
deafness, 277
defining, 280–282
dementia, 289
diethylstilbestrol, 258
diffuse control system, 274
dimensions, 278–279
dyslexia, 281
Edinburgh Handedness Battery, 279
Edinburgh Handedness Inventory, 257, 258, 260, 262–263
eye color, 282–283, 283t
hypopigmentation, 275, 282–284
immune system, 275
intermediate handedness, 258
Lateral Preference Inventory, 279, 280
laterality, 279–280
laterality quotients, 258, 260
laterality score, 258, 260–262
lupus erythematosus, 281
measurement, 259–260, 278–279
and occupation, 257, 258
as pathological marker, 273–275
pigmentation, 276, 277
premature gray hair, 289
scoring methods, 258, 260–263
self-described handedness, 260
testosterone, 275, 290
thyroiditis, 289
Hashimoto's thyroiditis, 146
Hecaen, Henry, 55
Heilman, Kenneth, 128–131
Helper cell, testosterone, 290
Hemispatial inattention, 127–133
History, 197
Hormone
    brain substrate, 234
    emotion, 233–234
    emotional disorder, 234, 235f
    epilepsy
        in men, 224–227
        reproductive dysfunction, 224
        reproductive endocrine disorder, 228, 229
        sexual dysfunction, 224
        therapy, 227
        in women, 228–233
    temporal lobe epilepsy, 234, 235f
Human language, origins, 120
Hyperconnection concept, 218–219
Hypergraphia, 32
    temporal lobe epilepsy, 215
Hypertrophic polyneuritis, 287
Hypopigmentation, handedness, 275, 282–284
Hypothalamopituitary axis, testosterone secretion, 226
Hypothalamus, 214
Hysteria, 37

I

Ideational apraxia, 179–180
Ideomotor apraxia, 172–177, 177, 178, 179
Immune system
    handedness, 275
    testosterone, 290–291
Immune system factor, fetus, 259
Infantile autism, 144
Inferior parietal lobe, left hemisphere lesion, 174
Inferior parietal lobule, 128, 129f
    polysensory cortical regions in monkey, 133
    spatial attention, 131
    unilateral neglect, 131
Information-processing system, aphasia, 171
Input praxicon, 178
Instrumentalities of speech, 80
Interictal behavior disorder, temporal lobe epilepsy, 36
Interictal syndrome, 32
Intermediate handedness, 258
International Neuropsychological Symposium, 53–55, 56
Intracranial bleeding, 37

J

Jackson, Hughlings, 207–208
Juvenile myoclonic epilepsy, 211

K

Kaplan, Edith, 115, 116
Kleine-Levin syndrome, 204–205
Kluver-Bucy syndrome, 28, 218
Korsakoff's amnestic syndrome, autism, 143

L

Language, 89
    epilepsy, 208–209
    Geschwind's anatomic model, 81–82
    seizure, 209
    Wernicke's area, 90–91
Language area, electrical stimulation, 208
Language disorder, autism, 144
Language-induced epilepsy, 209–211
Language-related cortex, leftward hemispheric asymmetry, 249–250
Lateral Preference Inventory, 279, 280
Laterality, handedness, 279–280
Lateralized dominance
    Geschwind-Behan-Galaburda hypothesis, 257, 258, 259, 266–267
    intrauterine functions, 259
Learned skilled movement, modular system, 177f
Learning, cerebral asymmetry, 250–253

Left dorsolateral frontal lesion, trimodal neglect, 130
Left frontal glioblastoma, 296
Left frontal operculum, 249
left hemiparesis, 135
Left hemisphere lesion
  aphasia, 172
  apraxia, 172, 173
  inferior parietal lobe, 174
Left parietal lobe, lesions anterior to, apraxia, 176
Left primary auditory area, embolic infarction, 6–7
Left supramarginal gyrus, apraxia, 174–175
Left temporoparietal region, 79
Left visual neglect, 135
Left-handedness. See Handedness
Lexical decision, 84–85
Liepmann, H., 171–173, 176, 179, 181
Limbic epilepsy, 32
Limb-kinetic apraxia, 171–172
Lupus erythematosus, handedness, 281
Lymphoblastoid cell, 287

M

Magnetic resonance imaging, autism, 153, 154
Medulla, decussation, 15–16
Memory, 39, 163–164
  epilepsy, 197
Menstrual cycle
  catamenial epilepsy, 230, 231f
  seizure, 196
  temporal lobe epilepsy, 196, 203–204
Mental state examination, attentional matrix, 45
Micropolygyria, planum temporale, 91
Mood disorder, reproductive endocrine disorder, 234, 235f
Motion vision, 121
Motor association cortex, 175f
Motor asymbolia, 118
Movement disorder, stuttering, 107
Movement representation, stores, 178
Multiple sclerosis, peripheral nerve involvement, 287, 288
Myelin basic protein, 287–288
Myelination, 117
Myoclonic epilepsy, 211–212

N

Naming
  contemporary approaches, 84–87
  distributed-processing models, 85
  naming ability, 120
Neglect
  contralateral limb, 130–131
  mechanisms, 128–129
  superior temporal sulcus, 132–133
Neglect syndrome, 128
Neocortical ectopia, 95
Neocortical language area, 118
Nervous system
  development, 243–244
  developmental anomaly, skin and its appendages, 24
  testosterone, 290–291
Neural crest, neuronal guide cell, 276
Neuroendocrinology
  epilepsy, 223–237
    overview, 223–224, 236–237
    temporal lobe epilepsy, associated emotional disorders, 234–236
Neurological examination, 197
Neurological modeling, 66–67
Neurological Unit at Boston City Hospital, 21
  Saturday morning case discussions, 21–24
Neuronal guide cell
  neural crest, 276
  pigment cell, 276
Neuronal synchrony, visual image integration, 122
Nominal aphasia, 80
Nonaphasic misnaming, 82–83, 133–134
  categories, 83
  diagnosis, 82–83
Nonverbal learning disability, 150, 151
Normal-pressure hydrocephalus, 37

O

Occipital lobe, cerebral asymmetry, 247
  gross anatomy, 247
  radiologic studies, 247
Olfaction
  Alzheimer's disease, 167
  dementia, 167–168
Optic aphasia, 85
Orbitofrontal cortex, 221, 221f
Organic brain syndrome, 164
Output praxicon, 178

P

Pandya, Deepak, 10–11
Paradigmatic diagram-maker, 65–66
Paranoia, temporal lobe epilepsy, 200
Paraphasia, 117
Parietal lobe
  cerebral asymmetry, 247–248
    cytoarchitectonics, 247
    radiologic studies, 248
  monkey vs. human, 131, 132f
Parkinson's disease, 17–18

Pathological hyperconnectivity, 199
Patients' rights, 57, 58
Perfect pitch, plana temporale, 252–253
Phobia, temporal lobe epilepsy, 201–202
Picture naming, mechanism, 84
Pigment cell, neuronal guide cell, 276
Pigmentation, handedness, 276, 277
Planum temporale
  asymmetry, 16
  micropolygyria, 91
  perfect pitch, 252–253
  testosterone hypothesis, 92–93
Polymodal association cortex, 120
Posterior fossa tumor, 36
Posterosuperior temporal lesion, 117
Postinfectious encephalomyelitis, 287–288
Praxis system, 178f
Prefrontal cortex, autism, 152
Pregnancy
  Asperger syndrome, 150, 151
  autism, 150, 151
  temporal lobe epilepsy, 204
Premature gray hair, handedness, 289
Presentism, 65
Primary emotion, 188
Primary motor cortex, 176
Progesterone
  adenosine, 232
  catamenial epilepsy, 231–232
  emotion, 234
  seizure, 231–233
Progestin, epilepsy, 233
Prosody, right hemisphere stroke, 183
Psychologic modeling, 66–67

R

Rare disorder, 23, 202
Reading, seizure, 209
Reduplicative paramnesia, 134
Religiosity, temporal lobe epilepsy, 215
Representation, aphasia, 171
Reproductive endocrine disorder
  anxiety, 234, 235f
  mood disorder, 234, 235f
Retrieval process, 86
Retrograde neuron labeling, 131
Right hemisphere
  affective gesture, 184
  affective prosody, 184
Right hemisphere infarction
  affective gesture, 185
  affective prosody, 185
  prosody, 183
Right hemisphere syndrome, emotion, 183–189
Right hemisphere-based learning disability, 150, 151

SUBJECT INDEX

Right middle cerebral artery territory infarction, acute confusional state, 136–137
Right parietal dominance, 123
Right parietotemporal lesion, trimodal neglect, 130
Right posterior sylvian infarction, auditory affective agnosia, 184
Right suprasylvian region, 183
Right-handedness. See Handedness

S

Schizophrenia, cerebral asymmetry, 251–252
  gross anatomy, 251
  radiologic studies, 252
Schizophrenia-like psychosis, epilepsy, 214–215
Schizophreniform behavior, temporal lobe epilepsy, 200
Scientific creativity, variables, 48–50
Seizure, 196
  aromatase inhibitor, 227
  arteriovenous malformation, 196
  autism, 144
  clomiphene, 227, 233
  gonadal steroid, 228–230
  language, 209
  menstrual cycle, 196
  progesterone, 231–233
  reading, 209
  speaking, 209
  testosterone, 227
  triggers, 196
  writing, 209
Selected Papers on Language and the Brain, 43
Selectivity, attention, 134, 138
Self-described handedness, 260
Semantic processing, two-stage model, 84
Semantic-category-specific dissociation, 85–86
Sense-modality-specific naming disorder, 84–87
Sensitivity, attention, 134, 138
Sensory cortex, 121
Serotonin, autism, 144
Sex steroid, 92
Sexuality, temporal lobe epilepsy, 215
Simple partial seizure, 198
Social cognition, autism, 152
Social emotion, 188
Spasmodic dysphonia, 110
Spatial attention, inferior parietal lobule, 131
Spatial skills, dyslexia, 252
Speaking, seizure, 209
Speech, characterized, 104–110
Speech acoustics, 102
Speech output, 104
Speech perception, 104

Stapedius reflex, stuttering, 102
Stereotactic radiofrequency lesion, 213
Stimulus-reward association, 128
Stocking-glove sensory loss, 32–33
Stroke
  acute dementia, 136
  confusional state, 136
Stuttering, 101–110, 209
  acquired, 106–107, 108
  association cortex, 103
  auditory masking device, 103
  in childhood, 103
  corrective strategies, 105, 107
  cybernetics, 106
  delayed auditory feedback, 104
  developmental, 107
  disorder of motor movement, 107–108
  disrupted cerebral laterality for language, 102
  dysfluence after cerebral compromise, 106–107
  fluency-evoking power of singing, 105
  gender, 103
  historical references, 103
  momentary instability in complex multiloop control system, 109
  movement disorder, 107
  prevalence, 103
  speech therapy, 107, 108
  stapedius reflex, 102
Subcortical matter, embolic infarction, 6–7
Superior temporal sulcus, 128, 129f
  neglect, 132–133
  polysensory cortical regions in monkey, 133
Supplementary motor area, 176–177
Suppressor cell, testosterone, 290
Synthesis, creativity, 48
Systemic metabolic disturbance, acute confusional state, 133

T

Tactile anomia, 83
Temporal limbic structure, hyperconnections, 218–219
Temporal lobe, 218
  cerebral asymmetry, 245–246
    cytoarchitectonics, 246
    frontal lobe, 246–247
    gross anatomy, 245–246, 246
    radiologic studies, 246
Temporal lobe epilepsy, 27, 32, 57, 58
  aggressiveness, 215, 218
  autonomic dysfunction, 198–199
  behavioral aspects, 195–205
  behavioral disorder, 199–202
  depression, 201
  drug reactions, 203

emotional disorder, 234, 235f
  examination, 195–199
  galvanic skin conductance responses to visual stimuli, 219f, 219–220
  history, 195
  hormone, 234, 235f
  hypergraphia, 215
  interictal behavior, 213–221
    change mechanism, 218–220
    testing, 215–218
  interictal behavior disorder, 36
  interictal personality changes, 39
  menstrual cycle, 196, 203–204
  neuroendocrinology, associated emotional disorders, 234–236
  paranoia, 200
  personality, 200
  phobia, 201–202
  polypharmacy, 203
  pregnancy, 204
  religiosity, 215
  schizophreniform behavior, 200
  sequence of symptoms, 195
  sexuality, 215
  treatment, 202–205
  vs. specific psychiatric syndromes, 218
Temporal lobe hamartoma, epilepsy, 197–198
Testosterone
  autoimmune disease, 290
  effects, 290
  epilepsy, 224
  fetus, 259
  handedness, 275, 290
  helper cell, 290
  immune system, 290–291
  nervous system, 290–291
  seizure, 227
  suppressor cell, 290
Testosterone hypothesis, planum temporale, 92–93
Testosterone secretion, hypothalamopituitary axis, 226
Teuber, Hans-Lucas, 53
Thalamus
  cerebral asymmetry, 249
    gross anatomy, 249
    language, 249–250
    left lateral posterior nucleus, 250
Theory of mind, autism, 152
Thyroiditis, handedness, 289
Todd's paralysis, 207
Tonsillar herniation, 36
Tourette's syndrome, cerebral asymmetry, 251
Transcortical aphasia, 117–118
Transcortical motor aphasia, 208
Trimodal neglect
  left dorsolateral frontal lesion, 130
  right parietotemporal lesion, 130

U

Unilateral neglect, 127–133
  acute confusional state, 135
  causes, 131
  human, 130
  inferior parietal lobule, 131
  monkeys, 130
  right hemisphere, 130
Unilateral tactile anomia, 83
Universality, attention, 134, 138
Utilization behavior, frontal lobe syndrome, 159

V

V1, 121, 122
  feedback connections, 121–122
V2, 121, 122
  feedback connections, 121–122
V3, 121, 122
V4, 121, 122
V5, 121, 122
V6, 122
Ventromedial hypothalamus, amygdala, 224
Vestibular stimulation, 147
Violent automatism, 213
Visual analysis
  parallel processing, 121
  serial model, 121
  top-down processing, 121
Visual association area, 121
Visual association cortex, 175f
Visual cortex, 121
  monkeys, 121
Visual hallucination, 195–196
  and good clinician, 167
Visual image integration, neuronal synchrony, 122
Visual pathway, amygdala, 221f
Vowel perception, 104–105

W

Wada test, affective prosody, 187–188
Water-drinking behavior, 202
Wernicke, Carl, 41–42, 117
Wernicke's aphasia, 91
Wernicke's area, 82, 175f
  language, 90–91
Western Aphasia Battery, 186
Word retrieval process, 84
Writing, seizure, 209

Y

Yakovlev, Paul, 17

Z

Zangwill, Oliver, 55, 116